AEROBIC
DANCE-EXERCISE
INSTRUCTOR MANUAL

AEROBIC DANCE-EXERCISE INSTRUCTOR MANUAL

NANEENE VAN GELDER
EDITOR

SHERYL MARKS
SUPERVISING EDITOR

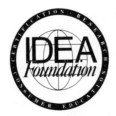

INTERNATIONAL DANCE-EXERCISE ASSOCIATION (IDEA) FOUNDATION

PUBLISHER

San Diego, California

Library of Congress Cataloging-in-Publication Data

Aerobic dance-exercise instructor manual.

   Includes index.
   1. Aerobic dancing—Study and teaching—Handbooks,
manuals, etc. 2. Aerobic exercises—Study and
teaching—Handbooks, manuals, etc. I. VanGelder,
Naneene. II. Marks, Sheryl.
RA781.15.A35   1987   613.7'1   87-80343
ISBN 0-9618161-0-4

First Edition, 1987
Reprinted, 1988
Reprinted, 1989

Published by
IDEA Foundation
6190 Cornerstone Court East
Suite 202
San Diego, CA 92121-4729
(619) 535-8227

ISBN 0-9618161-0-4
Printed in the United States of America

Design: MIKE YAZZOLINO
Production: YAZZ GRAPHIC DESIGN
Copy Editors: ROBIN WITKIN, NANCY STOCKWELL
Proofreaders: JANE FRUTTI, SUSAN LIPSON
Anatomical Illustrations: JAMES STAUNTON
Photographer: STEPHEN SIMPSON
Models: VALERIE COWAN, ROBERT BEJAR, LIZ LAPLANTE

Acknowledgements:
Special thanks to the IDEA Foundation staff : KIM CARL-
SON, VALERIE COWAN, DEBBY ELLISON, CASSIE SHAFER and
SHANNON TUTTLE.

To the entire IDEA, INC. staff for their support, especially
PETER DAVIS, PATRICIA RYAN and DEAN HAY for their professional guidance and encouragement.

The IDEA FOUNDATION gratefully acknowledges Reebok International Ltd. for their contribution to support the production of this book. Without their help, this project would not have been possible.

REVIEWERS

JULIE ANDERSEN, M.A.   Director of special projects for IDEA, Inc.; consultant with Selection Research, Inc.; IDEA Foundation certified.

◇ RAUL ARTAL, M.D.   Associate professor of obstetrics and gynecology, physical education, and exercise sciences at the University of Southern California, Los Angeles; coauthor of *Exercise in Pregnancy*.

MICHAEL S. BAHRKE, PH.D.   Sports psychology instructor at the U.S. Army Soldier Physical Fitness School, Fort Benjamin Harrison, Indiana.

◇ GINGER BANTA, M.A.   Official trainer for the YWCA–USA; IDEA representative, 1984–86.

JOHN L. BOYER, M.D.   Clinical cardiologist at the Alvarado Hospital Medical Center, San Diego.

MICHAEL BUONO, PH.D.   Assistant professor of physical education at San Diego State University.

◇ SUSAN CALHOUN.   Founder and director of Fitness Instructor Training Camps (Fitcamp); clinician for the International Council on Sport and Exercise Safety; IDEA Foundation certified.

NANCY CLARK, M.S., R.D.   Director of nutrition services for Sports Medicine Systems, Inc.; nutritionist for Sports Medicine Brookline; and author of *The Athlete's Kitchen*.

DEAN F. CONNORS, PH.D.   Former director of adult fitness at Central Michigan University.

◇ ♦ KATHIE DAVIS.   Executive director and cofounder of the International Dance-Exercise Association.

GERALD M. DWORKIN.   Consultant for Lifesaving Resources of Springfield, Virginia, specializing in first aid, CPR education, aquatics emergency management, and emergency medical services.

◇ ♦ PETER R. FRANCIS, PH.D.   Associate professor of physical education at San Diego State University; and biomechanics consultant for the US Olympic Committee.

DONNA M. GILLIEN, M.S.   Director of research and education at the Center for Sports Medicine of the Saint Francis Memorial Hospital, San Francisco.

♦ IDEA Foundation Board of Directors
◇ IDEA Foundation Committee on Standards and Certification in Dance Exercise.

◇ LAWRENCE A. GOLDING, PH.D., F.A.C.S.M. Director of the Exercise Physiology Lab at University of Nevada, Las Vegas; National YMCA physical fitness consultant; coauthor of *National YMCA Physical Fitness Program*; ACSM Preventive and Rehabilitation Certification Committee.

DAVID L. HERBERT, ESQ. Partner, Herbert, Treadon, Benson & Frieg, Attorneys at Law, Canton, Ohio; and associate professor at Kent State University.

WILLIAM G. HERBERT, PH.D., F.A.C.S.M. Director of the Cardiac Intervention Center; and director of the Laboratory for Exercise, Sport and Work Physiology at the Virginia Polytechnic Institute and State University, Blacksburg, Virginia.

◇ GWEN HYATT, M.S. Vice-president and director of education for Desert Southwest Fitness; IDEA representative, 1984–86; IDEA Foundation certified.

◇ NANCY KABRIEL, M.T.A. President of Rhythmic Aerobics, Inc.; member of the advisory board for SHAPE Magazine; consultant for Reebok, Ltd.; IDEA Foundation certified.

VICTOR L. KATCH, PH.D. Professor of kinesiology, and associate professor of pediatrics at the University of Michigan, Ann Arbor.

SARA KOOPERMAN, J.D. Attorney; owner of Sara's City Workout in Chicago; IDEA Foundation certified.

JANICE LETTUNICH, M.S. Instructor of physical education and director of the Donald B. Slocum Sports Medicine and Fitness Research Laboratory at the University of Oregon.

MYRA B. LURIE. Attorney with the law firm of Mathon and Rosensweig.

DANIEL J. LYNCH. Senior vice-president of Cardio-Fitness Corporation; and certified ACSM Program Director.

◇ MARY MAYTA. President of Fitness for Life International, Inc.; IDEA representative, 1984–86.

◇ LEORA MYERS, R.N. Founder of Creative Bodywork Center and F.I.T., San Francisco; member of California Governor's Council on Physical Fitness and Wellness; advisory committee member for the University of California, Santa Cruz, Fitness Instructor Certificate Program.

◇ GREG PHILLIPS, M.S. Exercise physiologist; director of health and fitness education for Jazzercise, Inc.; instructor for University of California at San Diego Extension, Instruction and Health Management.

◇ E. LEE RICE, D.O., F.A.A.F.P. Medical director of the San Diego Sports Medicine Center; team physician for the San Diego Chargers and USA men's and women's national volleyball teams; past president of the American Osteopathic Academy of Sports Medicine.

DOUGLAS H. RICHIE, JR., D.P.M. Sports podiatrist at the Seal Beach Podiatry Group; clinical instructor at the Los Angeles County–USC Medical Center; associate clinical professor at the California College of Podiatric Medicine.

CHARLENE SCHADE.   Fitness instructor for older adults at the Well-Being, a project of Scripps Memorial Hospital Foundation, and AMI Mission Bay Hospital Outreach Program; instructor for the San Diego Community Colleges; and coauthor of *Prime Time Aerobics*.

CHRISTINE VEGA, M.P.H.   Dietitian for the 11th USAF Contingency Hospital, Lockland Air Force Base, Texas; fitness instructor at University of California, Los Angeles, Extension and Los Angeles City College.

◇ GAIL L. WEAVER, M.S.   President of Lifetime Health and Nutrition Center; fitness programs coordinator for the University of California at San Diego, Extension.

JACK H. WILMORE, PH.D.   Margie Gurley Seay Centennial Professor in the department of physical education at the University of Texas, Austin; former director, Exercise and Sport Sciences Laboratory, University of Arizona; consultant to the President's Council on Physical Fitness and Sport; and author of 12 books.

CONTENTS

Foreword

Not long ago the only people exercising to music were ballerinas, square dancers, and Jack LaLanne. Now a familiar part of most people's vocabulary, words like "Jazzercise," "aerobics," and "dance exercise" didn't exist in the early 1970s. At that time I doubt anyone ever dreamed that within the next decade a billion dollar industry would develop, boasting over 20 million participants in a new form of exercise. I certainly didn't.

People often ask me if dance exercise is a passing fad. They question whether the dance-exercise industry will dwindle as the public's fascination with it fades. My response is that the day people decide health and fitness are no longer important, dance exercise will disappear. And you know what? I don't think that day will ever come!

I learned long ago that most people won't exercise if they don't enjoy it. Sure, some people can muster enough willpower and self-discipline to overcome their aversion to exercise—if they believe strongly in its benefits. The reason Jazzercise, and dance exercise in general, has been so successful is because it makes exercise *fun*. For many, dance exercise is the one form of exercise that is easy to enjoy. There's music, energy, variety, color, people, challenge, and—most importantly—results. Students keep coming back because they can see themselves and feel themselves becoming physically fit. And they're having a good time doing it.

Although there are still plenty of new students out there, gone are the days when an instructor only had to hang out a sign, print up two hundred fliers, and open the doors to lines of eager dance exercisers. Nor is looking good in a leotard or being an excellent dancer enough. Today's dance-exercise instructor shoulders the responsibility of teaching a thoroughly safe and effective class. To do so, she or he must stay abreast of new developments in the rapidly evolving fitness field. Dance-exercise instructors are now expected to relay important information accurately, such as methods for monitoring exercise intensity or technique and alignment reminders. There are courses to take, books and manuals to study, and magazines to read. Students look to us for answers: What should I look for in an aerobics shoe? What is the best way to lose weight? or How do I modify this exercise? Among the many hats the dance-exercise instructor now wears are teacher, coach, dancer-choreographer, health educator, performer, and friend, not to mention, business person. Regardless of the role, our success depends on our ability to connect with our students, drawing on our own creativity and imagination to make our classes as enjoyable as possible.

We should feel proud of our industry. We've gotten millions of people up and moving; people who otherwise may never have made fitness or dance a part of their lives. We've helped these millions commit to a healthier lifestyle, and in doing so, we've given them the chance to reap the wonderful benefits—both physical and mental—that come with that commitment. Through organizations like IDEA we've banded together to watch, listen, and learn from each other. In a relatively short time we've risen to the challenge of establishing our own standards of excellence, drawing on the knowledge and resources of the top fitness minds in the country.

This manual, the culmination of over two years of hard work by hundreds of individuals, represents the cooperative spirit that exists in the dance-exercise industry. In reading it, I know you will gain an incredible amount of useful, practical, and extremely valuable information. I hope you also gain, as I did when I read it, a feeling of pride in who you are and what you do. Dance exercise and fitness are here to stay.

JUDI SHEPPARD MISSETT
President, Jazzercise, Inc.

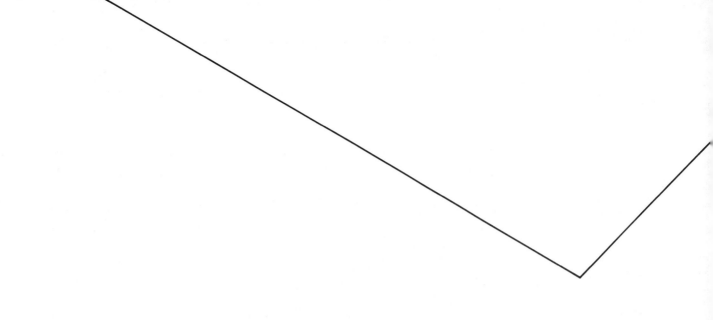

Foreword

A dance-exercise instructor is a leader, a role model, a teacher, and an adviser. Each role carries with it responsibilities that must be met for an instructor to become a true professional. To be the best you can be requires regular study and continued growth in the dance-exercise field and careful preparation for your classes.

Your students have entrusted their bodies to your care. They have the right to expect you to deal safely and effectively with them. Your students will come to you for information as well, so you need to know about exercise, nutrition, and other health-related topics.

As a role model, you exemplify what your students want to achieve and can achieve. You give them the willpower and motivation to improve their own lives. Seeing you regularly, listening to what you say, and receiving your encouragement gives them support and replenishes their spirit.

Refer to this manual frequently. The information it contains can help you achieve your goal of becoming the best instructor you can.

JACKI SORENSEN
Aerobic Dancing, Inc.

Introduction

Over the past several years, the dance-exercise industry has grown rapidly, not only in size, but also in scientific understanding of exercise and in professional expertise. As men and women, the athletic and the sedentary, the young and the old continue to flock to dance-exercise classes, it has become increasingly important that all instructors meet minimum professional standards. The recent industry-wide movement towards instructor certification is a sign that dance exercise is not just an industry concerned with health, but also a healthy industry eager to regulate itself.

The *Aerobic Dance-Exercise Instructor Manual* is a major contribution to the certification effort. It is the product of a process that began three years ago, when the IDEA Foundation formed a committee of experts and charged them with the task of determining the minimum level of knowledge an instructor must have to lead a safe and effective dance-exercise class. The committee worked for two years and published its consensus opinion in the form of a booklet entitled "Guidelines for the Training of Dance-Exercise Instructors" (included in Appendix B). After the publication of these guidelines, the IDEA Foundation formed another committee to develop a certification examination. Working with the Educational Testing Service, this committee wrote a series of test items directly related to the content areas contained in the guidelines. The first nationally-recognized certification exam was administered before the IDEA International Convention in 1986. Since then, more than 5,000 instructors have taken the exam, which is administered several times each year at more than 20 sites throughout the country.

Now, after 1 1/2 years of work by 21 contributors and 32 expert reviewers, *The Aerobic Dance-Exercise Instructor Manual* represents the third step in the IDEA Foundation's effort to foster a high degree of professionalism within the dance-exercise industry. The purpose of the book is to provide the basic information an instructor needs to conduct a typical dance-exercise class. Today's dance-exercise instructor is not only an exercise leader, but also an educator, a role model and a business person. Therefore, the text is organized into four parts which encompass all of these important roles.

Part I, Exercise Science, provides the scientific basis for the design of safe and effective classes. Part II, Screening, Testing and Programming, focuses on the actual teaching of a class, from health screening to modifying for individual needs. Part III, Injury Prevention and Emergency Procedures, reflects the industry's emphasis on providing exercise programs that are safe for most healthy participants. Part IV, Legal Issues, helps clarify an instructor's rights and responsibilities in such important areas as copyright law and legal liability. Many areas of specialization that require extensive education and training are not covered in this text. For example, neither rehabilitation programs for persons recovering from injuries or illnesses nor special programs for persons with arthritis or other medical conditions are addressed. Fitness tests requiring special equipment, such as hydrostatic weighing or graded exercise tests, are not discussed here because they are not part of a traditional dance-exercise setting. As this book stresses over and over again, instructors should always stay within the limits of their training and expertise and refer exercise participants with special needs to other programs or other health professionals.

The *Aerobic Dance-Exercise Instructor Manual* is designed to be used both as a text for instructors preparing for the IDEA Foundation's certification exam and as a reference for more experienced instructors. The IDEA Foundation Certification Committee also recommends that instructors consider taking additional supervised courses and training. The manual is organized in a logical sequence for the reader who wants to read the entire text. The chapters are also extensively cross-referenced for readers who prefer to focus on specific content areas. Key words and concepts from each chapter are highlighted in bold type and included in an extensive glossary at the back of the book. For instructors who wish to pursue their study of a certain area, most chapters contain a list of suggested reading. And a detailed index is provided to increase the book's value as a reference work.

It is important for the reader to realize that although this book contains the best information available at the time of publication, no body of information is ever complete, and in the field of dance exercise, new studies continue to expand our knowledge. In many areas, such as pregnancy and exercise, there remains considerable disagreement among the experts. Even in the crucial area of monitoring exercise intensity, the information in existing publications is often contradictory. Therefore, the ultimate responsibility for professional conduct remains with the individual instructor. The information contained here must be combined with training and experience, and guided by the instructor's common sense and concern for the health and well-being of all dance-exercise participants.

We hope this book will be a valuable starting point for those of you who are studying to become dance-exercise instructors and a thought-provoking perspective on the profession of dance-exercise. And we hope that all of you will go well beyond this book in your own professional development.

SHERYL MARKS
Executive Director, IDEA FOUNDATION

AEROBIC
DANCE-EXERCISE
INSTRUCTOR MANUAL

EXERCISE SCIENCE   PART I

The *Aerobic Dance-Exercise Instructor Manual* covers all facets of conducting a dance-exercise class, from health screening to copyright law. This first section of the book presents complex but essential material on the science of exercise. To design exercise programs that are safe, fun, and tailored to individual needs and goals, and to answer the questions posed by today's informed dance-exercise consumer, an instructor must have an understanding of the structure and function of the body. These chapters on exercise physiology, anatomy and kinesiology, and nutrition describe not only what happens during exercise, but also how and why. This information may not be easy to absorb in a single reading, however its relevance will become increasingly clear as the instructor applies it to the dance-exercise setting as described in Parts II and III. The reader may also find it helpful to refer back to these chapters for the rationale behind the various exercise recommendations and techniques discussed elsewhere in the text.

Exercise Physiology

Christine L. Wells

Christine L. Wells, Ph.D., a widely recognized authority on women and sports, is an author, lecturer, and professor of health and physical education at Arizona State University. She has been president of the Research Consortium of the American Alliance for Health, Physical Education, Recreation and Dance, a member of the Board of Trustees and Vice-President of Education of the American College of Sports Medicine, and a member of the IDEA Board of Advisors. Dr. Wells is the author of *Women, Sport and Performance: A Physiological Perspective,* published by Human Kinetics in 1985.

1

IN THIS CHAPTER:

- Bioenergetics of exercise: ATP, the phosphagen system, aerobic and anaerobic production of ATP, muscles and metabolism.

- The neuromuscular system: Types of muscular contractions, muscular response to training.

- The cardiovascular-respiratory systems: Carrying, delivering, and extracting oxygen.

- Responses to and benefits of aerobic exercise.

- Environmental considerations: Exercising in the heat, in the cold, and at high altitudes.

The versatility of human movement is staggering to consider. The construction of the body allows an extraordinarily wide range of possible movements requiring complex mechanisms of neuromuscular coordination. Knowledge of human anatomy enables us to understand which muscles and bones are used to perform specific movements. The human body is capable of movements requiring large bursts of energy over short periods, as well as movements requiring less energy sustained over a longer time. Knowledge of exercise physiology provides an understanding of these bodily functions. Aerobic-dance instructors (and other professionals dealing with physical fitness and human movement) should have a thorough understanding of exercise physiology and human anatomy. This chapter focuses on exercise physiology. The principles of anatomy and kinesiology are discussed in Chapter 2.

Exercise physiology is the study of how the body functions during exercise. Such knowledge provides the basis for understanding how the body functions at rest, how these functions change during exercise, and how the body adapts to exercise training. While the body is at rest, physiological functions are largely in a state of equilibrium or

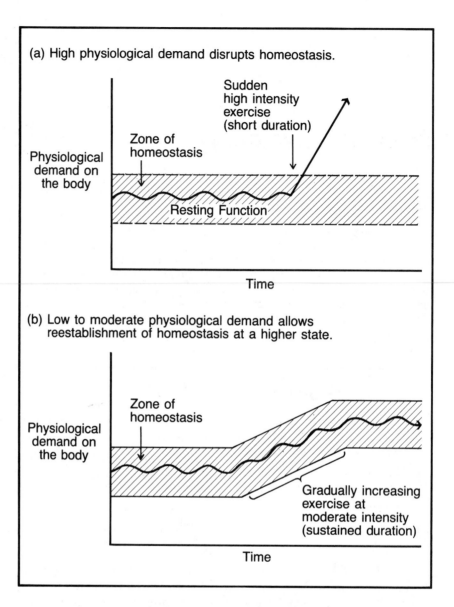

FIGURE 1–1 The concept of homeostasis

balance. This state of stability in the normal body is known as **homeostasis.** An easy way to envision homeostasis is to consider the concept of supply and demand: While at rest, the normal healthy body is functioning comfortably in that physiological demands are easily met. The body is experiencing little or no stress and feels comfortable. This is not to say, however, that bodily functions are static. Although often defined as a stable state, homeostasis is not a static or unchanging state; rather, it is a dynamic state of being that requires the continuous production of energy and removal of metabolic waste products.

Figure 1–1 illustrates that commencement of exercise disrupts the body's resting state of homeostasis. Movement patterns requiring a sudden burst of energy for relatively short periods are extremely stressful, placing such high metabolic demands on the body that the reestablishment of homeostasis at a higher level of function is impossible (Fig. 1–1a). Less stressful movement patterns requiring a moderate amount of sustained energy production, however, may allow the person to reestablish a new level of homeostasis (Fig. 1–1b). When exercise is terminated, physiological responses gradually return to the original level of resting homeostasis. A person's level of physical fitness largely determines the level of exercise intensity at which homeostasis can be reestablished; in other words, the physically fit person can establish relative homeostasis at a higher exercise intensity than the less fit person.

PHYSICAL FITNESS

Physical fitness is a complex concept that often means different things to different people. In this manual, **physical fitness** refers to an enhanced physiological or functional capacity that allows for an improved quality of life. As physiological or functional capacity increases, the capacity for exercise increases. In other words, a person can lift heavier weights or run farther or faster—in short, exercise more. Increased physical fitness is often reflected by physiological adaptations such as a lowered heart rate during a standardized exercise test or an improved ability to mobilize and use body fuels. **Quality of life** generally implies an overall positive feeling and enthusiasm for life, without fatigue or exhaustion from routine and required activities. A high level of physical fitness enables us to perform required daily tasks without fatigue, and thus participate in additional activities for personal enjoyment. For more athletically inclined persons, a high level of physical fitness implies optimal physical or motor performance.

There are several major components of physical fitness. Each component is of equal importance, and no one component should be emphasized over the others. Note that the five components defined below are health related as opposed to skill related. The development of a high degree of motor skill is sometimes confused with physical fitness, but these two attributes are not necessarily related to each other. A highly skilled person may have a low level of physical fitness, and the reverse may also be true.

1. **Muscular strength** is the force a muscle or muscle group can exert during contraction.

2. **Muscular endurance** is defined either as (a) the length of time a muscle or muscle group can continue to exert force without fatiguing, or (b) the number of times a muscle or muscle group can repeatedly exert force against a given resistance without fatiguing.

3. **Cardiovascular** or **cardiorespiratory endurance,** or **aerobic fitness,** is the capacity of the heart-lung system to deliver blood and, hence, oxygen to the working muscles during sustained exercise.

4. **Flexibility** refers to the range of motion possible about a joint. An adequate degree of flexibility is important to prevent injury and to maintain body mobility.

5. **Body composition** is the makeup of the body using a two-component model of lean body mass and body fat. **Lean body mass,** consisting of the muscles, bones, nervous tissue, skin, and organs, represents the metabolically active part of the body that makes a direct and positive contribution to energy production during exercise. Body **fat** or **adipose tissue** represents body tissue that stores energy for use during some forms of exercise, but otherwise does

not contribute directly to exercise performance. Body fat is further classified into essential body fat and excess body fat. **Essential body fat** is that amount thought to be necessary for maintenance of life and reproductive function; 3%–6% body fat* is generally thought to be essential for men, and 8%–12% for women. Excess body fat, or storage fat, is contained in the fatty depots or fat pads found both under the skin (subcutaneous fat) and internally. A large amount of excess body fat is referred to as **obesity.** While body fat levels change with age, the percentage of body fat can be maintained at a suitable level throughout a lifetime.

BIOENERGETICS OF EXERCISE

Body cells require a continuous supply of energy in order to function. Ultimately, the food we eat supplies this energy. However, our cells do not directly use the energy released from the food we eat, rather they need a chemical compound called **adenosine triphosphate** or **ATP.** ATP is the immediately usable form of chemical energy needed for cellular function, including muscular contraction. The foods we eat are made up of carbohydrates, fats, and proteins. The process of digestion breaks down these nutrients into their simplest components (glucose, fatty acids, and amino acids, respectively), which are absorbed into the blood and transported to metabolically active cells such as muscle, nerve, and liver cells. There, on location, these components either enter a metabolic pathway to produce ATP, or they are stored in body tissues for later use. Some of the ATP formed is used immediately to carry on cellular function, and some is stored in the cells for future use. Most food energy is stored in some other form, however, because the body's storage capacity for ATP is quite limited. Excess carbohydrates can be stored as glycogen in muscle or liver cells, and fats that are not immediately used for energy production can be stored as adipose tissue (fat depots). In contrast, relatively little of the protein we eat is used for energy production. Instead, it is used primarily for the growth or repair of cellular structures, or it is excreted in our waste products. Figure 1–2 illustrates this process.

ATP—The Immediate Energy Source

ATP is a complicated chemical structure made up of a substance called adenosine and three simpler groups of atoms called phosphate groups. Special high-energy bonds exist between two of the phosphate groups. Breaking the terminal phosphate bond releases energy that the cell uses directly to perform its cellular function. The specific cellular function performed depends on the cell type. In a muscle cell, the breakdown of ATP results in mechanical work known as muscular contraction. All "biological work" requires the breakdown of ATP. (See Fig. 1–3.)

ATP can be stored in the cells. The largest stores are found in the cells with the highest metabolic activity—in other words, in those cells that need ATP most. In comparison with other kinds of cells, muscle cells are capable of storing relatively high levels of ATP. Even so, the immediately available energy is extremely limited—sufficient for only a few seconds of muscular work. Therefore, ATP must be continuously

*Percent body fat refers to the percentage of total body weight.

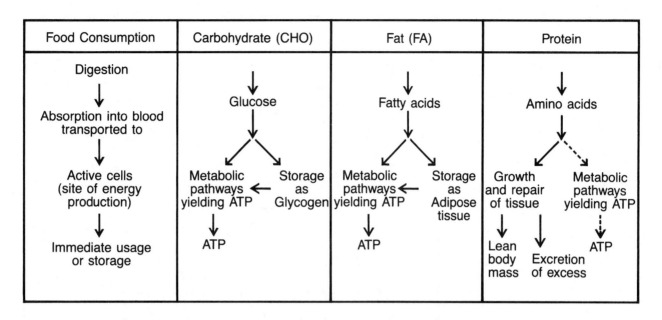

Food Consumption	Carbohydrate (CHO)	Fat (FA)	Protein
Digestion ↓ Absorption into blood transported to ↓ Active cells (site of energy production) ↓ Immediate usage or storage	Glucose ↓ Metabolic pathways yielding ATP ← Storage as Glycogen ↓ ATP	Fatty acids ↓ Metabolic pathways yielding ATP ← Storage as Adipose tissue ↓ ATP	Amino acids ↓ Growth and repair of tissue ⇢ Metabolic pathways yielding ATP ↓ ↓ ⇣ Lean body mass Excretion of excess ATP

FIGURE 1–2 Foods consumed ultimately produce the chemical energy required for cellular function.

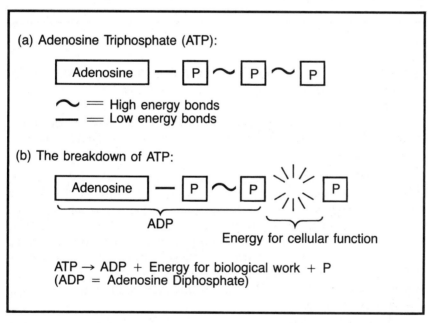

(a) Adenosine Triphosphate (ATP):

Adenosine — P ~ P ~ P

∼ = High energy bonds
— = Low energy bonds

(b) The breakdown of ATP:

Adenosine — P ~ P ⚡ P

ADP   Energy for cellular function

ATP → ADP + Energy for biological work + P
(ADP = Adenosine Diphosphate)

FIGURE 1–3 The ATP molecule

resynthesized to sustain muscular contraction for more than a few seconds. ATP can be resynthesized in several ways—immediately with creatine phosphate, anaerobically, or aerobically.

THE PHOSPHAGEN SYSTEM. **Creatine phosphate** (CP) is another high-energy phosphate compound found in close association with ATP. Together, these compounds are referred to as the **phosphagens.** When the high-energy phosphate bond in CP is broken down, the released energy is immediately used to resynthesize ATP from the available products of ATP breakdown. Consequently, as rapidly as ATP is broken down for muscular contraction, it is reformed from ADP (adenosine diphosphate) and P (the third phosphate group broken off from ATP) by the energy released from the breakdown of CP. This process is shown

AEROBIC DANCE-EXERCISE INSTRUCTOR MANUAL

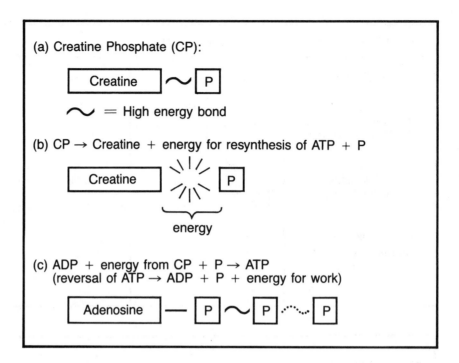

(a) Creatine Phosphate (CP):

Creatine ~ P

~ = High energy bond

(b) CP → Creatine + energy for resynthesis of ATP + P

Creatine   P

energy

(c) ADP + energy from CP + P → ATP
    (reversal of ATP → ADP + P + energy for work)

Adenosine — P ~ P ···· P

FIGURE 1-4 The immediate re-synthesis of ATP by CP

in Figure 1–4. The total amount of ATP and CP stored in the muscle is very small, and thus the amount of energy available for muscular contraction is extremely limited. In fact, there is probably enough energy available from the phosphagens for only about 10 seconds of all-out exertion. However, this energy is instantaneously available for muscular contraction.

ANAEROBIC PRODUCTION OF ATP.   The anaerobic production of ATP is required when energy is needed to perform activities requiring large bursts of energy over slightly longer periods. Here, mechanical work (muscular contraction) is performed so rapidly or intensely that the cardiorespiratory system cannot supply enough oxygen to the working muscles to meet the demand, and ATP must be produced in the absence of oxygen. Since **anaerobic** means without the presence of oxygen, the anaerobic production of ATP requires that ATP be formed without the availability of oxygen.

The anaerobic production of ATP is called **anaerobic glycolysis.** This metabolic pathway occurs within the cell and involves the breakdown of glucose (or glycogen, the storage form of glucose) to ATP with the liberation of lactic acid (LA) as a metabolic by-product:

$$\text{Glucose} \rightarrow 2\ \text{ATP} + 2\ \text{LA} + \text{heat}.$$

This formula indicates that 1 unit of glucose—the digested component of carbohydrate foods, or glycogen—breaks down without the presence of oxygen to yield 2 units of ATP and 2 units of lactic acid. Some energy is always lost in metabolic processes. This lost energy is represented in the formula by heat.

The formation of **lactic acid** poses a significant problem because it is associated with muscle fatigue. If the removal of lactic acid by the circulatory system cannot keep pace with its accumulation in the active muscles, temporary muscular fatigue occurs with painful symptoms usually referred to as "the burn." Thus, anaerobic glycolysis can only be used to a limited extent during sustained activity.

AEROBIC PRODUCTION OF ATP.   The aerobic production of ATP is used for activities requiring sustained energy production. Since **aerobic** means in the presence of oxygen, aerobic metabolic pathways require a continuous supply of oxygen. Without oxygen, these mechanisms fail and ATP is no longer produced. In the aerobic metabolism of carbohydrates, **glucose** (or glycogen) is broken down in the presence of oxygen (O_2) to yield 38 units of ATP, carbon dioxide (CO_2), water (H_2O), and heat:

$$\text{Glucose} + O_2 \rightarrow 38\ \text{ATP} + CO_2 + H_2O + \text{heat.}$$

This metabolic pathway, called **aerobic glycolysis,** occurs within the mitochondria, specialized structures within the cell. **Mitochondria** contain specific (oxidative) enzymes needed by the cell to utilize oxygen. Therefore, this highly efficient metabolic process—note the large amount of ATP produced for each unit of glucose oxidized—is limited mainly by the cardiorespiratory system's ability to deliver oxygen to the active tissues.

Aerobic pathways are also available to break down **fatty acids** for the production of ATP:

$$\text{Fatty Acid} + O_2 \rightarrow {>}100\ \text{ATP} + CO_2 + H_2O + \text{heat.}$$

This metabolic pathway, called **fatty acid oxidation,** also occurs within the mitochondria and requires a continuous supply of oxygen (as does the aerobic metabolism of glucose). The aerobic metabolism of fat yields a large amount of ATP, and therefore, fat is said to have a high caloric density. A calorie is a unit of heat energy. Fat yields 9 **kilocalories*** of energy per gram compared to 4 kilocalories of energy per gram of glucose. In other words, fat provides an excellent source of stored energy.

During rest, the body uses both glucose and fatty acid for energy production via aerobic pathways. The cardiorespiratory system can easily supply the oxygen necessary for this low level of energy metabolism. With exercise, however, supplying the required oxygen quickly enough becomes more difficult. Because glucose metabolism utilizes less oxygen than fatty acid metabolism, the body will use more glucose for energy production and less fat as exercise intensity increases. Significant amounts of fatty acid will only be used to produce energy when relatively low-intensity exercise is sustained over a long period (20 minutes or more), because the sympathetic nervous system must stimulate the release of fatty acids into the blood from fat storage sites (adipose tissue) before fatty acid oxidation can occur. In summary, with low-intensity, long-duration exercise, aerobic metabolism uses fatty acids as the fuel source. With higher intensity–shorter duration exercise, the primary fuel source for aerobic metabolism is glucose.

ATP and the Continuum of Human Movement

The human body is capable of brief, powerful movements as well as sustained, slower (less powerful) movements. Sprinting, jumping, and throwing are examples of brief, high-intensity movement. Walking and

---

*One thousand calories equals one kilocalorie (kcal).

jogging are characteristic of sustained, low-intensity movement. Of course, many movements fall somewhere between these extremes.

Often sports and dance combine movements requiring powerful jumps or sprints with slower, less intense movements. This continuum of human movement is almost ideally matched with the continuum of energy production. Extremely intense, powerful muscular contractions require a metabolic system that provides energy instantaneously, and the rate of energy production must be extremely high. Obviously this rate cannot be maintained for long periods, and therefore, the total amount of energy produced over a sustained period is relatively low. (The total amount of energy produced is called capacity.) Extremely intense exercise requires a metabolic system, then, that can supply energy at a very high rate.

The phosphagen system is such a metabolic system, but the system's capacity is low (i.e., the total energy production over a sustained period is very limited). Slightly less intense work can be sustained somewhat longer. For example, sprinting a quarter mile would require a metabolic system capable of supplying energy rapidly—not as fast as the phosphagen system, but more rapidly than required for slow, sustained activities. Such a metabolic system is provided by anaerobic glycolysis, which can supply energy at a high rate and has a higher capacity than the phosphagen system. The aerobic metabolism of ATP— aerobic glycolysis and fatty acid oxidation—is appropriate for slower, more sustained activities such as jogging and aerobic dance-exercise that are performed over a much longer time. This system has a high capacity for total energy production, but a low rate of energy production because it cannot supply energy rapidly.

Metabolic pathways are not mutually exclusive; at any instant, these pathways are working simultaneously to produce the ATP required for our bodily functions. The physiological demands of the movements determine which metabolic system predominates. It is the relative proportion of energy derived from each system that is important.

Comparison of Anaerobic and Aerobic Production of ATP

The metabolic pathways differ in several ways. While the phosphagens are available for immediate use, the total energy production is extremely limited. The primary advantage of anaerobic glycolysis is that it can be mobilized almost instantaneously since oxygen is not required; however, compared with aerobic pathways, relatively little ATP is formed per unit of glucose substrate utilized (i.e., 2 units of ATP are formed for every unit of glucose used). In addition, since lactic acid, a substance highly associated with fatigue, occurs as a by-product, the primary limiting factor is the amount of lactic acid that a person can tolerate before exhaustion. Finally, since only glucose (or glycogen) can be used as a substrate, a secondary limiting factor is substrate depletion.

Aerobic metabolism is a much slower pathway because it requires a continuous supply of oxygen to the metabolically active cells. However, since the by-products of aerobic metabolism (carbon dioxide and water) do not cause fatigue, this pathway is limited only by substrate (glycogen) depletion, which probably will not occur until 2 or more hours of continuous exercise have passed. Finally, the aerobic production of ATP is more efficient because it yields a considerably higher amount of ATP per unit of substrate (glucose or fat) used. The only disadvantage of aerobic glycolysis or fatty acid oxidation is that the rate of ATP production is limited by the rate of oxygen delivery to the

Table 1–1

COMPARISON OF ANAEROBIC AND AEROBIC SYSTEMS OF ATP PRODUCTION

ANAEROBIC SYSTEMS	RATE OF ATP PRODUCTION	SUBSTRATE	CAPACITY OF SYSTEM	MAJOR LIMITATION	MAJOR USE
Phosphagens (stored ATP & CP)	Very rapid rate	Creatine phosphate (CP)	Very limited ATP production	Very limited supply of CP	Very high-intensity, short-duration sprint activities. Predominates during activities of 1–10 seconds.
Anaerobic glycolysis (GLU → ATP + LA)	Rapid metabolic rate	Blood glucose Glycogen	Limited ATP production	Lactic acid by-product causes rapid fatigue	High-intensity, short-duration activities. Predominates during activities of 1–3 minutes.

AEROBIC SYSTEMS	RATE OF ATP PRODUCTION	SUBSTRATE	CAPACITY OF SYSTEM	MAJOR LIMITATION	MAJOR USE
Aerobic glycolysis	Slow metabolic rate	Blood glucose Glycogen	Unlimited ATP production	Relatively slow rate of oxygen delivery to cells	Lower intensity, longer duration, endurance activities. Predominates during activities longer than 3 minutes.
Fatty acid oxidation	Slow metabolic rate	Fatty acids	Unlimited ATP production	Relatively slow rate of oxygen delivery to cells	Lower intensity, longer duration, endurance activities. Fatty acid oxidation predominates after about 20 minutes of continuous activity.

mitochondria by the cardiorespiratory and vascular systems. Table 1–1 presents a comparison of the aerobic and anaerobic systems of ATP production.

Muscles and Metabolism

Our muscles are composed of several kinds of fibers that differ in their ability to utilize the metabolic pathways. **Fast twitch (FT) fibers** do not have a finely developed oxygen delivery system, but they are equipped with an outstanding capacity for ATP and CP storage and a high capacity for anaerobic glycolysis. Therefore, fast twitch fibers are specialized for anaerobic metabolism. They are used (recruited) predominantly for rapid, powerful movements such as jumping, throwing, and sprinting.

Slow twitch (ST) fibers, on the other hand, are exceptionally well equipped for oxygen delivery and have a high quantity of aerobic or oxidative enzymes. Although they do not have a highly developed mechanism for either ATP and CP storage or anaerobic glycolysis, ST fibers have a large number of mitochondria and, consequently, are particularly well designed for the aerobic metabolic pathways of aerobic glycolysis and fatty acid oxidation. These fibers are recruited primarily for low-intensity, longer duration activities such as walking, jogging, and swimming.

Persons who excel in activities characterized by sudden bursts of energy, but who tire relatively rapidly, probably have a high percentage of fast twitch fibers. Persons who are best at lower intensity, endurance activities probably have a large percentage of slow twitch fibers. Most people have roughly equal percentages of both fiber types. There are also a number of "intermediate" muscle fibers that have a fairly high capacity for both fast anaerobic and slow aerobic movements.

Muscle fiber distribution (fast twitch, intermediate, or slow twitch) is determined by genetic makeup. This is not to say, however, that metabolic capacity is unresponsive to activity lifestyle. All three types of muscle fibers are highly trainable; that is, they are capable of adapting to the specific metabolic demands placed on them. If a person regularly engages in low-intensity endurance activities, improvement is seen in aerobic capacity. Although all three types of muscle fibers will show some improvement in aerobic ability, the ST fibers will be most responsive to this kind of training and will show the largest improvement in aerobic capacity. If, on the other hand, short-duration, high-intensity exercise like interval training is pursued, other metabolic pathways will be emphasized, and the capabilities of the FT fibers to perform anaerobically will be enhanced. ST fibers will be less responsive to this kind of training.

It is important for physical fitness professionals to have a thorough understanding of the different metabolic systems in order to prescribe specific exercise programs that will enable participants in their classes to achieve desired results. As we've discussed, exercise intensity and duration is directly related to the continuum of metabolic pathways and movement patterns. For example, prescribing quick, explosive movements specific to the use of phosphagens and anaerobic glycolysis will have little effect if the goal of the exercise program is to develop cardiorespiratory endurance. This principle, known as **exercise specificity,** is probably the single most important principle to understand.

THE NEUROMUSCULAR SYSTEM

Dance-exercise instructors need to understand how a motor skill is executed. To do so requires a basic appreciation of the neuromuscular system, which includes both the nervous system and the skeletal muscle system. The nervous system is responsible for coordinating movement. It is possible for a person to have well-developed muscles and still have poor coordination.

Basic Organization of the Nervous System

The basic anatomical unit of the nervous system is the **neuron,** or nerve cell. There are two kinds of neurons, sensory and motor. **Sensory neurons** convey electrical impulses from sensory organs in the periphery (such as the skin) to the spinal cord and brain (called the central nervous system). **Motor neurons** conduct impulses from the central nervous system (CNS) to the periphery. Because the motor neurons carry electrical impulses from the CNS to the muscle cells, they signal the muscles to contract or to relax and, therefore, regulate muscular movement. The endings of the motor neuron connect or synapse with muscle cells in the periphery of the body. This motor neuron–muscle cell synapse is called the **motor end plate.** (Fig. 1–5 shows a motor neuron and motor end plate.) The basic functional unit of the neuromuscular system is the **motor unit,** which consists of one motor neuron and the muscle cells that it innervates. Motor units are arranged according to muscle fiber type. A neuron capable of conducting nervous impulses very rapidly will synapse with the cells of fast twitch muscle fibers. The cells of slow twitch muscle fibers will be controlled by somewhat slower conducting neurons.

Basic Organization of the Muscular System

The skeletal muscle cell is a complicated organ and is described only briefly here. Basically, the muscle is entirely surrounded by connective tissue that extends from the tendon, which connects the muscle to the bone. Various sublayers of connective tissue divide each muscle into bundles of individual muscle cells. The connective tissues provide an important element of strength and structural integrity to the muscular system and are thought to be involved with delayed muscle soreness.

An individual muscle cell is composed of many threadlike protein strands called myofibrils (see Fig. 1–6), which contain the contractile proteins. The basic functional unit of the myofibril is the sarcomere. Within the sarcomere are two protein myofilaments: the thick myofilament is myosin, and the thinner myofilament is actin. The myosin and actin myofilaments are arranged to interdigitate in a prescribed, regular way, revealing a pattern of alternating light and dark bands or striations within the sarcomere. Tiny projections called cross-bridges extend from the myosin myofilaments toward the actin myofilaments.

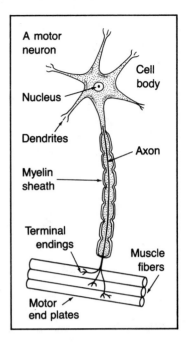

FIGURE 1–5 Basic anatomical structure of a neuron (or nerve cell) and motor end plate

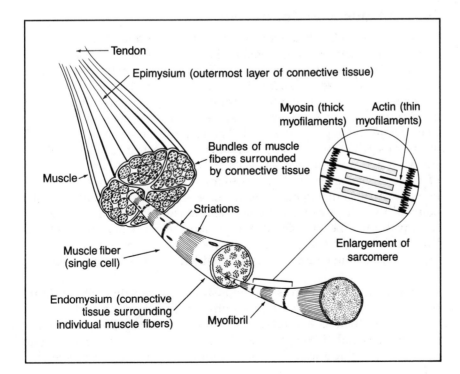

FIGURE 1–6 Muscle organization

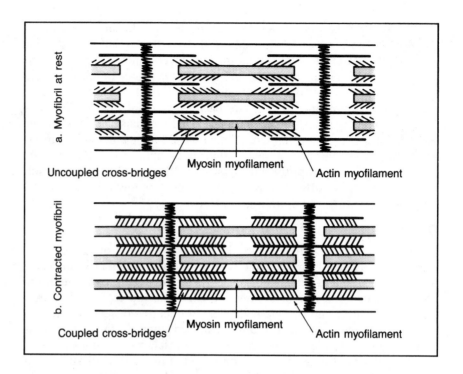

a. Myofibril at rest

Uncoupled cross-bridges   Myosin myofilament   Actin myofilament

b. Contracted myofibril

Coupled cross-bridges   Myosin myofilament   Actin myofilament

FIGURE 1-7 The sliding filament theory

According to the sliding filament theory, muscular contraction occurs when the cross-bridges extending from the myosin myofilaments attach (or couple) to the actin myofilaments and pull them over the myosin myofilaments. As the cross-bridges produce tension, the muscle shortens. The actual muscle shortening occurs as the actin myofilaments are pulled toward the center of the sarcomere, and the sarcomere shortens (see Fig. 1-7). The coupling of myosin and actin and the shortening process depend on the breakdown of ATP for energy.

Types of Muscular Contraction

What has been described above is one form of **isotonic muscular contraction.** The actin myofilaments slide over the myosin myofilaments toward the center of the sarcomere. Each sarcomere in a stimulated myofibril is reduced in length. The muscle visibly shortens, and joint movement occurs. Tension (or force) develops throughout the muscle as it contracts, but the tension changes with the total length of the muscle and the angle of the joint. The greatest force can be generated at the muscle's optimal length—the length of greatest strength—where the actin and myosin myofilaments are aligned so the largest number of cross-bridges between the myofilaments can be activated simultaneously. At all other lengths, fewer cross-bridges are simultaneously coupled to actin myofilaments and less tension can be developed by the myofibril. The change in muscle tension with muscle length is illustrated in Figure 1-8(a). This form of isotonic muscle contraction is also called **concentric** contraction, which means shortening muscle contraction.

Eccentric contraction is the opposite of concentric contraction in that the muscle is developing tension as it lengthens against a resistance (rather than as it shortens against a resistance). This movement is sometimes called "negative work." A typical eccentric contraction occurs in lowering a weight to the beginning position, resisting a move-

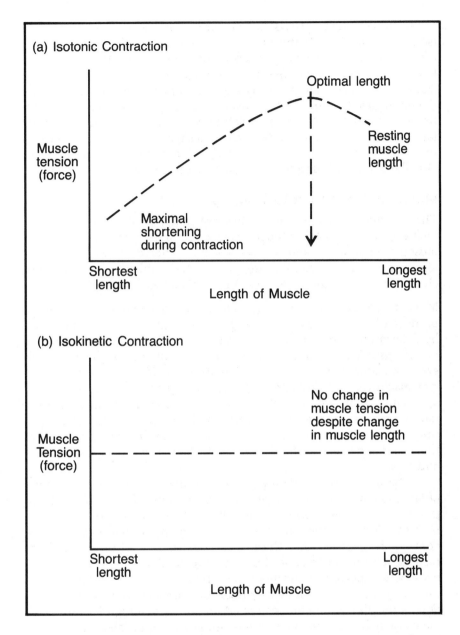

FIGURE 1–8 The length-tension
curve during contraction

ment, or moving with gravity. Walking down stairs is an example of negative work. In typical weight-lifting movements, eccentric contractions usually follow concentric contractions.

Isometric muscle contraction occurs when muscle shortening and joint movement does not occur. During this type of muscular contraction, the tension developed within the muscle does not change because the muscle length does not change. An example of an isometric muscle contraction is holding a weight at arm's length or attempting to move an immovable object (i.e., exerting force outward against a door frame). The actual amount of tension developed by a muscle is directly related to the number of motor units stimulated by the nervous system. For example, more motor units will be stimulated to overcome a 10-lb resistance than a 2-lb resistance. Since no joint movement occurs, this type of contraction is sometimes referred to as a static contraction.

Isokinetic contractions, in outward appearance, look much like isotonic contractions. In this kind of contraction, however, tension within the muscle does not change even though the muscle length changes (shortens or lengthens). (See Fig. 1–8b.) To accomplish an isokinetic contraction, special equipment is required to alter the resistance offered the muscle as it contracts at a constant velocity. This approach is sometimes referred to as "accommodating resistance" or "variable resistance" exercise. Isokinetic exercise enables maximal tension to develop in a muscle throughout its entire range of motion; with isotonic exercise, the muscle can develop maximal tension only at its optimal length.

Muscular Response to Training

Three components of physical fitness warrant more discussion because they are directly related to the neuromuscular system. Muscular strength, muscular endurance, and flexibility can be altered with regular exercise if some basic principles are applied. Let's consider how the principle of specificity applies to these three components of physical fitness.

MUSCULAR STRENGTH.   Strength refers to the maximal tension or force produced by a muscle or muscle group. Strength is usually measured by determining how much weight can be lifted in a single effort. The one-repetition maximum (1 RM) test is determined through a trial-and-error procedure using either free weights (barbells and weights) or special machines (e.g., dynamometers, Hydra-gym, Nautilus, Universal apparatus). Most often 1 RM tests are completed for the following muscle groups: (a) the bench press for the muscles of the chest and upper arms; (b) the arm curl for the muscles on the anterior aspect of the upper arms; and (c) the leg press for the muscles of the upper legs and hips.

After testing, training programs can be developed to enhance muscular strength. To improve strength, training intensity should be high, the number of **repetitions** of each lift or movement should be kept relatively low, and the movements should be performed carefully at a controlled speed so that there is a consistent application of force throughout the movement. Good posture and body mechanics are extremely important. Movements requiring strength are performed primarily by the fast twitch muscle fibers and are anaerobic; that is, muscular strength-training movements do not require a high level of aerobic capacity because the movements use anaerobic metabolism. Because strength training is relatively stressful on the connective tissues and muscular structure of the body, it is usually recommended that heavy strength training be performed only about 3 times per week. It is important that the muscles and supporting structures be given time to recover sufficiently between workouts although there is considerable disagreement about the length of time.

In summary, training to improve strength is characterized by the following principles:

1. High resistance is used—often the weight equivalent to the 6–10 repetition maximum, or the maximum weight that can be lifted 6–10 times.

2. Few repetitions are performed—usually about 5–7 per set for 3 **sets**—so muscles and joint structures are not overstressed.

3. Movements are controlled and deliberate—emphasizing the movement speed appropriate to the skill for which increased strength is being developed.

After physical training, the physiological system that has been stressed alters its state of homeostasis; that is, it adapts to the demands that have been placed on it. These adaptations result in a higher functional capacity, an improved ability to meet physical demands. However, none of these adaptations or changes in physiological response to exercise are permanent. According to the **reversibility principle,** training adaptations will gradually decline if not regularly reinforced by a "maintenance" exercise program. Strength training causes the following adaptations to occur in the neuromuscular system:

1. *Muscular hypertrophy* is a general increase in the size or diameter of muscle cells. Specifically, muscular hypertrophy is the result of an increase in the muscle's content of contractile proteins. In other words, there is a proliferation of myosin and actin myofilaments within the trained myofibrils. Since strength training is largely performed by the fast twitch fibers, these are the fibers most capable of hypertrophy. People with unusually large, muscular builds very likely have a high percentage of fast twitch fibers. Generally, women do not experience muscular hypertrophy to the same extent as men because the male hormone testosterone is important in synthesizing the contractile proteins. Nevertheless, women will increase substantially in strength in response to a progressive strength-training program. Muscular hypertrophy is not required for improvement in strength. With muscle disuse, as in paralysis, muscle atrophy or wasting occurs.

2. *Metabolic alterations in the strength-trained muscles* include an enhancement of the phosphagen system, which means that the strength-trained muscle fibers are capable of storing a larger supply of ATP and CP and of the enzymes important for their breakdown.

3. *Other changes occur* that enhance the action of the fast twitch motor units; however, these changes are beyond the scope of this manual.

MUSCULAR ENDURANCE.   Endurance refers to the ability to repeatedly contract a muscle or muscle group against resistance. Tests of muscular endurance usually involve selecting a fixed percentage of the maximum strength, for example, 70% of the 1 RM, and counting the number of repetitions that can be completed without resting. Sit-up or pull-up tests are examples of muscular endurance tests, not of strength tests as often thought. It is usually recommended that muscular endurance training be completed 3–5 times per week for maximum results. This form of training is most specific to aerobic metabolism and slow twitch muscle fibers and motor units.

Training programs specific for muscular endurance should employ the following principles:

1. Moderate resistance is used.

2. Many (20–50) repetitions are completed because this is the aspect of performance being developed.

3. Speed of contraction is maintained at the same rate required for muscular endurance in performance.

AEROBIC DANCE-EXERCISE INSTRUCTOR MANUAL

4. Training frequency is usually 3–5 times per week.

After muscular endurance training, these neuromuscular adaptations are seen:

1. *Increased vascularity*, in which blood supply and, consequently, oxygen delivery is enhanced to the myofibrils.

2. *Increased concentrations of oxidative enzymes*, which extract oxygen from the blood, in the specific muscles trained. Increased concentration of oxidative enzymes coupled with increased vascularity means that the aerobic capacity of the trained muscles has improved.

3. *Enhanced glycogen storage* delays fatigue because more metabolic substrate (fuel) is available.

These neuromuscular changes are specific to the slow twitch muscle fibers and motor units, and are of particular relevance to dance exercise. Although dance exercise does not adhere precisely to the training principles mentioned earlier, regular participation in dance exercise generally enhances muscular endurance.

FLEXIBILITY. Flexibility refers to the range of motion possible about a joint over which a muscle or group of muscles span. Flexibility is often related to age; young children are usually extremely flexible, while the elderly generally have lost much of the flexibility they had as younger adults.

Range of motion can be limited by the bony structure of a joint, the ligamentous structure of a joint, or the musculotendinous structure of the muscle(s) spanning the joint. The bony structure of a joint is, of course, a self-limiting factor that cannot be altered. In addition, a joint ligament (the fibrous band connecting bones) or joint capsule should never be stretched because to do so would lead to an unstable joint (joint laxity) and an increased risk of joint injury. Therefore, the only desirable way that range of motion can be altered is by gently stretching the musculotendinous structures controlling the movement of the joint. Sometimes these structures can become extremely taut, causing a reduction in the normal range of motion.

Although at times flexibility exercises are ignored, flexibility is thought to be related to the incidence of acute muscle injury due to strenuous exercise and also to delayed muscle soreness. As a result, there is renewed interest in improving flexibility. Acute muscle injuries such as muscle pulls or tears are more likely to occur if the muscle fibers or surrounding tissues are so taut and inflexible that a sudden stretch causes tissue injury. The exact cause of delayed muscle soreness, which occurs 24–48 hours after strenuous exercise, is not known. Minute tissue damage could explain delayed muscle soreness, or muscle soreness could be caused by local muscular spasms (the "spasm theory") that reduce muscle blood flow, resulting in pain. Another prominent theory is that damage to surrounding connective tissue liberates hydroxyproline (or other substances) commonly seen with delayed muscle soreness. Whatever the exact cause, delayed muscle soreness appears to be particularly associated with the eccentric phase of a contraction. Stretching exercises performed before and after an exercise session help to prevent soreness and also to relieve soreness when it does occur.

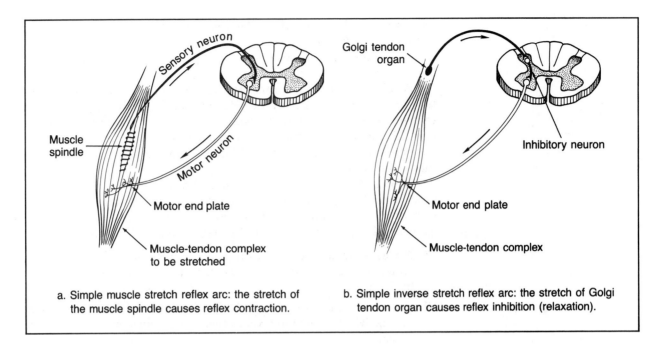

a. Simple muscle stretch reflex arc: the stretch of the muscle spindle causes reflex contraction.

b. Simple inverse stretch reflex arc: the stretch of Golgi tendon organ causes reflex inhibition (relaxation).

There are two types of stretching to increase flexibility: static stretching and dynamic or ballistic stretching. **Static stretching** involves holding a static (nonmoving) position so that the specified joint is immobilized in a position that places the desired muscles and connective tissues passively at their greatest possible length. A static stretch position is typically held for 10–30 seconds but should be held for 30–60 seconds to achieve optimal results. Static stretching is best characterized as low-force, long-duration stretching, and has repeatedly been shown to produce good results with little muscle soreness. In fact, static stretching is commonly used to reduce muscle soreness. Little risk of physical injury exists if static stretching is performed as just described.

Dynamic or **ballistic stretching** is characterized by jerking, bobbing, or bouncing motions representing relatively high-force, short-duration movements. Ballistic stretching motions, while seemingly effective, actually invoke the **stretch reflexes** that oppose the desired stretching. Muscle stretch reflexes are involuntary motor responses controlled by the **muscle spindle,** a sensory organ located within the muscle. When a muscle spindle is stimulated, an impulse is propagated over a sensory nerve fiber. The nerve fiber synapses in the spinal cord with a motor neuron that returns to the muscle containing the muscle spindle (see Fig. 1–9a). This reflex results in the suddenly stretched muscle responding with a corresponding contraction; the amount and rate of this contraction varies directly with the amount and rate of the movement causing the initial stretch. Ballistic stretching, then, seems to evoke the opposite physiological response—an increase in muscle tension—from that desired from a stretching exercise.

A firm static stretch, on the other hand, invokes an inverse stretch reflex by stimulating another sensory organ (with a higher threshold level) called the **Golgi tendon organ.** When stimulated, this organ causes an inhibition not only of the muscle whose muscle spindle was stretched, but also of the entire muscle group (see Fig. 1–9b). Static stretching,

FIGURE 1–9 The muscle spindle and simple stretch reflex

then, seems to bring about a reduction in muscle tension, which is the desirable physiological response. In addition, static stretching is safer because it does not impose a sudden, possibly injurious force upon the tissues.

A third type of stretching, proprioceptive neuromuscular facilitation or PNF, is a relatively new technique originally developed for rehabilitative purposes in physical therapy. PNF involves statically stretching a muscle immediately after maximally contracting it. As yet, controlled experiments using PNF have found no advantage over regular static stretching techniques.

General flexibility exercises should be part of every physical fitness exercise program. Gentle stretching exercises should be included in every warm-up and cool-down phase of an exercise session. Some general principles specific to the enhancement of flexibility include:

1. A very easy general warm-up (such as walking and swinging the arms) should precede stretching exercises to increase blood flow to the area.

2. Stretching exercises should be performed without bouncing or jerking, which may injure connective tissues and stimulate the stretch reflex.

3. Attempts to stretch a muscle or muscle group beyond the normal range of motion should never be made.

4. Excessive resistance should never be used. All stretching should be done gently and only to the extent that muscle tension is perceived, but muscle pain does *not* occur.

5. Instructors should understand that their students will vary greatly in flexibility. Everyone is not equally flexible or equally responsive to flexibility training.

After specific flexibility training, the muscles and connective tissues adapt by elongating slightly, thus increasing the range of motion.

THE CARDIOVASCULAR-RESPIRATORY SYSTEMS

Cardiorespiratory endurance was defined earlier as the capacity of the heart and lung systems to deliver blood and, hence, oxygen, to the working muscles during sustained exercise. The oxygen is necessary, of course, to produce the ATP necessary to perform low- to moderate-intensity levels of exercise for long periods. The production of ATP requires metabolic systems with a relatively unlimited capacity to produce ATP at a slow rate. (See Table 1–1.) In other words, physical activities classified as cardiovascular endurance activities (aerobic) require aerobic metabolism, specifically aerobic glycolysis (carbohydrate as substrate) or fatty acid oxidation (fatty acids as substrate). Aerobic exercise depends largely, then, on the interaction of the cardiovascular system and the respiratory system to provide oxygen to the active cells so that carbohydrates and fatty acids can be converted to ATP for muscular contraction. These two systems are also important for the removal of metabolic waste products such as carbon dioxide and lactic acid, and for the dissipation of the internal heat produced by metabolic processes.

Let's consider how these systems accomplish these tasks. Basically, there are three primary factors:

1. Getting oxygen into the blood—a function of the oxygen-carrying capacity of the blood and respiratory ventilation.

2. Delivering oxygen to the active cells—a function of cardiac output.

3. Extracting oxygen from the blood to complete the metabolic production of ATP—a function of the oxidative enzymes located in the active cells.

Oxygen-Carrying Capacity

The oxygen-carrying capacity of blood is determined primarily by two variables, the hemoglobin content of the blood and the ability to ventilate the lungs adequately. **Hemoglobin** (Hb) is a protein molecule in red blood cells that is specifically adapted to bond (carry) oxygen molecules. Persons with low hemoglobin concentrations cannot carry as much oxygen in their blood as persons with high hemoglobin concentrations. Anemia (less than 12 gm of Hb per 100 ml of blood), although relatively rare, definitely limits the blood's oxygen-carrying capacity. In most healthy persons, however, the oxygen-carrying capacity of the blood is not a limiting factor in the performance of aerobic exercise.

Respiratory ventilation is a function of the depth of each breath (the tidal volume) and the respiratory rate (respiratory frequency). With exercise, both tidal volume and respiratory frequency increase. Certain respiratory diseases may limit the ability to load oxygen onto the red blood cells. Persons with asthma (constriction of breathing passages) or emphysema (loss of normal elasticity of lung tissues) cannot move enough air through their lung tissues (hypoventilation) to interface adequately with the blood flowing through these tissues (**perfusion**). As a result, the blood leaving the lungs is not sufficiently loaded with oxygen.

At high levels of exercise, hyperventilation may occur. More air is breathed in and out through the lung passages than is necessary for the existing metabolic rate (i.e., more air is supplied than is needed by the body). Carbon dioxide is "blown off" faster than it is produced metabolically, resulting in a condition known as hypocapnia, which is a lowering of normal blood levels of carbon dioxide. Hypocapnia may be triggered by emotional excitement or fear, and is sometimes seen in the inexperienced exerciser. Symptoms include dizziness, lightheadedness, bluing of the lips, and tingling of the fingers.

Oxygen Delivery

The second important factor in cardiovascular-respiratory endurance, the delivery of blood to the active cells, is a function of **cardiac output.** Cardiac output is the product of stroke volume (the quantity of blood pumped per heartbeat) and heart rate (beats per minute):

$$\text{Cardiac output} = \text{SV} \times \text{HR}$$

A full explanation of how cardiac output is regulated is beyond the scope of this manual. Basically, **stroke volume** is a function of the amount of blood filling the heart during its resting or diastolic period, and the force of the contraction of the heart during its contraction or systolic period. Static exercise (as in isometric exercise) or holding the breath while contracting the chest muscles (the **Valsalva maneuver**) increases thoracic pressure, hinders venous return of blood to the heart and reduces stroke volume. On the other hand, rhythmic exercise characterized by alternate contraction and relaxation of muscle groups favors the venous return of blood to the heart and enhances stroke volume. The higher the stroke volume for any given level of cardiac output, the lower the heart rate needs to be. Because the heart gets more rest with a slower heart rate, delivery of blood is more efficient with a higher stroke volume and a lower heart rate. Outstanding endurance athletes usually have very high stroke volumes and rather low, corresponding heart rates compared to sedentary persons.

Because we have a limited quantity of blood (about 5–6 liters), all cells in our body are not perfused with blood at once. Blood is distributed according to metabolic need. At rest, our cardiac output level is low (about 5–7 liters per minute depending on body size). Essential organs such as the brain, heart, lungs, liver, and kidneys receive most of the blood, while secondary functions receive relatively low quantities. When eating a meal, our intestinal tract temporarily receives more blood to enhance digestion and absorption. While sunbathing, skin blood flow increases so overheating does not occur.

As the exercise level increases, blood flow patterns change according to metabolic need. As the blood flow to our muscles (to produce ATP for contraction) and to our skin (to dissipate the metabolic heat produced) increases, the amount of blood flowing to less active organs such as the kidney and intestinal tract decreases. In this instance, we conserve water (less urine is formed) and slow down digestion. However, because our muscles need so much oxygen to carry on their work, the net effect is a tremendous increase in cardiac output. One of the most significant factors in cardiovascular endurance, which represents the ability to perform aerobic exercise, is cardiac output. The greater the capacity to increase cardiac output, that is, to deliver oxygen to the active muscle cells and to dissipate the internal heat of metabolism, the greater the capacity for endurance (aerobic) performance.

Blood pressure is very important in blood flow distribution because it drives the circulatory system. Blood pressure is influenced by many factors. Basically, blood pressure is a function of the force generated by the heart during its contraction phase (systole), and the force generated by the vessels on the blood flowing through them. Just as the strength of heart contraction can vary, some blood vessels (notably the smaller arteries called arterioles) can contract (vasoconstriction) or relax (vasodilation), and thus alter their resistance to blood flow. This variable is important in determining patterns of blood flow. For example, during exercise, vasoconstriction occurs in the vessels of inactive organs (such as the intestine), and vasodilation occurs in vessels of active organs (muscles), thus redirecting blood flow to areas of the body where it is directly needed.

Oxygen Extraction

The third important factor in cardiovascular-respiratory endurance is the extraction of oxygen from the blood at the cellular level for the actual production of ATP. The amount of oxygen extracted is largely a function of muscle fiber type and the availability of specialized oxidative enzymes in the mitochondria. As discussed earlier, the slow twitch muscle fibers are specifically adapted for oxygen extraction and utilization due to their high levels of oxidative enzymes. The slow twitch fibers are where oxygen is actually used by the cells to produce ATP.

RESPONSES TO AEROBIC EXERCISE

Aerobic exercise—whether aerobic dance-exercise, jogging (running), cycling, swimming, cross-country skiing, or walking (striding)—is best characterized as (a) rhythmic large muscle activity (i.e., alternating muscle contraction and relaxation) that usually moves the body from one place to another, and (b) low- to moderate-intensity exercise that can be performed continuously without undue respiratory distress.

Such movement patterns depend on oxidative or aerobic metabolic pathways that require oxygen in order to use the potential energy contained within carbohydrate or fatty acid substrates for ATP production to drive muscular contraction. The other metabolic pathways (the phosphagen system and anaerobic glycolysis) are used only minimally to produce energy for muscular activity. Physiological responses to aerobic exercise (a) provide oxygen to the metabolically active cells, (b) rid the body of metabolic waste products (excess carbon dioxide), and (c) dissipate the internal heat produced during energy production.

The body at rest is in a state of dynamic equilibrium known as homeostasis. More specifically, the respiratory ventilation, cardiac output, blood pressure, and blood flow distribution patterns are adequately meeting the body's metabolic needs. In terms of bioenergetics, the cardiovascular-respiratory-metabolic systems are providing and using a relatively small quantity of oxygen to produce the ATP required by the body's active cells. In terms of oxygen consumption ($\dot{V}O_2$), the body is in steady state, meaning that the delivery and utilization of oxygen is meeting metabolic demands, and aerobic systems are providing the energy required.

When aerobic exercise begins, the body rapidly responds to increase the quantity of oxygen required to produce the ATP necessary to meet the higher metabolic demand. Cardiac output must increase to deliver more blood to the active muscle cells. To meet this requirement, heart rate, stroke volume, and systolic blood pressure increase immediately. Diastolic blood pressure either remains constant or decreases. Respiratory ventilation must increase to load more oxygen onto the red blood cells as they release the carbon dioxide produced by the oxidation of glucose at the muscle level.

In Figure 1–10, these responses are graphically illustrated. The bolder line indicates the level of oxygen consumption required at rest (left-hand side) and the sharp increase that occurs with commencement of exercise (upward arrow). The line quickly returns to the resting level when exercise is abruptly stopped (downward arrow). The actual oxygen consumption that results from these physiological responses is indicated by the sloping line in the figure. Notice that the actual oxygen consumption momentarily does not meet the physiological demand (requirement) for oxygen. A physiological **oxygen deficit** occurs (left-hand side of Figure 1–10).

The physiological responses that occur with commencement of exercise take approximately 2–4 minutes to meet the increased metabolic demands for oxygen adequately. During this time, the other metabolic systems (capable of producing energy more rapidly) produce the

AEROBIC DANCE-EXERCISE INSTRUCTOR MANUAL

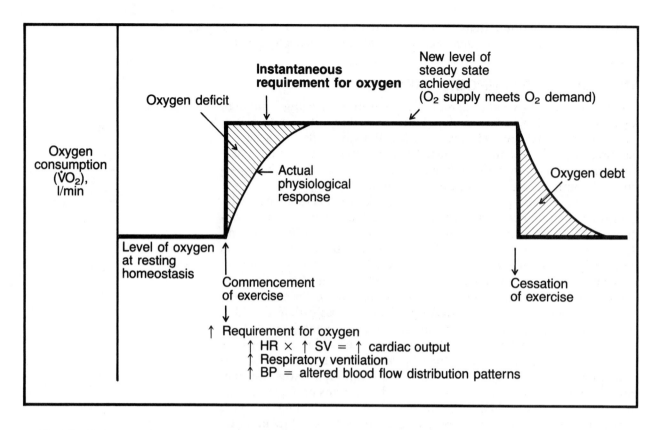

FIGURE 1–10 Oxygen consumption during aerobic exercise

energy needed to carry out the exercise; the phosphagens are depleted, and a small amount of lactic acid is formed. When the cardiorespiratory systems have adequately responded, a new level of oxygen consumption is achieved. If the exercise intensity is not too high relative to cardiovascular endurance, a new level of steady state is achieved as shown in Figure 1–10.

With cessation of exercise, the requirement for oxygen abruptly returns to the initial resting level. Again, however, the body responds more slowly. As cardiac output, blood pressure, and respiratory ventilation return to resting levels, oxygen consumption slowly declines as well. This temporarily elevated level of oxygen consumption, called **oxygen debt,** "pays back" the oxygen deficit. The energy produced during this time is used to replenish the depleted phosphagens, to eliminate accumulated lactic acid, and to restore homeostatic conditions.

If exercise intensity is so high that the body cannot depend predominantly on aerobic pathways for ATP production, then the oxygen deficit and corresponding oxygen debt are extremely high, and exercise cannot be performed for more than a few minutes. Figure 1–11 shows diagrammatically the oxygen consumption pattern during anaerobic (high-intensity) exercise. Extreme dyspnea (respiratory distress) and muscle pain (the "burn" of lactic acid or oxygen deficiency) are experienced. With high-intensity exercise, anaerobic metabolic pathways must be relied on heavily for ATP production. The result is phosphagen depletion, high levels of lactic acid, and fatigue. A homeostatic steady state cannot be achieved, and the recovery period is prolonged in proportion to the duration of exercise.

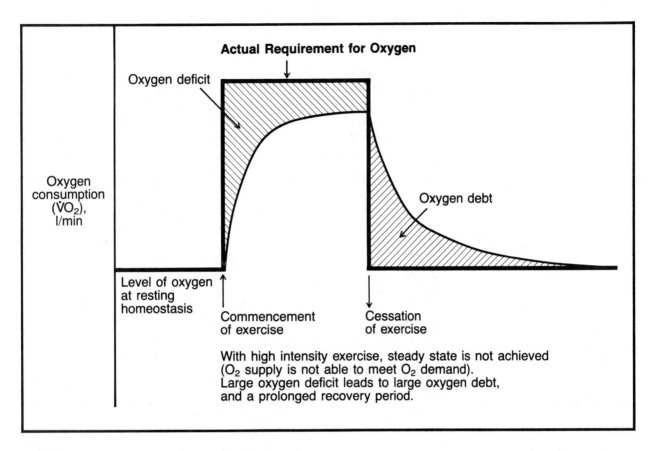

FIGURE 1–11 Oxygen consumption during anaerobic exercise

Guidelines for Improving Cardiovascular-Respiratory Endurance

As for improving muscular strength and muscular endurance, there are three basic variables to consider when developing an exercise program to improve cardiovascular-respiratory endurance:

1. Exercise intensity—how hard to exercise.
2. Exercise duration—how long to exercise.
3. Exercise frequency—how often to exercise.

The following general recommendations are based on thorough investigations of these variables:

1. *Exercise intensity should be approximately 50%–85% of maximal oxygen consumption (also referred to as maximal functional capacity).* Below this range, little if any training stimulus is achieved. Above this range, the exercise stress becomes more anaerobic than aerobic, and the principle of exercise specificity is violated. Because measuring maximal oxygen consumption is so costly and time consuming, target heart-rate zones have been established that adequately estimate exercise **intensity** in terms of maximal oxygen consumption. For aerobic exercise, heart rate is a fairly reliable indicator of how hard the body is working. The target zone of 50%–85% of maximal oxygen consumption is roughly equivalent to 60%–80% of the maximal heart rate reserve. Maximal heart rate declines after approximately 25 years of age. To obtain an estimate of maximal heart rate (HR max), subtract the person's age from 220. For example, a 30-year-old has a maximal attainable heart rate of about 190 (220 − 30 = 190), and a 65-year-old has a maximal attainable heart rate of about 155 (220 − 65 = 155). To calculate heart rate reserve subtract resting heart rate from HR max. The target heart-rate zone for aerobic exercise for the 30-year-old, with a resting heart rate of 70, would be 142–166. For the 65-year-old, with a resting heart rate of 80, the target heart-rate zone would be 125–140. (See Chapter 9 for a discussion of heart-rate monitoring techniques.)

2. *Exercise duration may vary from 15 to 60 minutes, depending on the population.* The aerobics component of most dance-exercise classes is 20–30 minutes. Duration refers to the actual time that the person is within the target heart-rate zone and does not include a warm-up or cool-down period. Of course, if a student is incapable of 20 minutes of continuous exercise when first beginning an exercise program, this guideline can be set as a goal. Exercise duration over about 40 minutes in the target heart-rate zone is more than most people need to achieve excellent cardiovascular endurance. However, someone who is training to compete in ultraendurance events needs to train in the target heart-rate zone for very long periods.

3. *Exercise frequency should be a minimum of 2–3 times per week.* Two aerobic-exercise sessions per week performed within the target heart-rate zone for 20 minutes at each session is probably a minimum guideline. A totally sedentary person will probably experience a training stimulus with such a routine, but a more fit person will need to exercise more frequently—perhaps 3–4 times per week. Little additional benefit is achieved by exercising more than 5 times per week.

Any program designed to improve cardiovascular endurance should apply the concept of progressive overload. **Overload** refers to the level of stress imposed on the physiological systems involved. For training adaptation to occur, the system must be systematically stressed slightly more than it is accustomed to. Applying the concept of progressive overload to cardiovascular endurance means increasing the exercise intensity, or the exercise duration, or the exercise frequency. Usually, it is best to vary the method of applying progressive overload. Using jogging or running as an example, start with a specified distance and pace. After 2 weeks, increase the distance by about 10%. After another 2 weeks, increase the pace slightly. When fully accustomed to the new distance and pace, then increase the distance again. The principle is the same for aerobic dance-exercise. A progressive overload program might involve the use of carefully designed dance-exercise routines that require slightly higher exercise intensity each week.

The concept of progressive overload pertains to the use of interval training, as well as to continuous training. More specifically, however, **interval training** involves exercise at high-intensity levels (80%–100% of maximal heart rate) for relatively brief periods (usually 10 seconds to 5 minutes) with intervening rest or relief (walking, jogging) periods to allow the heart rate to decline. Often the exercise periods are "anaerobic" rather than "aerobic." For athletic training, interval training may offer an advantage because the faster pace may more accurately simulate competitive conditions. Generally, however, continuous exercise at lower levels of intensity is safer and more specific to the goals of general health enhancement and physical fitness. Continuous training is less stressful to the musculoskeletal system and, therefore, more appropriate for middle-aged and older adults.

Warm-Up and Cool-Down

The period of exercise at the desired target heart rate should be preceded by a warm-up of about 5–10 minutes. The warm-up should include stretching and limbering exercises to prepare the musculotendinous system for the exercises to be performed. Static stretching—holding a steady stretch with the desired muscles at their greatest possible length—is beneficial to joints and muscles and helps to prevent injuries and muscle soreness. Warm-up activities should also include large muscle movement to raise the heart rate, blood pressure, cardiac output, and respiratory ventilation gradually to intermediate levels so that these mechanisms are not suddenly taxed. A proper warm-up can reduce the incidence of exercise-induced cardiac abnormalities such as arrhythmias.

It is also important to cool down gradually after a period of vigorous exercise. Stopping exercise abruptly after a vigorous workout may trap a large quantity of blood in the muscles or lower parts of the body. As a result, an insufficient amount of blood circulates back to the brain or heart, which may cause dizziness or faintness. It is best to provide a series of movements during the cool-down period that allows the muscles and cardiovascular-respiratory system to reduce their elevated levels of activity gradually. A gradual cool-down usually aids in the removal of accumulated lactic acid and may prevent cardiac arrhythmias following strenuous exercise. When heart rates are near resting levels, muscle stretching and limbering exercises should again be performed to reduce the risk of developing delayed muscle soreness.

Use of Hand or Ankle Weights with Aerobic Exercise

Adding extra weight to the body during exercise increases the amount of work done and, in effect, increases exercise intensity—a fact long recognized by members of the armed services, backpackers, and hikers. Centering the extra weight as directly over the center of gravity as possible appears to minimize the effect. The devastating effect of carrying additional weight in the form of extra-heavy boots is immortalized by a common backpacking adage: An extra pound on the feet is equivalent to 4 pounds in the pack.

During aerobic exercise, the addition of hand and ankle weights adds to the weight of the total mass that must be moved, requiring the production of more energy. This weight must also be swung back and forth by relatively small muscle groups, contributing even more to the total energy production. The increased work is usually manifested by a higher exercise heart rate. At best, the use of hand and ankle weights contributes to increased muscle tone and muscular endurance (not muscular strength). If excessive weight is used, however, undesirable postural changes may occur, resulting in excess body strain. The extra weight also adds to impact stress on ankles, knees, hips, and the lower back.

HEALTH BENEFITS OF AEROBIC EXERCISE FOR HEALTHY PARTICIPANTS

Regular exercise, particularly aerobic exercise, enhances a person's physiological or functional capacity and enables him or her to achieve an improved quality of life. With a heightened physiological reserve, the regular stresses and strains of life, whether physical or psychological, are taken in stride. More specifically, the musculotendinous and skeletal systems are maintained at a moderately high level of strength and endurance. Although aerobic exercise improves muscle tonus (firmness) and general body flexibility, it is not specific to the development of high levels of muscular strength and endurance. To develop high levels of muscular strength and endurance, weight training must be added to regular aerobic exercise. Recent studies have shown that weight-bearing exercise promotes improved bone density, an extremely important consideration in the prevention of osteoporosis after age 50–60.

The benefits of aerobic dance exercise are most specific to the cardiovascular and respiratory systems. A regular program of aerobic dance exercise significantly improves the efficiency with which the body performs. Hand in hand with improvement in aerobic performance is improved cardiac efficiency (increased stroke volume, lowered resting heart rate), improved breathing capacity (improved tidal volume, increased capacity for respiratory ventilation), and improved capacity for dissipating metabolically produced heat. Further, regular participation in a progressive dance-exercise program enhances the body's ability to use oxygen for the production of ATP (oxygen consumption). These benefits are similar to those achieved with a jogging or cycling program. Generally, these physiological benefits occur with a well-planned 12-week period of dance exercise performed 3 times per week.

A long-term program of aerobic exercise produces favorable changes in body composition—an increase in lean body mass (muscle mass) and a decrease in body fat.

Numerous studies on the psychological benefits of aerobic exercise have also shown that persons who regularly perform aerobic exercise have increased vigor and decreased depression scores on basic psychological tests. Students of aerobic dance exercise claim to be invigorated by the music and the exercise.

HEALTH BENEFITS OF AEROBIC EXERCISE FOR PERSONS WITH CHRONIC DISEASE

A well-planned aerobic exercise program can provide health benefits to persons with chronic diseases such as adult-onset diabetes, arthritis, obesity, asthma, and coronary heart disease.

Living with *adult-onset diabetes* often requires a complete lifestyle revision, including losing body fat, reducing stress, and learning to monitor blood glucose levels. Exercise enables carbohydrates to be used more effectively by promoting glucose uptake from the blood and, thereby, reducing the need for insulin among diabetics requiring its use. Severe exercise, however, may induce hazardously low blood glucose levels. Research has shown that regularly performed moderate exercise can help a diabetic maintain normal blood glucose levels, but the guidance of a physician is necessary. The diabetic needs to understand the interactions among exercise, glucose uptake, insulin, and carbohydrate consumption. A regular program of physical activity may help diabetics lose body fat, reduce tension and anxiety, and deal with stress.

Arthritis (osteoarthritis) is a gradual, progressive degeneration of joint structures that causes painful movement and sometimes severe aches and pains. The notion that severe exercise early in life contributes to the incidence of arthritis later on has recently been debunked. There is no association between exercise and the incidence of arthritis, other than the tendency for arthritic pain to occur in areas of the body that experienced earlier athletic injury. Persons with mild arthritic pain generally respond well to mild levels of exercise. Maintenance of flexibility and moderate levels of muscular strength and endurance is important; movement should not be avoided because of general aches and pains. However, movements involving high-impact stress on knees, hips, and the lower back should be avoided. Low-intensity, slow aerobic-dance movements are more productive than higher intensity movements requiring considerable jumping or hopping.

Obesity, or overfatness, has become a severe nutritional and health-related problem in the industrialized world. Low-intensity aerobic exercise is the best method for obese persons to use energy and expend calories. The most effective way to lose body fat is strict dietary control to lower caloric intake and aerobic exercise to generate increased caloric output (energy production). Dieting alone is not as effective. While severe dieting can lead to weight loss, the loss is frequently from the lean body mass (mainly the muscles) rather than from the fat mass of the body. Low-intensity, long-duration exercise allows the fatty acids from the adipose tissue depots to be used as energy substrate (fatty acid oxidation). Higher intensity exercise utilizes carbohydrate stores, not body fat stores, as the substrate for energy production. The mobilization of fatty acids from adipose tissue is a slow process requiring about 20 minutes of exercise; therefore, long-duration exercise is specifically prescribed for fat reduction.

Asthma occurs when the bronchi (large breathing passages) become constricted (bronchospasm). Although exact causes are unknown, the onset of symptoms is related to irritants such as tobacco smoke, animal dander, and cold air. The labored breathing that occurs when the bronchi constrict discourages asthmatics from exercising. Some people experience exercise-induced asthma (EIA); the most widely accepted hypothesis is that airway cooling causes the bronchospasm. Nevertheless, an exercise program for asthmatics is not contraindicated. Asthmatics can learn to recognize symptoms and employ proper self-care steps to control the condition. A very gradual warm-up may prevent EIA. Asthmatics should be encouraged to exercise and to have brochodilator medications readily available if symptoms become severe. Research has shown that increased aerobic fitness raises the exercise level at which asthmatic symptoms occur.

Coronary heart disease is partial or total closure of the coronary arteries resulting in symptoms or signs of reduced or occluded coronary blood flow. The American Heart Association has identified a number of factors that increase the risk of cardiovascular disease. The three primary risk factors are hypertension (elevated blood pressure), cigarette smoking, and high blood cholesterol levels. Secondary risk factors include family history of heart disease, physical inactivity, obesity, diabetes, being male, age over 65, and a high level of emotional stress. Obviously, little can be done to change the family health history, but lifestyle changes can significantly alter aspects of the other risk factors. Regular participation in a well-planned aerobic exercise program has been shown to reduce high blood pressure, serum cholesterol levels, body fat levels, and emotional stress.

ENVIRONMENTAL CONSIDERATIONS WHEN EXERCISING

One physiological function that is closely regulated is body temperature. Since most mechanisms used to maintain body temperature are directly or indirectly related to the cardiovascular system, exercising under extreme environmental conditions adds significantly to cardiovascular stress.

Exercising in the Heat

Considerable metabolic heat is produced during exercise. To reduce this internal heat load, venous blood is brought to the skin surface (peripheral vasodilation) to be dissipated to the cooler environment. Sweating also occurs; sweat glands secrete extracellular water onto the skin where the water evaporates. This evaporative process cools the body. If environmental conditions are favorable, these mechanisms will adequately prevent the body temperature from rising more than about 2 degrees during heavy exercise.

When exercising in the heat, however, dissipating internal body heat is difficult and external heat may accrue from the environment as well. In an attempt to cool the body, extensive vasodilation reduces the venous return of blood to the heart, and profuse sweating results in considerable loss of body water. The result is greatly elevated cardiovascular stress; as stroke volume is reduced, heart rates rise. If the lost fluids are not replenished, dehydration eventually results, and blood volume declines. Again, this condition is manifested by very high heart rates.

Air Temperature (°F)	Danger Zone (% RH)
70	80
75	70
80	50
85	40
90	30
95	20
100	10

The most stressful environment for exercising combines heat and humidity. When the air contains a large quantity of water vapor, sweat will not evaporate readily. Since it is this evaporation process that cools the body, adequate cooling will not occur in very humid conditions. The intensity of exercise lasting 30 minutes or more should be reduced whenever relative humidity (% RH) and air temperature create a dangerous situation. Careful heart rate monitoring is particularly important in a hot, humid environment. See the temperature/humidity guideline on the previous page. (See Chapter 14 for a further discussion of heat-related syndromes.)

It is important not to impede heat loss from the body. When exercising in the heat, never wear anything or do anything that will interfere with heat loss.

1. *Always wear lightweight, well-ventilated clothing.* Cotton materials are cooler; most synthetics retain heat. Wear light-colored clothing if exercising in the sun; white reflects heat better than other colors.

2. *Never wear impermeable or nonbreathable garments.* The notion that wearing nonbreathable leggings while performing dance exercise will result in fat loss from the legs is a myth. Wearing impermeable clothing is a dangerous practice that could lead to significant heat stress and heat injury.

3. *Replace body fluids as they are lost.* Drink lots of fluids (preferably water) at regular intervals while exercising. Don't wait until thirst occurs because thirst is not an adequate indicator of the need to replace body fluids.

4. *Recording daily body weight is an excellent way to prevent accumulative dehydration.* For example, if 5 pounds of body water is lost after aerobic exercise, this water should be replaced before exercising again the next day. Exercise should be curtailed until the body is adequately rehydrated.

5. *Heat acclimatization can occur quickly.* Begin exercise in the heat gradually. Exercise for a short period each day for a week. Discomfort will decrease noticeably as the week progresses.

Exercising in the Cold

Generally, few temperature-regulation problems occur when exercising in cool environments. The environmental conditions favor the loss of internal body heat, and the body remains cool and refreshed while exercising. Following exercise, however, chilling can occur quickly if the body surface is wet with sweat and vasodilation continues to bring body heat to surface tissues. Therefore, when it is cool, put on warm-up clothing (including a hat) to retain body heat immediately after exercising.

Temperature regulation can become a problem when exposure is prolonged or when the body core temperature cannot be maintained. Under these conditions, a general vasoconstriction results in an elevation in central blood volume. The kidneys increase urine production and the blood becomes more concentrated. To prevent dehydration while exercising, this lost body fluid must be replaced.

The following guidelines govern exercising in the cold:

1. *Wear several layers of clothing.* By layering clothing, garments can be removed and replaced as needed. When exercise intensity is high, remove outer garments. Then, during periods of rest, warm-up, cool-down, or low-intensity exercise, put them back on. Head covering is also important because considerable body heat radiates from the head.

2. *Allow for adequate ventilation of sweat.* Sweating during heavy exercise can soak inner garments. If evaporation does not readily occur, the wet garments will continue to drain the body of heat during rest periods, when retention of body heat is important.

3. *Select garment materials that allow the body to give off body heat during exercise, and retain body heat during inactive periods.* For example, cotton is a good choice for exercising in the heat because it soaks up sweat readily and allows evaporation; for those same reasons, though, cotton is a poor choice for exercising in the cold. Even when wet, wool garments help maintain body warmth. When wind chill is a problem, nylon materials are good for outer wear. Since water vapor cannot permeate nylon, however, inner garments can become quite wet. Remove outer garments during exercise and replace them during rest periods.

4. *Replace body fluids in the cold, just as in the heat.* Urine production increases in the cold, making fluid replacement important.

Exercising at Higher Altitudes

At moderate to high altitudes, the partial pressure* of oxygen in the air is reduced. Because there is less pressure to drive the oxygen molecules into the blood in the lungs, the oxygen-carrying capacity of the blood is reduced. Therefore, a person exercising at high altitudes will not be able to deliver as much oxygen to the exercising muscles, and exercise intensity will have to be reduced (compared to sea level). Generally, respiratory distress is the dominant symptom, and recovery from exercise is delayed. Persons who usually exercise at sea level may develop a headache when exercising at higher altitudes. This headache will eventually subside.

Remember: The usual level of exercise intensity will be more difficult to perform. For best results, reduce exercise intensity to a comfortable level. A more gradual warm-up and cool-down period is also desirable.

It generally takes longer to acclimatize to altitude than to heat or cold. Some adaptations occur within about one week, but other physiological adaptations may take several months.

SUMMARY

This chapter is designed to provide the dance-exercise instructor with basic principles of exercise physiology. Considerable space is devoted to the presentation of aerobic and anaerobic metabolism because the principle of specificity clearly dictates that physiological adaptations are specific to encountered stresses. The exercise instructor must understand the various methods of applying stress (training) and the physiological results. Exercise programming is becoming more and more exacting. Too often the exercising public falls victim to the poor advice of exercise teachers, coaches, and other "experts," who fail to apply the concept of exercise specificity because they simply do not understand basic principles.

A large amount of information has been given in a relatively small amount of space. The emphasis has been on basic understanding rather

---

*Partial pressure is the pressure of each gas in a multiple gas system—in this case, air, which is composed of nitrogen, oxygen, and carbon dioxide.

than on detailed explanation. Students of this material are strongly encouraged to seek further knowledge of exercise physiology and the principles of physical fitness and human movement through more advanced study.

SUGGESTED READING

Anderson, B. *Stretching*. Bolinas, Calif.: Shelter Publishers, 1980.

Beaulieu, J. E. *Stretching for All Sports*. Pasadena: The Athletic Press, 1980.

Fox, E. L. *Lifetime Fitness*. Philadelphia: Saunders College Publishing, 1983.

Fox, E. L. *Sports Physiology*. 2nd ed. Philadelphia: Saunders College Publishing, 1984.

Getchell, B. *Physical Fitness: A Way of Life*. 3rd ed. New York: Wiley, 1983.

Katch, F. I., and W. D. McArdle. *Nutrition, Weight Control, and Exercise*. 2nd ed. Philadelphia: Lea & Febiger, 1983.

Sharkey, B. J. *Physiology and Physical Activity*. New York: Harper & Row, 1975.

Sharkey, B. J. *Physiology of Fitness*. 2nd ed. Champaign, Ill.: Human Kinetics Publishers, 1984.

Skinner, J. S. *Body Energy*. Mountain View, Calif.: Anderson World, Inc., 1981.

Anatomy and Kinesiology

Ellen Kreighbaum

Ellen Kreighbaum, Ph.D., is a professor of physical education with a specialization in biomechanics at Montana State University in Bozeman. Coauthor of *Biomechanics: A Qualitative Approach for Studying Human Movement,* a textbook now in its second edition, Dr. Kreighbaum also writes on lower-extremity alignment and the biomechanics of gymnastics.

2

IN THIS CHAPTER:

- Components of the cardiovascular system, pulmonary system, and nervous system.
- The skeletal system: skeletal structure, the articulations, the link system and its movements.
- The muscular system: properties of muscle tissue, how muscles effect movement, muscles of the upper extremity, muscles of the lower extremity, muscles of the vertebral column and pelvis.

- Postural alignment of the trunk: ideal posture, anteroposterior pelvic tilt, pathological postures.
- Postural alignments of the lower extremity: ideal alignment, misalignments, maladies.
- Center of gravity, balance, and stability.
- Building an exercise program: two-joint muscles, method of analysis.

The human body can run, jump, kick, throw, and perform a variety of movements because of the way in which the muscles are attached to the skeletal system. Think of the skeleton as a puppet and the muscles as the strings that pull on the bones to make them move. The muscles receive the energy they need to work properly from the blood, which is given oxygen by the pulmonary system, pumped by the heart, and circulated through a system of vessels. The network of nerves affects each and every muscle fiber, stimulating the muscles to contract. This chapter will discuss the structure and function of five important systems—the cardiovascular system, the pulmonary system, the nervous system, the skeletal system, and the muscular system— and will explain how these systems produce the body movements used in dance exercise.

THE CARDIOVASCULAR SYSTEM

The cardiovascular system, composed of the heart and its blood vessels, supplies the energy needed by the muscles, nerves, and brain to produce and control body movement. The heart pumps blood to the

AEROBIC DANCE-EXERCISE INSTRUCTOR MANUAL

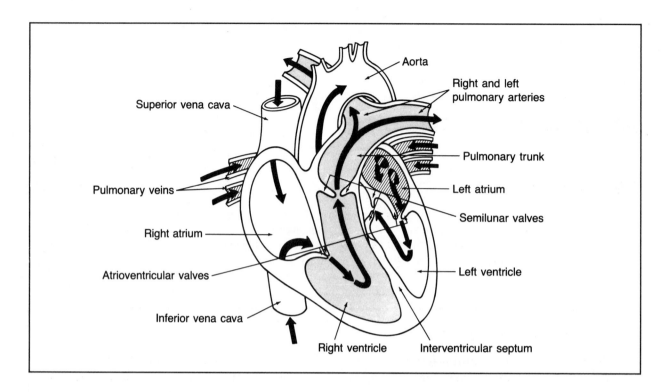

Superior vena cava

Pulmonary veins

Right atrium

Atrioventricular valves

Inferior vena cava

Aorta

Right and left pulmonary arteries

Pulmonary trunk

Left atrium

Semilunar valves

Left ventricle

Right ventricle   Interventricular septum

FIGURE 2–1 Anatomy of the heart and pathways of the blood (Courtesy of Burgess Publishing Co.)

lungs to receive oxygen. The oxygenated blood returns to the heart and is then pumped to the rest of the tissues. Blood vessels called **arteries** carry oxygenated blood from the heart to the tissues, and vessels called **veins** return the deoxygenated blood to the heart. Figure 2–1 illustrates the anatomy of the heart and its connecting veins and arteries and maps the direction of blood as it flows through the heart to the lungs and out to the tissues.

The heart is made up of four chambers: two superior chambers called **atria** (left and right), and two inferior chambers called **ventricles** (left and right). Oxygenated blood from the lungs enters the left atrium through the pulmonary vein and is pushed through a valve into the left ventricle, where the blood is forced out of the heart through the aorta. The aorta is the main vessel through which the oxygenated blood passes to the tissues. The aorta branches "downstream" to smaller vessels called arteries, including the two coronary arteries that supply oxygen to the heart muscle itself. The arteries divide into smaller, more numerous vessels called **arterioles,** which in turn divide into the smallest units, **capillaries.** At the capillary level the exchange of oxygen and nutrients occurs, and the tissues release their waste products to the bloodstream. After the blood passes through the capillary network and the oxygen is exchanged, the deoxygenated blood is sent back toward the heart through the veinules, which converge into veins, and finally into the superior and inferior vena cava where it enters the right atrium of the heart. From the right atrium the blood is forced into the right ventricle, out through the pulmonary artery, and into the lungs for oxygenation.

The heart is a muscle and becomes stronger with use. As the heart tissue strengthens, the heart becomes a more forceful pump; that is, with every contraction the heart sends more blood to its destination.

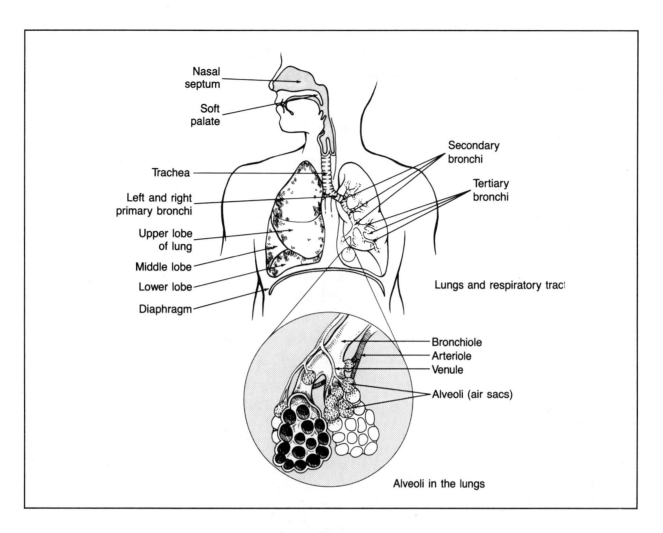

Nasal septum

Soft palate

Trachea

Left and right primary bronchi

Upper lobe of lung

Middle lobe

Lower lobe

Diaphragm

Secondary bronchi

Tertiary bronchi

Lungs and respiratory tract

Bronchiole
Arteriole
Venule

Alveoli (air sacs)

Alveoli in the lungs

FIGURE 2–2 Anatomy of the pulmonary system (Courtesy of Burgess Publishing Co.)

Thus, a strong heart does not have to contract as frequently to fulfill its responsibility. A stronger heart muscle is a major benefit of aerobic exercise.

The blood vessels also remain healthier if worked harder and used more. Blood vessels that are not worked can lose their elasticity and become clogged. The number of capillaries can diminish if the tissues that they supply are not taxed regularly. Regular performance of endurance exercise causes the cardiovascular system to develop increased numbers of capillaries, thus enabling a more efficient and extensive exchange of essential nutrients.

THE PULMONARY SYSTEM

The lungs fill the blood with oxygen and carry off carbon dioxide to the atmosphere. Air, inhaled through the nose and mouth, passes through the trachea and enters the **primary bronchi** and its subdivisions, the secondary and tertiary bronchi. The tertiary bronchi further divide, ending finally in the **bronchioles** that supply the air to the lung's **alveoli,** or air sacs. (The anatomy of the pulmonary system is shown in Figure 2–2.) The oxygen and carbon dioxide exchange takes place between the alveoli and the capillaries located in the walls of the alveoli. Pulmonary veins transport the newly oxygenated blood into the left atrium

Aerobic Dance-Exercise Instructor Manual

of the heart, while carbon dioxide, a waste product, is expired through the same series of passageways that carried the inhaled air.

THE NERVOUS SYSTEM

Visualize the nervous system as the computer that controls all functions of the human body. Input to this human computer is through **receptors** in the tissues that respond to changes in the external environment. The receptors are like keys on a computer keyboard. When a keyboard is stimulated by pressure or touch, the computer responds. The receptors of the human computer, called **afferent neurons,** transmit impulses to the brain or spinal cord. These receptors are stimulated

FIGURE 2–3 Map of the spinal nerve pathways (Courtesy of Burgess Publishing Co.)

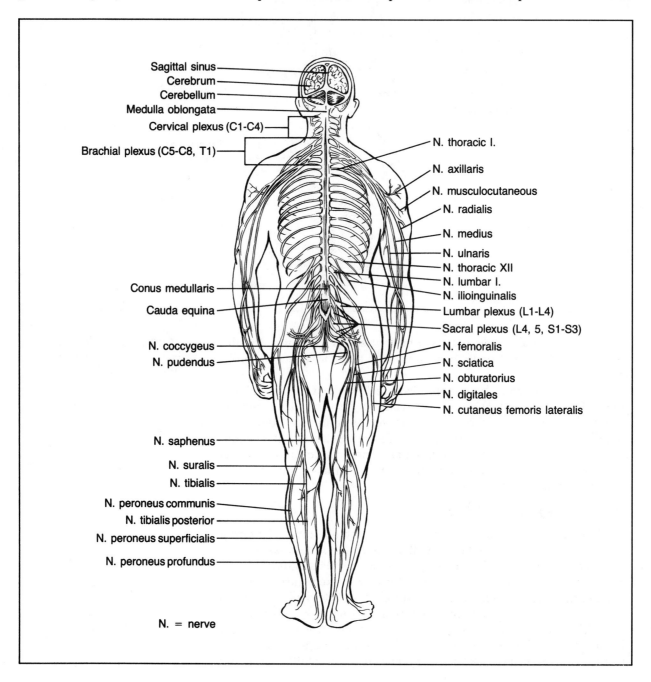

Sagittal sinus

Cerebrum

Cerebellum

Medulla oblongata

Cervical plexus (C1-C4)

Brachial plexus (C5-C8, T1)

N. thoracic I.

N. axillaris

N. musculocutaneous

N. radialis

N. medius

N. ulnaris

N. thoracic XII

N. lumbar I.

N. ilioinguinalis

Conus medullaris

Cauda equina

Lumbar plexus (L1-L4)

Sacral plexus (L4, 5, S1-S3)

N. coccygeus

N. pudendus

N. femoralis

N. sciatica

N. obturatorius

N. digitales

N. cutaneus femoris lateralis

N. saphenus

N. suralis

N. tibialis

N. peroneus communis

N. tibialis posterior

N. peroneus superficialis

N. peroneus profundus

N. = nerve

by the senses of sight, sound, smell, touch, taste, as well as the sense of position and movement of the body parts.

Of primary interest to the exercise instructor are the responses of the brain and spinal cord that stimulate the motor neurons. The motor neurons are called **efferent neurons** and branch out to the muscles, causing them to contract or relax.

The nervous system consists of the central nervous system, composed of the brain and the spinal cord, and the peripheral nervous system, consisting of pairs of nerve branches from the central nervous system. These pairs of spinal nerves are the pathways over which the stimulus and response impulses travel. Figure 2–3 provides a simplified map of the spinal nerve pathways. There are 12 pairs of cranial nerves that supply impulses to the brain and 31 pairs of spinal nerves. The spinal nerves are divided into sections corresponding to the sections of the vertebral column: 8 cervical pairs, 12 thoracic pairs, 5 lumbar pairs, 5 sacral pairs, and 1 coccygeal pair. The pairs of nerves branching from the vertebral column continually divide and radiate out into all areas of the body and its extremities.

As the spinal nerves branch out, they continue to subdivide until they reach the end of the nervous pathway and integrate with the muscle. The last single nerve fiber has branches that attach to the skeletal muscle fibers, allowing the electrical impulses to reach the site where they stimulate a chemical reaction in the muscle that initiates muscular contraction. A motor unit, which consists of the last single nerve cell body and its associated muscle fibers, is the smallest functional unit of the neuromuscular system.

Many motor units exist within a single muscle. The more muscle fibers stimulated by a single motor unit, the fewer motor units per muscle, and the more gross the movement. The fewer muscle fibers stimulated by a single motor unit, the more motor units per muscle, and the more precise the movement. Therefore, muscles used for fine motor tasks such as accuracy skills will have fewer muscle fibers associated with each motor unit. Muscles used for gross motor tasks, such as forceful movements, will have more muscle fibers associated with each motor unit.

THE SKELETAL SYSTEM

The skeleton has several important functions: (a) to protect the vital organs and soft tissues within the body, (b) to support the soft tissues, (c) to serve as the factory for making red blood cells, (d) to serve as a reservoir for minerals, particularly calcium and phosphate, and (e) to provide attachments for skeletal muscles to produce a system of levers upon which the muscles act to make movements possible.

This section describes the structure of the skeletal system, defines specific reference terms, describes the types of articulations that permit movement of the skeleton, discusses how the integrity of the system is maintained, describes the system of levers on which muscles act to effect movement, and defines the skeletal system as a "link system" for movement analysis.

Skeletal Structure

Structurally the human skeleton is divided into two general areas: the central **axial skeleton,** which includes the head, neck, thorax, and

AEROBIC DANCE-EXERCISE INSTRUCTOR MANUAL

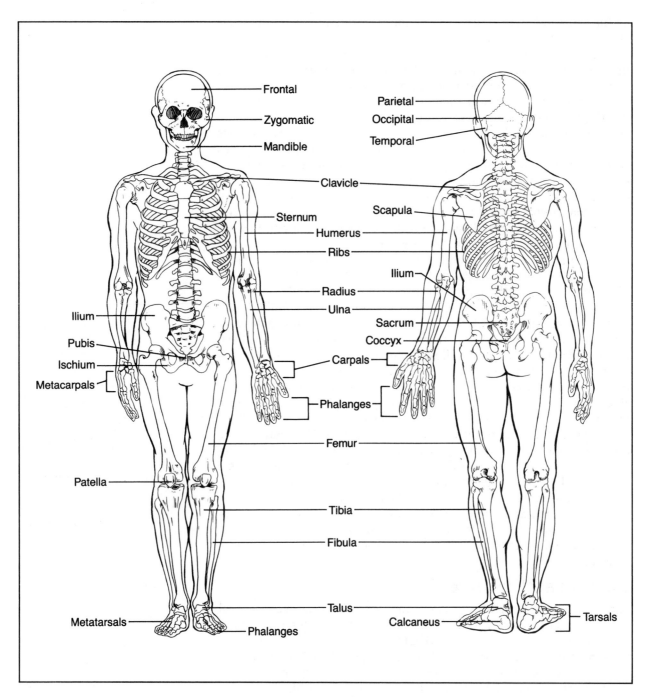

FIGURE 2–4 Major bones of the skeletal system (Redrawn from Kreighbaum and Barthels 1985, 21–22)

vertebral column; and the extremities, or **appendicular skeleton,** which includes the pelvis and the bones of the upper and lower extremities. A rendering of the skeleton, identifying the important bones, is presented in Figure 2–4.

The vertebral column is divided into five functional units; the **cervical,** or neck, has 7 bones; the **thoracic,** or upper back, has 12 bones from which the ribs arise; the **lumbar,** or lower back, has 5 bones; the **sacrum** has 5 bones that are fused into a single unit; and the **coccyx,** or tailbone, has 4 bones. The sections of the vertebral column are illustrated in Figure 2–5.

Of greatest importance to the dance-exercise instructor are the lumbar and the cervical areas. The lumbar vertebrae, which are the largest vertebrae in the back, can be easily injured during trunk-strengthening exercises, particularly if the abdominal muscles are weak. The cervical vertebrae can be injured when body **weight** is placed on the neck area, and the thoracic area can be injured when the thoracic vertebrae are forced into an extreme forward-bending posture. For example, the plough exercise should not be used under any circumstances because of the inherent danger to both the cervical and thoracic areas (see Fig. 2–6). Further discussion of potential musculoskeletal injury due to exercise will be presented later in this chapter and in Chapter 11.

Skeletal Reference Terms

When standing erect with feet forward and palms facing forward, the body is in the **anatomical position.** The front of the body or segment is called **anterior** and the back is the **posterior.** **Lateral** refers to the outside of the body or body segment and **medial** refers to the inside. Thus, the lateral side of the elbow is that side away from the body and the medial side of the elbow is that side closest to the body when the body is in anatomical position. Lateral and medial also define movement. **Lateral flexion** of the vertebral column is the bending or tilting of the trunk to the side, either to the right or to the left. **Medial rotation** is the rotation of the body part toward the body as in medial rotation of the thigh at the hip joint.

A **superior** body part lies above another part, and an **inferior** body part lies below another. The body lying face up is **supine;** the body lying face down is **prone.** Two movement terms originate from the words "supine" and "prone"—supination, when the palm is facing forward or upward, and pronation, when the palm is facing backward or downward. Supination and pronation occur in the forearm and in the foot.

Dorsal refers to the top as in the top of the foot; **plantar** refers to the bottom as in the bottom of the foot. **Proximal** is the end of a bone or a muscle of the extremities that is located closest to the body; **distal** is the end located farthest from the trunk. These terms will be used to describe the motions of specific body segments.

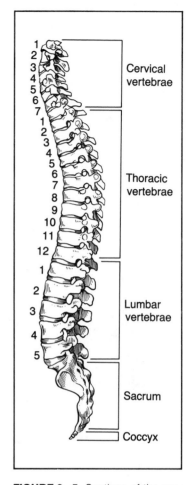

FIGURE 2–5 Sections of the vertebral column (Redrawn from Kreighbaum and Barthels 1985, 22)

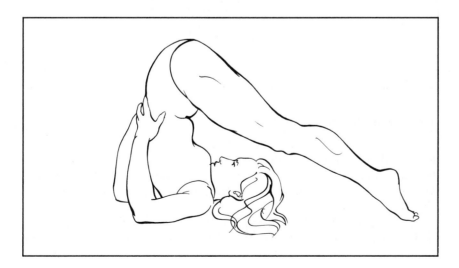

FIGURE 2–6 The plough: an ill-advised exercise

AEROBIC DANCE-EXERCISE INSTRUCTOR MANUAL

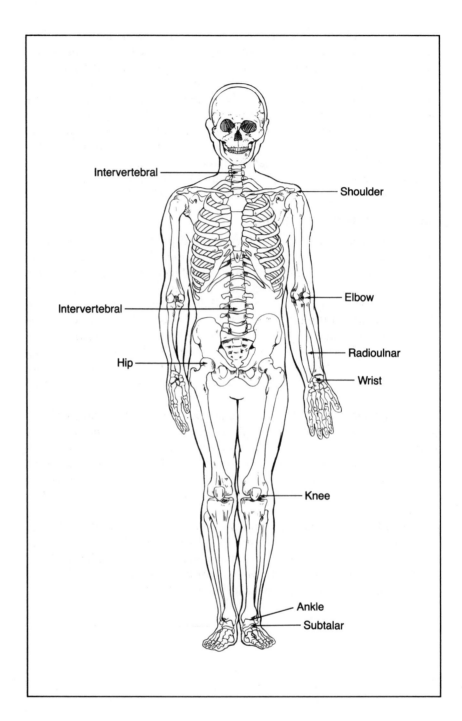

FIGURE 2–7 Articulations of the skeleton (Redrawn from Kreighbaum and Barthels 1985, 22)

The Articulations

The bones that constitute the skeletal system are joined together at **articulations** or joints of the body. All movements of the skeletal system take place at the articulations. The names and locations of the articulations that are most important to dance-exercise instructors are shown in Figure 2–7.

Each articulation is held together by **ligaments,** the strong tissues that connect one bone to another. The number and strength of the ligaments surrounding articulations vary. Some articulations, such as

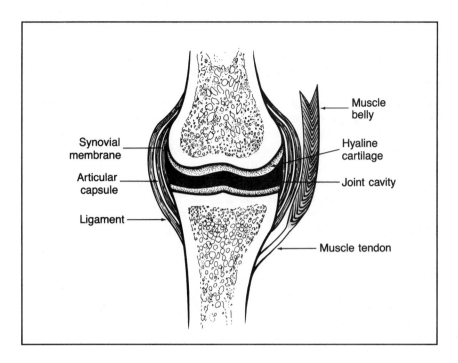

FIGURE 2–8 Structure of a typical diarthrodial articulation

the hip and ankle, have numerous strong ligaments holding them together; others, such as the shoulder and knee, have fewer and smaller ligaments surrounding them. Articulations with weaker ligamentous arrangements must rely on the strength of the muscles surrounding them to maintain their integrity under stress.

Types of Articulations

There are three major types of articulations in the body: synarthrodial articulations are classified as immovable, amphiarthrodial articulations are classified as slightly movable, and diarthrodial articulations are classified as movable. Diarthrodial articulations are the most important articulations in exercise analysis.

In the **synarthrodial** articulation, two bones are "fused." For example, in an adult the skull bones are fused at the sutures and, barring any forceful impact, will not move relative to each other.

The **amphiarthrodial** articulations are joined by fibrocartilage, which is dense connective tissue. The articulations between the sacrum of the vertebral column and the ilium of the pelvis (the sacroiliac joint) are amphiarthrodial. Slight movement does occur between the bones, but the movement serves mainly to absorb shock. During pregnancy, hormones allow the fibrocartilage to become more pliable and thus enable the pelvic cavity to accommodate the fetus. Often the amphiarthrodial articulations are injured in the exercising adult because, as the body ages, fibrocartilage loses its resilience and shock cannot be absorbed adequately. The most frequent injuries occur at the intervertebral articulations and the sacroiliac joints.

Diarthrodial articulations are the most prevalent and the most important in exercise analysis. These articulations, which move due to the voluntary contractions of the skeletal muscles, make movement possible. A typical diarthrodial articulation is shown in Figure 2–8. Hyaline cartilage—the smooth, elastic substance found on the ends of chicken bones—covers the adjoining ends of the bones. The cartilage's main functions are to absorb shock and to provide a relatively frictionless surface over which the bones can move. The joint cavity provides a space for the movement of the bones and houses the synovial fluid, a fairly thick material that lubricates the hyaline cartilage. The viscosity of the synovial fluid may change with activity, which, if true, would lend some credence to the use of warm-up activities as a way to ease the movability of the joints.

The synovial membrane surrounds the joint cavity but does not cover the hyaline cartilage. Filled with nerve endings, the membrane is sensitive to changes within the capsule and to pressure from foreign objects such as bone chips that may be lodged within the capsule. Outside the synovial membrane is the articular capsule, which surrounds the articulation like a collar and helps hold the bones together. Ligaments, located on the outside of the capsule, hold the two bones together. **Tendons,** also on the outside of the capsule, are connective tissues that attach the muscles to the bone. Not all muscles have tendinous attachments. Some muscle fibers, such as those of the serratus anterior, the trapezius, the deltoid, and the gluteus maximus, attach directly to the bone.

The several types of diarthrodial articulations are named according to the type of movement they allow.

1. Hinge joints permit motion only in one plane of motion.
2. Pivot joints allow turning around the long central axis of the segment.
3. Gliding joints allow movement in all directions.
4. Saddle joints allow movement in two planes of motion; one bone "sits" in the articular surface of the other.
5. Condyloid joints allow movement in two planes of motion.
6. Ball-and-socket joints allow movement in three planes of motion; one bone has a concave surface into which the spherical end of the adjacent bone fits (Langley 1978). The planes of motion are discussed further in the following section.

Maintaining the Integrity of the Skeletal System

Mobility of the musculoskeletal system is the degree to which an articulation is allowed to move before being restricted by surrounding tissues. Mobility is determined by the articulation's **range of motion (ROM),** or flexibility. **Stability** of an articulation is the ability of the skeletal framework to absorb shock and withstand motion without injury to the joints and their surrounding tissue (Kreighbaum and Barthels 1985). During exercise, the participant should attempt to enhance mobility (increase flexibility) while maintaining stability (increase strength) so chance for injury, such as straining a muscle or dislocating a joint, is minimized.

Several types of tissues are used in holding the skeletal system together: bone tissue, ligaments, muscles and their associated tendons.

BONY STABILITY. While many long bones in the body articulate with the end of the next bone without any cohesive structure, some bones have hooks or knobs that come together with the articulating bone to form an attachment. The strongest bony articulations are the elbow, the hip, and the ankle. The humerus has a hingelike structure at its distal end called the trochlea. The olecranon process at the proximal end of the ulna is a hooklike structure that fits around the trochlea and forms a fairly stable bony articulation. The pelvis has a concave socket into which the sphere-shaped head of the femur fits to form a fairly stable bony arrangement for the hip. The distal end of the tibia is concave in shape and fits over the saddlelike talus bone of the foot. Dislocations of the elbow, hip, and ankle are rare, partly because of the stability of these bony arrangements.

The shoulder, the intervertebral joints, and the knee have weak bony articulations. The articulations between the vertebrae and between the distal end of the femur and the proximal end of the tibia at the knee are barely more than the ends of two bones butting up against each other. These articulations must rely on strong ligaments and muscles to maintain their integrity. Thus, dislocations of the shoulder and tearing of the knee ligaments are caused by forces that could not be counteracted by the existing structures. Exercise instructors should keep in mind the importance of strengthening the muscles surrounding the shoulder, the vertebral column, and the knee, and incorporate exercises for these areas into their routines.

LIGAMENTOUS STABILITY.   Ligaments are strong tissues that connect one bone to another. Ligaments attach to one bone, cross one or more articulations, and attach to another bone on the other end. The ligaments crossing the hip articulation are the strongest in the body.

Generally, ligaments are not subjected to extreme forces during exercise routines unless the muscles cannot prevent an articulation from moving beyond its safe range of motion. Warm-up exercises that are joint specific enhance blood flow to surrounding structures, increase the area temperature, and thus allow the ligaments to stretch farther without injury. For this reason, it is important to engage in joint-specific warm-up exercises before initiating vigorous and forceful movements.

Unfortunately, ligaments do not have a vascular system of their own and do not repair themselves once their tissue has been torn or stretched excessively. A ligament that has been torn or stressed beyond its ability to recoil remains loose and nonfunctional until repaired by a physician. Thus, it is an old exercise dictum that it is better to break a bone than to tear a ligament; the bone will mend to a state stronger than the original whereas the ligament will not.

MUSCULOTENDINOUS STABILITY.   Frequently the proximal ends of muscles attach directly to the bone; however, the distal ends commonly become tendons before attaching to the bone. Tendons are strong ligamentous-like material. These musculotendinous structures cross articulations as do ligaments and help hold together the articulations. Muscle tissue strength is particularly important in the shoulder and the knee articulations because the bony and ligamentous arrangements around these joints are simply not strong enough to maintain the integrity of the joint under stress.

The angle at which the muscle tendon pulls on the bone affects the success of the tendon in stabilizing the articulation. As a general rule, the smaller the angle of attachment between the muscle, or muscle tendon, and bone, the greater the muscle's contribution to stabilizing the articulation. Figure 2–9 illustrates the angle of attachment at the

AEROBIC DANCE-EXERCISE INSTRUCTOR MANUAL

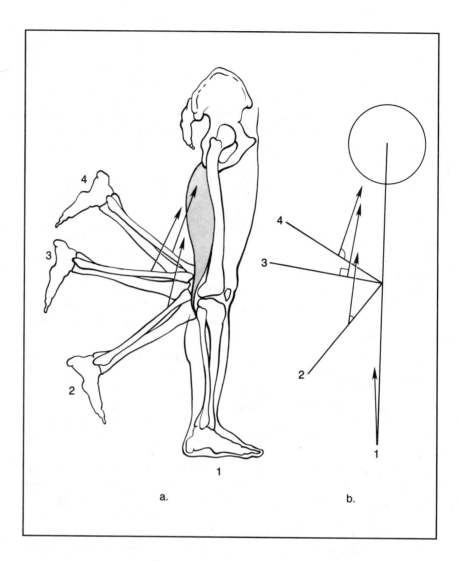

FIGURE 2−9 Hamstrings' angle of attachment to the bone in four positions (Redrawn from Kreighbaum and Barthels 1985, 173)

a.   b.

knee of the hamstring group. The hamstrings' angle of attachment changes as the knee is flexed. Figure 2−9(a) shows the musculoskeletal arrangement for the knee at four different angles. In Figure 2−9(b) a stick drawing represents the bones and the angle of muscle pull. Note that at position 1 the muscle angle is approximately 25 degrees to the bone; at position 2 the angle is approximately 35 degrees; at position 3 the angle is 90 degrees; and at position 4 the angle is 105 degrees to the bone. Thus, the contracting muscle group will contribute most to holding the knee articulation together when the knee angle is 180 degrees and the muscle-bone angle is the smallest. The muscle group will contribute least to holding the knee articulation together when the knee is flexed to 160 degrees and the bone angle is greatest. (The bone-muscle angle should not be confused with the joint angle; in this example, the joint angle decreases as the bone-muscle angle increases.)

Some bone-muscle angles never achieve an angle greater than 30 degrees or 40 degrees and therefore the muscle always helps to stabilize the articulation it crosses. Generally, tendons are in the best position to stabilize an articulation when the joint is in anatomical position. Muscle angles will be discussed further later in this chapter.

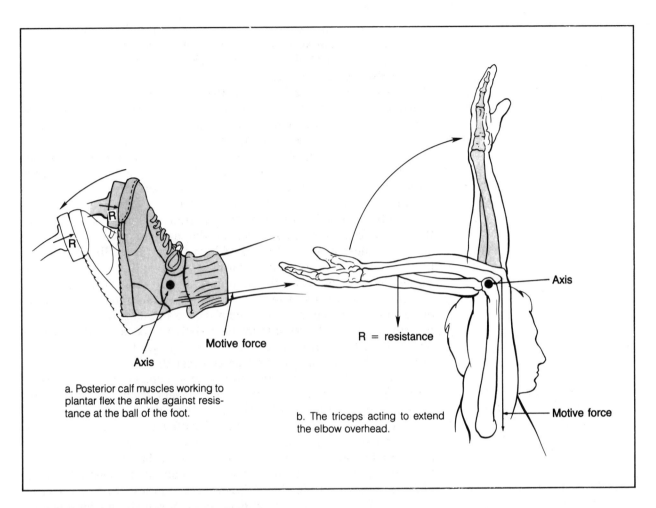

a. Posterior calf muscles working to plantar flex the ankle against resistance at the ball of the foot.

b. The triceps acting to extend the elbow overhead.

R = resistance

Axis

Motive force

Axis

Motive force

The Musculoskeletal Lever System

The long bones of the body, the articulations that connect the long bones, and the muscles that cross those articulations form a mechanical lever system that allows movement to take place. A lever system consists of four parts: (a) a rigid body to serve as the lever, (b) a fulcrum or axis around which the lever rotates, (c) a force applied to the lever that causes motion, and (d) a force applied to the lever that resists motion. In the body, the long bones serve as the lever, the articulations serve as the fulcrum or axis, and the muscles and the force of gravity or other external force serve as the motive and resistive forces. Thus, the muscle pulls on the bone causing the bone and any external load attached to it to rotate around the axis. In this example, the muscle is the motive force. Gravity can also cause motion as when lowering a weight to the floor. When gravity causes the motion, it becomes the motive force; and the muscle force, resisting that motion with an eccentric contraction, is the resistive force.

In Figure 2–9 the fulcrum is at the knee joint, the leg and foot serve as the lever, the hamstrings provide the motive force to lift the leg and foot, and the weight of these segments is the resistive force.

The lever system can be arranged in three ways. In a first-class lever, such as a teeter-totter, the fulcrum is between the motive force and the resistive force. First-class levers in the musculoskeletal system

FIGURE 2–10 Examples of first-class levers in the musculoskeletal system (Redrawn from Kreighbaum and Barthels 1985, 182)

are rare. Two examples are the gastrocnemius and the soleus acting to plantar flex the foot against a resistance at the ball of the foot and the triceps acting to extend the elbow overhead (see Fig. 2–10).

The second-class levers are arranged so the fulcrum is at one end of the lever, the motive force is at the other end of the lever, and the resistive force is in between the two. A wheelbarrow and a rowboat are examples. When serving as the motive force, muscles rarely act as second-class levers. The total body serves as a second-class lever, however, when a push-up is done from the floor. The fulcrum is at the toes, the body is the lever, the weight of the body acting at the center of gravity is the resistive force, and the reaction force of the ground pushing up at the hands is the motive force.

In a third-class lever system, the fulcrum is at one end of the lever, the motive force is in the middle, and the resistive force is at the other end. Most muscles act as third-class levers when providing the motive force for moving a bone. The previous example of the hamstrings moving the leg and foot is an illustration of a third-class arrangement.

The arrangements of lever systems allow for advantages in force or advantages in speed of movement. For example, if the motive force is farther from the fulcrum than the resistive force, as in second-class levers, then the motive force has an advantage; that is, less motive force must be applied to move a greater resistive force. If, on the other hand, the resistive force is located a greater distance from the fulcrum than the motive force, as in third-class levers, then a greater motive force is needed to move a lesser resistive force.

Since most muscles act as third-class levers when providing the motive force, they are at a great disadvantage in force; that is, a muscle must provide far more force to move an object than the object weighs. It is not uncommon for the elbow flexor muscles to need 80 pounds of force to move a 10-lb object. However, third-class levers do have an advantage in range of motion and speed of movement. If a muscle must provide 8 times the amount of force to lift a resistance, then that resistance will move 8 times farther than the muscle needs to shorten. The resistance will move farther than the muscle moves and thus it will also move faster. For example, the hamstrings must provide far more force to move the leg and foot than they weigh. Notice, however, that as the knee is flexed the foot moves a greater linear distance than does the attachment of the hamstrings. Therefore, third-class levers, which include most muscles, have a disadvantage in force but an advantage in range of motion and speed of movement.

As with the stabilizing function of muscles discussed in the previous section, the effectiveness of the muscle to move a bone changes as the bone-muscle angle changes. The most effective position is when the bone-muscle angle is closest to 90 degrees. Notice in Figure 2–9 that the hamstrings' angle changes as the knee angle changes. When the knee is extended, the bone-muscle angle is approximately 20 degrees. In position 3, where the angle is 90 degrees, the hamstrings are most effective in moving the resistance, in this case, the leg and foot. Most muscles cannot achieve an angle of 90 degrees, and thus, the bone-muscle angle closest to 90 degrees is the angle at which they are most effective.

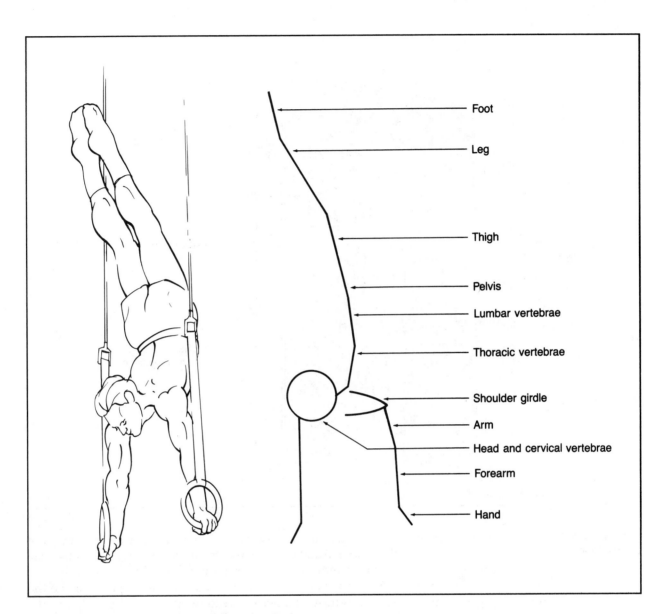

FIGURE 2–11 Major segments in the body's link system (Redrawn from Kreighbaum and Barthels 1985, 36)

Foot

Leg

Thigh

Pelvis

Lumbar vertebrae

Thoracic vertebrae

Shoulder girdle

Arm

Head and cervical vertebrae

Forearm

Hand

The Link System and Its Movements

The skeletal system is a system of segments linked together at their articulations; thus, the body is called a "link system." For the exercise instructor, the body is best described by eleven segments or links: the head and neck, the thoracic vertebrae, the lumbar vertebrae, the pelvis, the thigh, the lower leg, the foot, the shoulder girdle, the arm, the forearm, and the hand (see Fig. 2–11). The movement of the links in the system takes place at the articulations of the segments. Each articulation is restricted to movement in one, two, or three planes of motion— the **sagittal** (which divides the body into right and left parts), the **frontal** (front and back), and the **transverse** (upper and lower)—shown in Figure 2–12.

Table 2–1 lists the articulations important in movement analysis, the type of diarthrodial articulation, the number of planes in which

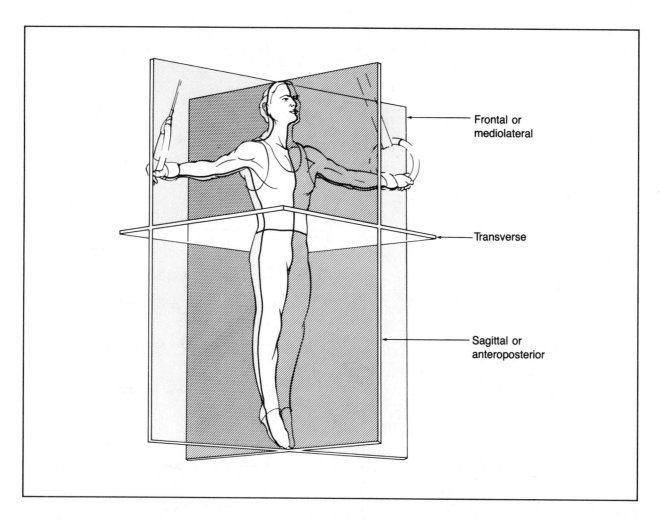

Frontal or
mediolateral

Transverse

Sagittal or
anteroposterior

FIGURE 2–12 The body's three
planes of motion

movement is possible, and the movements that can be performed at
each articulation. As shown in the table, several articulations may
perform a single movement pair. A **movement pair,** for example flexion-extension, is the movement away from anatomical position and the
movement that returns the body part to its anatomical position in the
same plane. For this reason, a general definition of each of these movements is in order. Figures 2–13 through 2–15 illustrate the various
movements of the link system. Refer to these figures while reading the
following sections.

FLEXION-EXTENSION/HYPEREXTENSION.   **Flexion** is a movement that
decreases the angle at an articulation, and **extension** is the return
movement that increases the angle at an articulation. Thus, flexion-
extension is termed a movement pair, that is, a movement and the
opposite movement that returns the body part to anatomical position.
When the body is in anatomical position, all articulations are extended
(except at the ankle joint where the foot is in a neutral position during
anatomical position and is neither flexed nor extended). Flexion of the
vertebral column is the movement of the trunk bending forward, thus
decreasing the angle of the vertebral column from the 180 degrees in
anatomical position to possibly 90 degrees. Extension is the return
movement to anatomical position. Flexion of the vertebral column is

Table 2–1

ARTICULATIONS AND THEIR MOVEMENTS

ARTICULATION	TYPE OF ARTICULATION	NUMBER OF PLANES	POSSIBLE MOVEMENTS
Cervical, Thoracic, Lumbar vertebrae	Gliding	3	Flexion-extension Right-left lateral flexion Right-left rotation
Sternoclavicular	Gliding	2	Elevation-depression Protraction-retraction
Shoulder	Ball and socket	3	Flexion-extension Abduction-adduction Medial-lateral rotation Transverse abduction– transverse adduction
Elbow	Hinge	1	Flexion-extension
Radioulnar	Pivot	1	Pronation-supination
Wrist	Condyloid	2	Flexion-extension Radioulnar flexion
Hip	Ball and socket	3	Flexion-extension Abduction-adduction Medial-lateral rotation Transverse abduction– transverse adduction
Knee	Modified hinge	2	Flexion-extension Medial-lateral rotation (possible only when flexed)
Ankle	Hinge	1	Dorsi-plantar flexion
Subtalar	Gliding	1	Inversion-eversion

a separate movement from flexion of the hip. When the vertebral column flexes, the pelvis stays in anatomical position rather than tipping forward.

Hyperextension is extension beyond the anatomical position. A back bend is an example of hyperextension of the vertebral column. Articulations that can flex-extend and hyperextend are the cervical, thoracic, and lumbar vertebrae, the shoulder, the elbow, the wrist, the hip, the knee, and the ankle (Fig. 2–13, a–g).

Related to flexion-extension is a movement specific to the vertebral column called lateral flexion. The trunk leaning to the right or to the left is termed right lateral flexion or left lateral flexion (Fig. 2–14a).

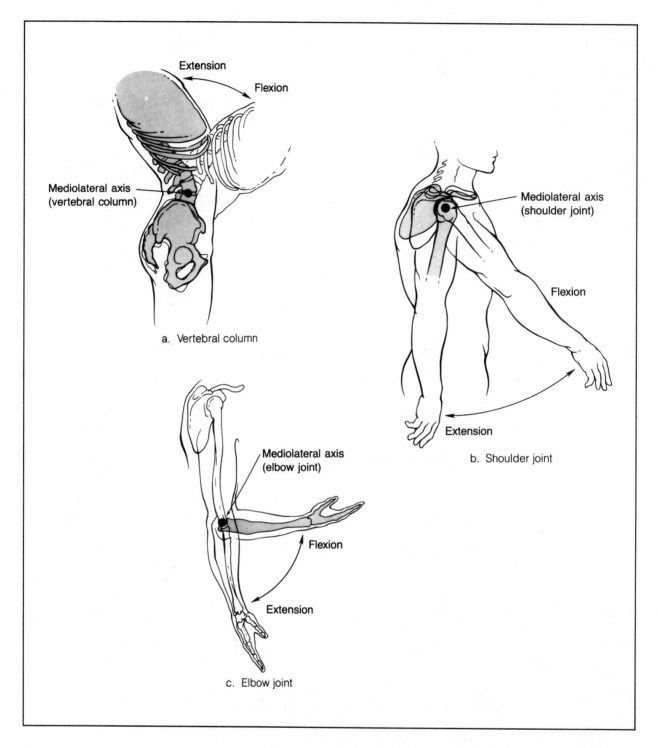

FIGURE 2–13 Segmental movements in the sagittal plane (Redrawn from Kreighbaum and Barthels 1985, 43–44)

ABDUCTION-ADDUCTION.   **Abduction** is the movement of a segment to the side, away from the midline of the body. Its opposite movement, **adduction,** is the movement of a body part toward the midline of the body. For example, raising the arm out to the side is called abduction of the shoulder (Fig. 2–14b). The return movement back to the anatomical position is adduction. Shoulder and hip articulations (Fig. 2–14c, d) allow the abduction-adduction movement pair.

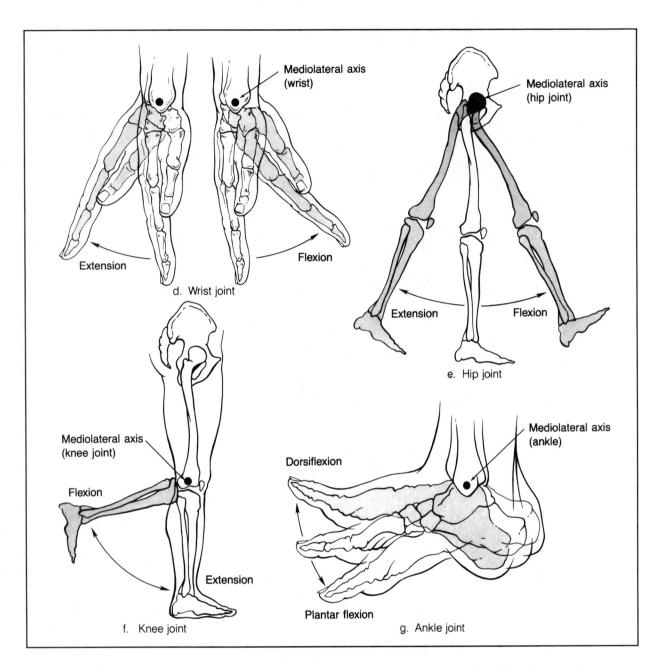

d. Wrist joint

e. Hip joint

f. Knee joint

g. Ankle joint

FIGURE 2–13 (cont'd)

A related movement is transverse abduction-adduction. If the arm is abducted at the shoulder, it can then move across the chest toward the midline of the body, transverse adduction, and return to a position out to the side, transverse abduction. The shoulder and hip articulations allow these movements.

MEDIAL-LATERAL ROTATION. When a body segment rotates around itself, the movement is called either medial-lateral rotation, as when the arm rotates at the shoulder articulation, the thigh rotates at the hip articulation, and the leg rotates at the knee articulation (see Fig. 2–15a and 2–15b), or right-left rotation, as when the head rotates at the cervical vertebrae and the trunk rotates at the thoracic and lumbar vertebrae (see Fig. 2–15c).

AEROBIC DANCE-EXERCISE INSTRUCTOR MANUAL

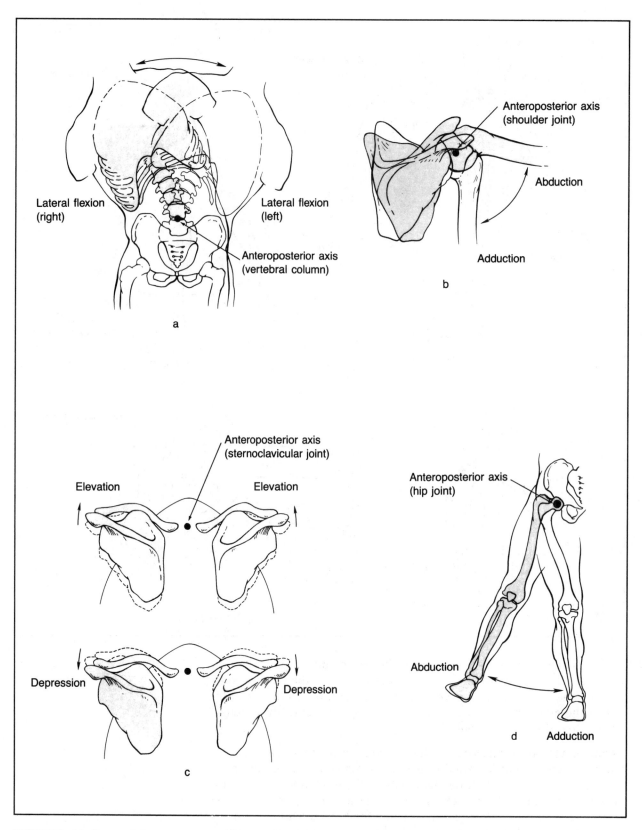

FIGURE 2–14 Segmental movements in the frontal plane (Redrawn from Kreighbaum and Barthels 1985, 45–46)

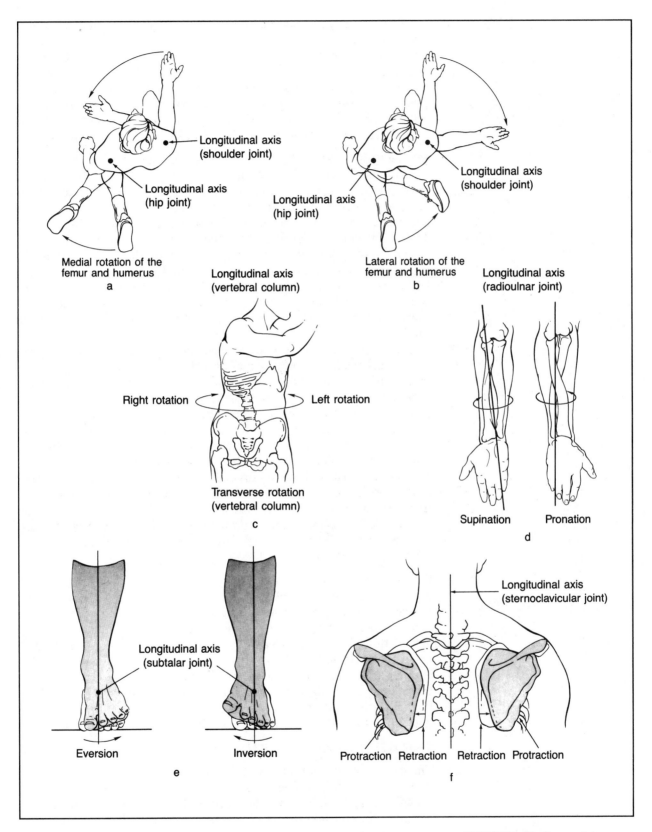

FIGURE 2–15 Segmental movements in the transverse plane (Redrawn from Kreighbaum and Barthels 1985, 47–48)

The movement of a segment in a circular pattern is **circumduction.** The shoulder, hip, wrist, and vertebral joints allow this motion. Therefore, the head and neck, the trunk, the upper and lower extremities, and the hand can perform circumduction. The motion is produced by using flexion, lateral movements, and extension in a series. For example, if the head and neck were flexed forward, laterally flexed to the right, hyperextended, laterally flexed to the left, and returned to the forward flexed position, the head and neck would be circumducted.

MOVEMENTS OF THE WRIST AND ANKLE ARTICULATIONS. Because of the unique nature of the human skeletal system, several articulations have unique movements. The movement of the forearm in turning the palm is termed **supination** when the palm faces forward or upward and **pronation** when the palm faces backward or downward (Fig. 2–15d). These movements take place between the radius and the ulna of the forearm, not at the elbow. The wrist allows the hand to move to the right or left and toward or away from the body. Although appearing to fit the definition of abduction and adduction, the movements at the wrist are called **radial flexion** or deviation, when the hand moves toward the radius or thumb side, and **ulnar flexion** or deviation, when the hand moves toward the ulnar or little-finger side.

Since the foot is in a neutral position when the body assumes anatomical position, the ankle allows the foot to **dorsiflex** when the foot is pulled up toward its dorsal side, or shin, and **plantar flex** when the foot moves toward the plantar surface (bottom) of the foot. (The terms "extension of the foot" for plantar flexion and "flexion of the foot" for dorsiflexion are also used.) The subtalar articulation allows the foot to rotate around itself so the plantar surface tends to face the midline of the body, as in turning the ankle. This movement at the subtalar articulation is called **inversion** of the foot. Rotation of the foot to the outside so the plantar surface tends to face away from the midline of the body is called **eversion** of the foot at the subtalar articulation (Fig. 2–15e). These movements do *not* occur at the ankle joint; if forced to occur at the ankle joint, these movements would damage the surrounding ligaments.

PRONATED/SUPINATED FOOT. The terms "pronation" and "supination" are frequently used to refer to the foot. Technically, supination and pronation movements do not occur at any single articulation, but are instead a combination of movements at both the ankle and the subtalar articulations. Figures 2–16 and 2–17 illustrate a pronated and a supinated foot, respectively. *Pronation* of the foot occurs when the ankle is dorsiflexed and the subtalar joint is everted; the ankle collapses to the medial side. *Supination* of the foot is a combination of plantar flexion of the ankle and inversion of the subtalar articulations simultaneously; the ankle falls to the outside as in "turning the ankle."

THE MUSCULAR SYSTEM

The muscular system provides the forces that cause the bones to move. A muscle is attached to at least two bones and crosses one or more articulations between its proximal and distal attachments. This section describes the special properties of muscle tissue, explains how muscles effect movement, and discusses the muscle groups that cause motion of the articulations of the upper and lower extremities, the vertebral column, and the pelvis.

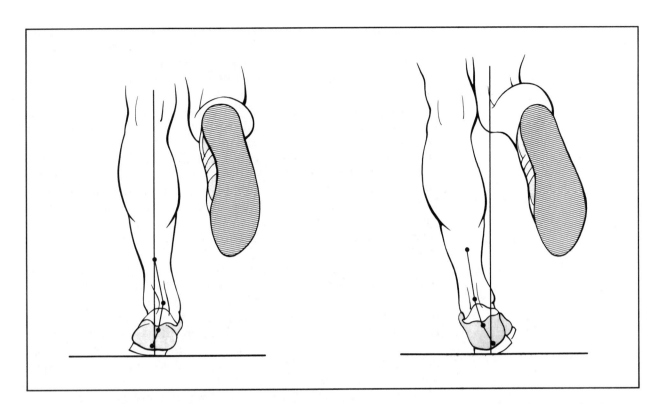

Properties of Muscle Tissue

Muscle tissue has four functional properties: (a) contractility, it can contract or shorten; (b) distensibility, it can distend or stretch; (c) elasticity, it can return to its original shape after being stretched; and (d) irritability, it can respond to electrical stimuli. Of these four properties, contractility and distensibility are probably the most important for exercise instructors to understand.

CONTRACTILITY OF MUSCLE TISSUE.   When irritated or stimulated by an electrical impulse from the nervous system, muscle tissue attempts to shorten or contract. Tension, or a pulling force, is produced at each end of the muscle where it attaches to the bones. Each end tries to move toward the middle of the muscle, pulling with it the bone to which it is attached. If the resistance of the bone is not too great, one or both ends of the muscle and the attached bones will move toward the middle of the muscle. Hence, movement takes place at the articulation, and the segment(s) is flexed or extended or rotated depending on the location of that muscle relative to that bone.

The force with which a muscle contracts depends on the number of muscle fibers stimulated, the strength of the nervous stimulation, the type of muscle fibers stimulated, and the length of the muscle at the time of stimulation. Obviously, the greater the number of muscle fibers stimulated and the stronger the nervous stimulation, the stronger the muscle contraction. A muscle is composed of three basic types of fibers: slow twitch, fast twitch, and intermediate (fast-twitch oxidative). Each fiber type is associated with certain contractile characteristics. Slow twitch fibers are endurance fibers. Although they have less strength and are relatively small, these fibers have dense capillary networks and therefore are resistant to fatigue. Slow twitch fibers are the "dark meat" in poultry. Fast twitch fibers are larger and stronger

FIGURE 2–16 (*left*) A pronated foot

FIGURE 2–17 (*right*) A supinated foot

and contract in an explosive manner, but their small capillary supply means they fatigue quickly. Fast twitch fibers are the "white meat" in poultry. Intermediate fibers are a compromise: they are large and strong, contract quickly, and have a good blood supply, but they still fatigue more quickly than slow twitch fibers.

Each person and each muscle within a person has a different combination of the three types of fibers. Some people have muscles that are fairly high in slow twitch fibers and thus are better at endurance activities. Others have higher concentrations of fast twitch fibers and are better at strength and explosive activities, but their muscles tire easily. Although current theory holds that muscle fiber types cannot be changed, the muscle's oxidative aerobic capacity can be enhanced through training; thus a muscle consisting predominantly of fast twitch fibers can increase its endurance capacity through endurance (aerobic) training.

As muscles shorten or contract, they will attempt to effect change in all articulations they cross. A muscle can be **uniarticulate,** that is, cross one articulation; **biarticulate,** cross two articulations; or **multiarticulate,** cross more than two articulations. If the muscle crosses two articulations between its proximal and distal attachments, both articulations will attempt to display the appropriate movement when the muscle tries to shorten. If only one articulation is crossed, then only that articulation will be affected.

Exercise instructors need to know which muscles are one-, two-, and three-joint muscles, because the exercises used to strengthen a multiarticulate muscle may be quite different from the exercises used to strengthen a uniarticulate muscle. For example, the hamstring muscles originate on the posterior of the pelvis, cross the hip joint and the knee joint, and insert on the posterior part of the bones of the leg below the knee. When these muscles contract, they will cause the hip joint to extend and the knee joint to flex. Working the muscle only over the hip joint or only over the knee joint will not effectively strengthen the hamstrings. To work the entire hamstring group, extend the hip *and* flex the knee against resistance. Figure 2–18(a) illustrates the forces at the proximal and distal ends of the hamstrings during hip extension and simultaneous knee flexion. Figure 2–18(b) illustrates the stretching the hamstring group undergoes when the opposite movements—hip flexion and knee extension—are performed simultaneously. Analyzing exercises in terms of strengthening or stretching uni-, bi- and multiarticulate muscles will be discussed later in this chapter.

DISTENSIBILITY OF MUSCLE TISSUE AND TENDONS.   Muscle fibers and their associated tendons can be stretched or lengthened and will return undamaged to their original length, if the stretching or lengthening is not too great. This ability is called **elasticity;** that is, the muscle tissue displays a property similar to that of a rubber band; it is elastic and returns to its original shape after being stretched. However, if a muscle or its tendon or a ligament, is stretched beyond its limit, it will remain extended. This point beyond which the tissue will not return to its original length is called the **elastic limit.** Pulling a muscle or spraining an ankle occurs when muscles, tendons, and ligaments reach their elastic limits. Because muscle tissue can heal itself, an overstretched

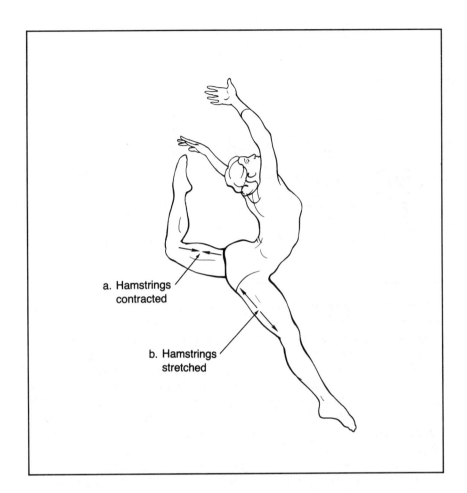

a. Hamstrings
contracted

b. Hamstrings
stretched

FIGURE 2–18 Contracting and stretching a biarticulate muscle (Redrawn from Kreighbaum and Barthels 1985, 222)

muscle can usually repair itself unless torn from its attachment to the bone. A ligament, however, does not have that ability; medical help is required to put the ligament back in working order.

Flexibility exercises attempt to stretch a muscle and its tendon without exceeding its elastic limit. The most appropriate flexibility exercises are slow stretching exercises because they stretch the tissue without forcing it beyond a safe limit. Fast bouncing or ballistic stretching exercises may force the articulation beyond the elastic limits of its tissues and cause injury.

As with the strengthening exercises, flexibility exercises must be designed to accommodate the uni-, bi-, or multiarticulate muscle. The hamstrings were used earlier as an example of strengthening a two-joint muscle. Remember that a two-joint muscle crosses two articulations. The hamstring group crosses the posterior hip and knee joints. The muscle must be stretched over both joints simultaneously, or one end of the muscle will lengthen while the other end shortens and there will be no net stretch. Thus, to stretch the hamstrings, flex the hip to stretch the hamstrings as a hip extensor and *at the same time* extend the knee to stretch the hamstrings as a knee flexor (see Fig. 2–18b).

How Muscles Affect Movement

Analyzing a particular exercise for its muscular components first requires an understanding of how and why the segments or links of the body

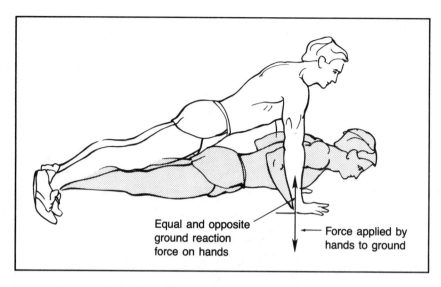

Equal and opposite
ground reaction
force on hands

Force applied by
hands to ground

FIGURE 2-19 Push-up

move the way they do. This section is very important for designing an exercise program. The segments of the body move because a net force on them causes them to move; however, many different types of forces can cause a body part to move. For example, gravitational force, muscle force, an external object, or another person can influence the movement of the body part. If you hold your arm out to the side (abduction) and the abductor muscles suddenly relax, your arm will fall back to the side (adduction). The adduction of the arm is not caused by muscles at all, but instead by the force of gravity acting on the mass of the arm in a downward direction. Gravity always acts downward toward the center of the earth. Thus, when a body part moves downward toward the floor, gravity usually is causing that motion. If you move your arm back out to the side again (abduction), the body part is moving away from the earth, and muscles or some other force (a partner, for example) is causing the arm to be abducted.

When analyzing an exercise to determine the muscles involved, an instructor must not rely solely on a knowledge of what the muscles are designed to do. That is, if the elbow is flexing, it is not always the flexor muscles that are causing the motion.

The procedure for muscular analysis begins by observing the movement. Using a push-up as an example, the exerciser starts in a prone position lying on the floor. The first part of the exercise is to push the body away from the floor (see Fig. 2–19).

1. *Determine what segments are moving and what movements they are displaying.* The shoulder girdle is protracting, the shoulder joint is flexing, and the elbow is extending.

2. *Ask yourself what force is causing the movement.* The body is moving away from the ground so it could not be gravitational force. There is no external object or partner causing the person to move upward. Therefore, the muscles that cross those articulations must be causing the movement. The forces that are causing the body to move upward are the shoulder girdle protractors, the shoulder joint flexors, and the elbow extensors. When muscles contract and cause the body part to move, the muscles are contracting **concentrically,** that is, they are shortening as they contract.

During the second part of the exercise, the exerciser allows the body to return to the starting position. Decide which joints are moving and what their movements are. Notice that the shoulder girdle is retracting, the shoulder joint is extending, and the elbow is flexing. Be cautious; do not be fooled into thinking that those associated muscles are working. What is causing the body to return to the floor? It is not the muscles but gravity that is pulling the body back down. However, if gravity were the only force acting on the body, the body would crash to the floor. Obviously, the exerciser wants to control or resist those movements so there is no chance of injury. The only muscles that can resist the movement caused by the application of another force are muscles that cause a motion *opposite* to the motion being performed. Therefore, the shoulder girdle protractors resist shoulder girdle retraction, shoulder joint flexors resist shoulder joint extension, and elbow extensors resist elbow flexion. These muscles are contracting **eccentrically,** or lengthening against a resistance. In summary, if muscles are causing the joints to move, then the muscles that cause the motion are the ones being worked. If another force, such as gravity, is causing the motion of the joints, then the muscles being used are the muscles opposite to the motion.

In the push-up, then, the same muscles are being used on the way up and on the way down. In fact, whenever calisthenics are performed—that is, when gravity and the body's weight are used as a resistance—this rule is true: Movements away from the ground use the same muscle groups as the movement itself. Movements toward the ground use the opposite muscle groups to the movement being performed.

During the performance of an exercise, some body parts that should remain stable tend to move. For example, during the push-up, the trunk tends to sag or hyperextend. The hyperextension of the trunk is caused by the force of gravity acting on it. To prevent hyperextension of the trunk caused by gravity, contract the muscles that cause the movement opposite to the undesirable movement. The vertebral column flexors (abdominals) are used to prevent the trunk from hyperextending. Whenever muscles are used to prevent a motion, as in this example, they are contracting statically, or **isometrically,** and are not shortening or lengthening as they contract.

Any force on the body can act to move a body part, to resist a body part's movement, or to stabilize a body part so it will be difficult to move. It is important to know which function muscles are performing to determine which muscles or muscle groups are being used.

Muscles of the Upper Extremity

The muscles of the upper extremity cause movement of the following articulations: the sternoclavicular, the shoulder, the elbow, the radioulnar, and the wrist joints.

MUSCLES OF THE SHOULDER GIRDLE.   The shoulder girdle consists of the clavicle, which makes up the anterior portion of the shoulder, and the scapula, which makes up the posterior portion. The clavicle articulates with the sternum at the sternoclavicular joint; movement of the entire shoulder girdle takes place at that articulation. Most muscles that effect movement of the shoulder girdle attach to the scapula; however, two relatively small muscles attach to the clavicle. Because the

AEROBIC DANCE-EXERCISE INSTRUCTOR MANUAL

Figure 2–20

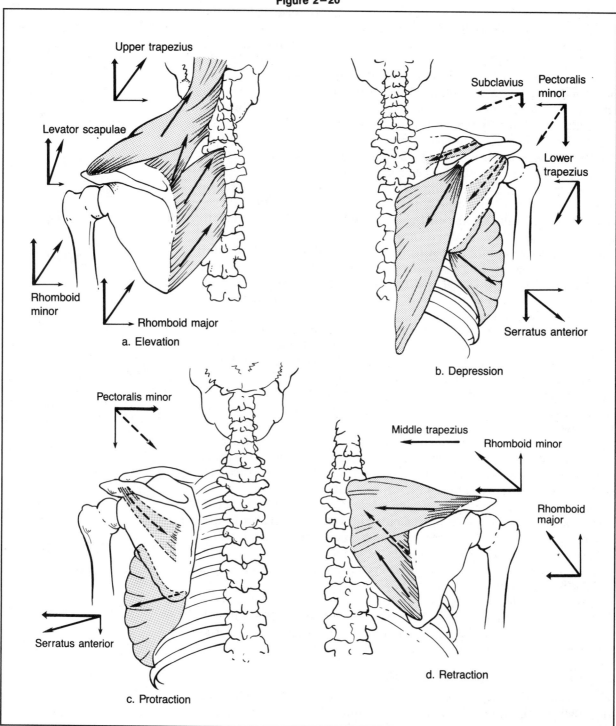

a. Elevation

b. Depression

c. Protraction

d. Retraction

FIGURE 2–20 Muscles effecting movements in the shoulder girdle (Redrawn from Kreighbaum and Barthels 1985, 196–97)

clavicle and scapula are joined at their lateral ends, muscles pulling on either one effects movement of both, that is, the entire shoulder girdle. Four main muscle groups effect movement of the shoulder girdle: the elevators, the depressors, the protractors, and the retractors. The individual muscles constituting these groups are shown in Figure 2–20(a)–(d).

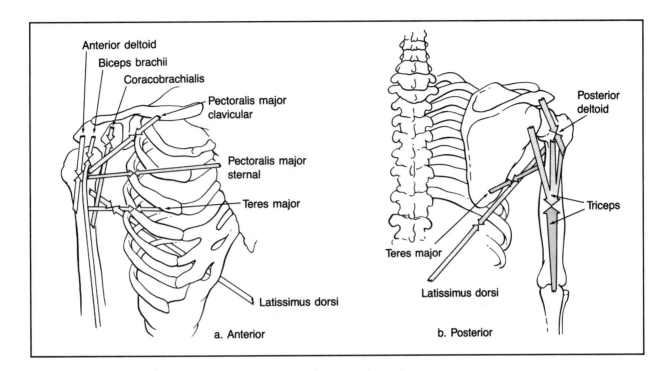

Anterior deltoid
Biceps brachii
Coracobrachialis
Pectoralis major clavicular
Pectoralis major sternal
Teres major
Latissimus dorsi

a. Anterior

Posterior deltoid
Triceps
Teres major
Latissimus dorsi

b. Posterior

FIGURE 2–21 Anterior and posterior muscles of the shoulder joint (Redrawn from Kreighbaum and Barthels 1985, 201)

The shoulder girdle elevation muscles, shown in Figure 2–20(a), are the upper section of the trapezius, the levator scapulae, the rhomboid major, and the rhomboid minor. The illustration indicates, by means of arrows, the direction in which these muscles pull on the scapula to elevate it.

The shoulder girdle depression muscles, which cause the scapula to depress, are shown in Figure 2–20(b). These muscles are the subclavius, the pectoralis minor, the lower section of the trapezius, and the serratus anterior.

The shoulder girdle protraction muscles—the pectoralis minor and the serratus anterior—cause the scapula to protract (Fig. 2–20c).

The shoulder girdle retraction muscles, shown in Figure 2–20(d), cause the scapula to retract. These muscles are the middle section of the trapezius, the rhomboid major, and the rhomboid minor.

MUSCLES OF THE SHOULDER JOINT. The muscles surrounding the shoulder joint cause the following arm movements: flexion-extension, abduction-adduction, medial-lateral rotation, and transverse abduction-adduction. Figure 2–21(a) illustrates the muscles attached to the anterior portion of the humerus that work to flex the shoulder joint and transversely adduct the shoulder joint when it is abducted. The major muscles in this group are the anterior deltoid, the biceps, the coracobrachialis, and the clavicular portion of the pectoralis major. The arrows show the approximate locations of the proximal and distal attachments and the direction of muscle pull on the proximal and distal bones.

The muscles attached to the posterior portion of the humerus that work to extend the shoulder joint and transversely abduct the shoulder joint when it is abducted are shown in Figure 2–21(b). The primary muscles are the long head of the triceps, the posterior deltoid, the latissimus dorsi, and the teres major.

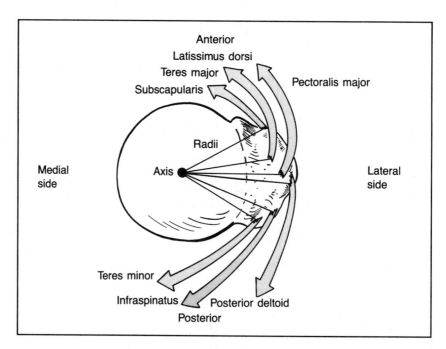

FIGURE 2–22 Medial and lateral rotation muscles of the shoulder joint (Redrawn from Kreighbaum and Barthels 1985, 202)

Figure 2–22 illustrates the muscles that cause medial and lateral rotation of the humerus. The medial muscles attach distally on the anterior side of the humerus and proximally somewhere on the trunk. The pectoralis major attaches proximally on the sternum; the teres major attaches on the scapula; the latissimus dorsi attaches on the vertebral column. The lateral muscles—the infraspinatus and the teres minor—attach distally on the posterior side of the humerus and proximally on the scapula.

The middle portion of the deltoid and the supraspinatus cause abduction of the shoulder joint (Fig. 2–23). Both muscles attach distally on the lateral portion of the humerus and proximally on the scapula.

The latissimus dorsi, the teres major, and the sternal portion of the pectoralis major cause adduction of the shoulder joint. The force of these muscles is directed downward toward the midline of the body when the arm is abducted.

MUSCLES OF THE ELBOW AND RADIOULNAR JOINTS.   Although the elbow and radioulnar joints are two separate joints, they are considered together here because their movements are frequently related. The movements of these joints are flexion and extension of the elbow and pronation and supination of the radioulnar joint. The anterior and posterior muscles of the elbow and radioulnar joint are illustrated in Figure 2–24(a) and (b), respectively.

There are three elbow flexor muscles: the biceps, the brachialis, and the brachioradialis. Of these, the biceps and the brachialis are the most influential.

The biceps is a two-joint muscle that effects flexion and transverse-adduction of the shoulder joint. Since the biceps also causes radioulnar supination, it is technically a three-joint muscle, effecting movement in the shoulder, the elbow, and the radioulnar joints. Therefore, any exercise to strengthen or stretch the biceps should use all three joints.

Although the biceps receives more attention, the brachialis is probably in a better position to contribute to the force of elbow flexion.

Anatomy and Kinesiology

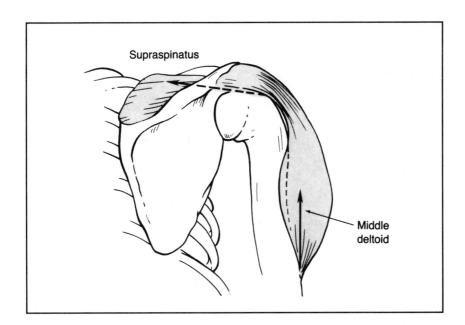

FIGURE 2–23 Abduction muscles of the shoulder joint (Redrawn from Kreighbaum and Barthels 1985, 203)

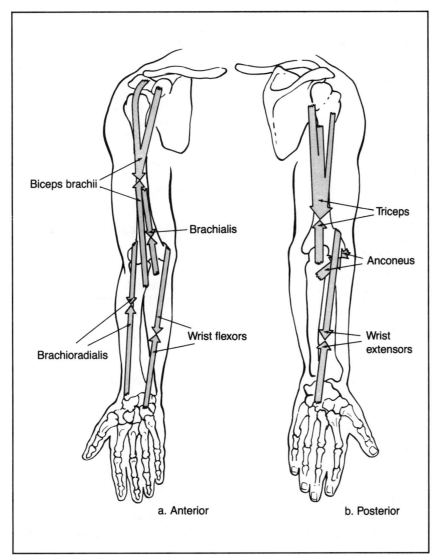

a. Anterior   b. Posterior

FIGURE 2–24 Anterior and posterior muscles of the elbow and radioulnar joints (Redrawn from Kreighbaum and Barthels 1985, 207)

Table 2-2

MAJOR MUSCLES OF THE UPPER EXTREMITY AND THEIR MOVEMENTS

MUSCLE	ARTICULATIONS CROSSED	MOVEMENT CAUSED
Sternocleidomastoid	Cervical	Cervical flexion Lateral flexion Rotation to the opposite side
Pectoralis major	Sternoclavicular Shoulder	Protraction Depression Adduction Transverse adduction Flexion (clavicular)
Trapezius	Sternoclavicular	Elevation (upper) Retraction (middle) Depression (lower)
Rhomboid major	Sternoclavicular	Elevation Retraction
Serratus anterior	Sternoclavicular	Depression Protraction
Deltoid	Shoulder	Flexion (anterior) Transverse adduction (anterior) Abduction (middle) Extension (posterior) Transverse abduction (posterior)
Biceps brachii	Shoulder Elbow Radioulnar	Flexion (long head) Flexion Supination
Coracobrachialis	Shoulder	Flexion Transverse adduction
Supraspinatus	Shoulder	Abduction
Infraspinatus Teres minor	Shoulder	Lateral rotation Transverse abduction
Latissimus dorsi Teres major	Shoulder	Medial rotation Extension
Triceps	Shoulder Elbow	Extension Transverse abduction Extension
Brachialis	Elbow	Flexion
Brachioradialis	Elbow Radioulnar	Flexion Supination-pronation to midposition
Wrist extensors	Elbow Wrist	Extension Extension
Wrist flexors	Elbow Wrist	Flexion Flexion

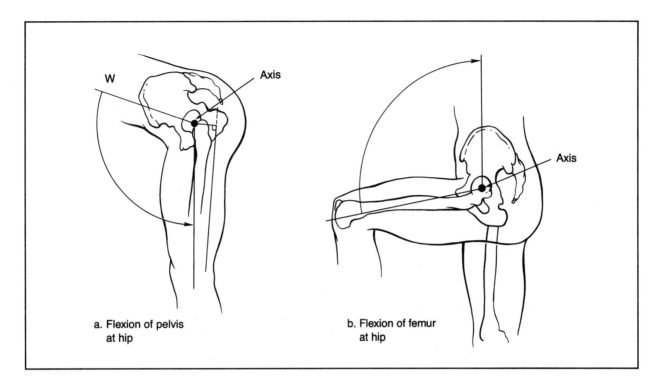

a. Flexion of pelvis at hip

b. Flexion of femur at hip

FIGURE 2-25 Flexing the hip by moving the pelvis and by moving the thigh

The brachialis, as a one-joint muscle, does not have to use part of its energy to attempt to cause movement in other joints. Most of the flexors of the wrist joint cross on the anterior side of the elbow and assist in flexing the elbow.

The main elbow extensor is the triceps. The triceps is a two-joint muscle that crosses the shoulder and the elbow. To strengthen or stretch this muscle effectively, the triceps must be worked over both shoulder and elbow joints. Most primary extensors of the wrist cross on the posterior side of the elbow and therefore help extend the elbow.

Table 2-2 lists the major muscles of the upper extremity, the number of articulations crossed, and the main movement function at each articulation.

Muscles of the Lower Extremity

Muscles of the lower extremity effect the movement of four basic articulations: the hip, the knee, the ankle, and the subtalar joints.

MUSCLES OF THE HIP JOINT.   The hip joint consists of the articulation of the pelvis and the femur. The movement of the pelvis or the femur can take place at the hip joint. When you flex forward while weight bearing and keeping the vertebral column extended, you are flexing your hip. You also flex your hip when you raise your femur upward as in climbing stairs. Remember, the muscles that cross an articulation attempt to cause movement of both bones to which they attach. Therefore when the muscles that cross the hip joint contract, the bone that is to remain stationary must be stabilized by other muscles. Figure 2-25(a) and (b) illustrates hip flexion both by moving the pelvis and by moving the femur.

The muscles crossing the anterior and medial portion of the hip are indicated by arrows in Figure 2-26. The hip flexor muscles are the rectus femoris of the quadriceps group and the iliopsoas. The iliopsoas is in a good position to pull the pelvis and vertebral column

AEROBIC DANCE-EXERCISE INSTRUCTOR MANUAL

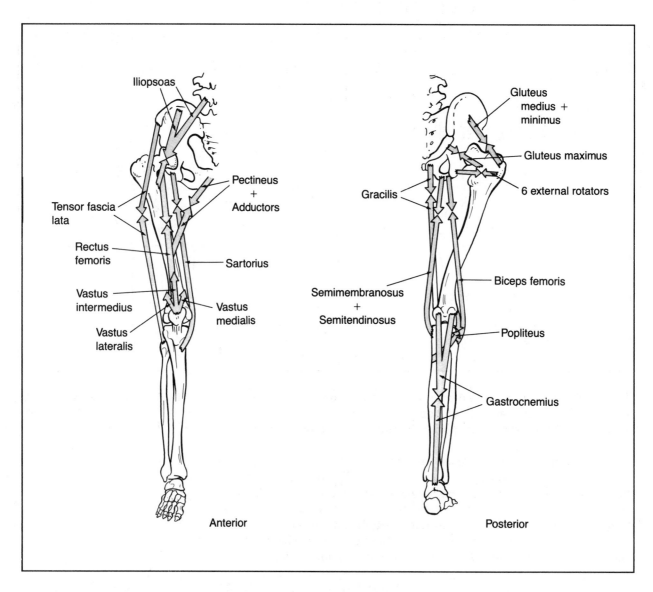

FIGURES 2–26 *(left)* Anterior and medial muscles of the hip and knee joints (Redrawn from Kreighbaum and Barthels 1985, 222)

FIGURE 2–27 *(right)* Posterior muscles of the hip and knee joints (Redrawn from Kreighbaum and Barthels 1985, 222)

forward and to lift the thigh into flexion. The only abductor on the anterior side is the tensor fascia lata. Because this muscle is directed outward slightly from its proximal to distal attachment, it will cause a slight medial rotation of the thigh when the pelvis is fixed. The tensor fascia lata is used to flex the thigh. The thigh's adductors shown in this anterior view of the thigh are the pectineus, the sartorius, and the three adductor muscles—the adductor magnus, the adductor brevis, and the adductor longus. The adductor muscles are indicated by one arrow in the illustration because they are located in the same vicinity.

The pectineus medially rotates and adducts the hip joint. The sartorius, the longest muscle in the body, flexes and laterally rotates the hip and also helps to flex the knee. Also called the "tailor's" muscle, the sartorius causes the lower extremity to move into a tailor's sitting position (sitting cross-legged). The adductor muscles mainly effect adduction.

The posterior hip joint muscles are shown in Figure 2–27. The main hip extensors are the three hamstring muscles: the biceps femoris, the semitendinosus, and semimembranosus. Although all of the hamstring muscles cause hip extension, note that the biceps femoris attaches distally to the lateral leg and the semitendinosus and semi-membranosus attach distally on the medial side of the leg. The location of these attachments becomes important when the knee is flexed and will be discussed in the next section.

The one adductor of the hip that can be seen on this posterior view is the gracilis. The abductors shown on the posterior view are the gluteus maximus, the gluteus medius, and the gluteus minimus. The gluteal muscles are located close to the hip joint on the lateral posterior side. The gluteus medius and gluteus minimus work to abduct the hip. The gluteus maximus helps abduct the hip and also functions as a strong hip extensor when the hip is flexed more than 60 degrees. For example, flexing forward when climbing enhances the use of the gluteus maximus because the muscle does not contribute as much during the last part of hip extension. The gluteus maximus, along with the six external rotators, work to laterally rotate the femur relative to the pelvis or, if weight bearing, laterally rotate the pelvis on the femur. The lateral rotation movement is used in ballet to toe out when the foot is free and to change direction toward the opposite side when weight bearing.

MUSCLES OF THE KNEE JOINT.   The muscles that effect movement of the knee joint are shown in the anterior and posterior views of the lower extremity in Figures 2–26 and 2–27. Any muscle that crosses the knee joint can effect the movement of the knee joint, although some muscles are in a better position than others.

The main muscles of knee extension are the four quadriceps muscles: the rectus femoris, the vastus medialis, the vastus lateralis, and the vastus intermedius. Of these muscles, only the rectus femoris crosses the hip joint. The three vasti muscles are attached to the femur on the proximal end and the patella on the distal end. The patella in turn attaches to the tibia. Thus, when the quadriceps muscles contract, they pull on the patella which, by way of the patellar tendon, pulls on the tibia causing the knee to extend. The main knee flexors are the muscles of the hamstring group with some assistance from the sartorius. Although the gastrocnemius also crosses the knee, it functions mainly to plantar flex the ankle.

Recall the distal locations of the hamstring attachments. The biceps femoris attaches to the lateral side of the leg, and the semi-muscles (semitendinosus and semimembranosus) attach to the medial side of the leg. When the knee is flexed, the bony structure enables the leg to rotate medially and laterally. The biceps femoris causes lateral rotation, and the semi-muscles and the popliteus cause medial rotation of the leg. Frequently, the strengths of the medial and lateral rotators are not balanced; the lateral rotator is usually stronger. Thus, when the knee is flexed against a resistance, the leg rotates outward simultaneously (see Fig. 2–28). This rotation should be prevented by strengthening the medial rotators.

MUSCLES OF THE ANKLE AND FOOT JOINTS.   The ankle and foot articulations are considered together because the positions and movements of the foot use all of these joints. The muscles acting on the ankle and foot are indicated by arrows in Figure 2–29.

AEROBIC DANCE-EXERCISE INSTRUCTOR MANUAL

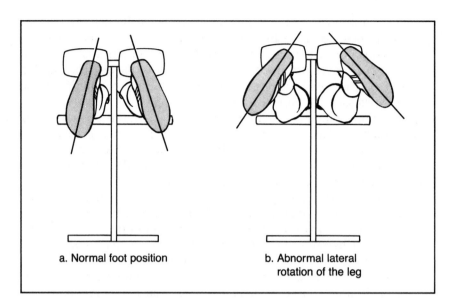

a. Normal foot position

b. Abnormal lateral rotation of the leg

FIGURE 2–28 Lateral rotation of the tibia with flexion of the knee (Redrawn from Kreighbaum and Barthels 1985, 229)

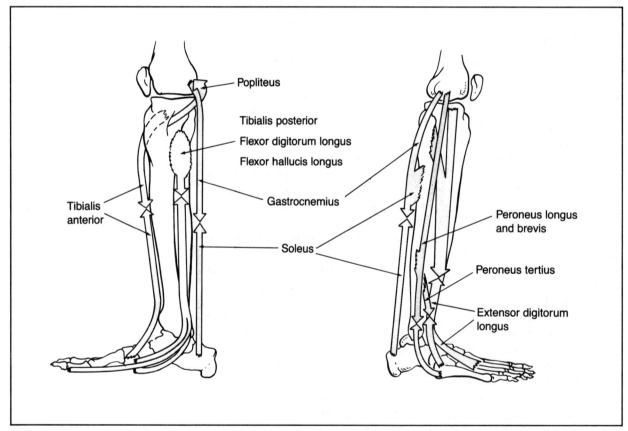

Popliteus

Tibialis posterior

Flexor digitorum longus

Flexor hallucis longus

Gastrocnemius

Tibialis anterior

Soleus

Peroneus longus and brevis

Peroneus tertius

Extensor digitorum longus

FIGURE 2–29 Muscles of the ankle and foot (Redrawn from Kreighbaum and Barthels 1985, 238)

The primary plantar flexors of the ankle are the muscles attached to the Achilles tendon: the gastrocnemius and the soleus. Recall that the gastrocnemius crosses both the knee, causing flexion, and the ankle, causing plantar flexion; therefore, to stretch this muscle, extend the knee while dorsiflexing the ankle joint. The soleus, on the other hand, only crosses the ankle, causing plantar flexion. To stretch the soleus, flex the knee to make the gastrocnemius "slack" while dorsiflexing the ankle. Otherwise, the gastrocnemius becomes taut before any stretching begins on the soleus, and the soleus will not be affected.

Assisting the Achilles tendon muscles to plantar flex the ankle are three medial muscles that pass from the foot around the medial malleolus of the tibia and up the posterior leg, and two lateral muscles that pass from the foot around the lateral malleolus of the fibula and up the lateral leg. The medial muscles—the tibialis posterior, the flexor digitorum longus, and the flexor hallucis longus (or the *Tom, Dick, and Harry* muscles)—plantar flex the ankle and invert the foot. These movements are associated with supination of the foot. The lateral muscles—the peroneus longus and the peroneus brevis—plantar flex the ankle and evert the foot.

The ankle has three main dorsiflexors: the tibialis anterior, the peroneus tertius, and the extensor digitorum longus. The tibialis anterior attaches distally on the medial side of the foot and proximally on the lateral side of the tibia. Thus, when the tibialis anterior contracts, it tends to dorsiflex the ankle and invert the foot. The peroneus tertius and the extensor digitorum longus both dorsiflex the ankle and evert the foot. The three dorsiflexor muscles are located in the anterior compartment of the leg.

Table 2–3 lists the major muscles of the lower extremity, the articulations crossed, and the major movements.

Muscles of the Vertebral Column and Pelvis

The vertebral column articulations consist of the intervertebral joints—the cervical, the thoracic, the lumbar, and the lumbosacral—and the sacroiliac, which is the articulation between the sacrum of the vertebral column and the ilium of the pelvis. Two primary muscle groups control the stability and the movement of these articulations: the erector spinae muscles along the posterior vertebral column and the abdominal muscles on the anterior of the vertebral column. The abdominal muscles are shown in Figure 2–30.

The main muscles used to flex the trunk are the rectus abdominis and the internal and external obliques. The rectus abdominis, attached proximally to the base of the sternum and distally to the pubic bone, flexes the vertebral column but does not cause rotation. The location of the internal and external obliques enables them to cause both flexion and rotation of the vertebral column. For example, sit-ups performed with a rotation component (touching the elbow to the opposite knee) use the internal and external oblique muscles.

The posterior muscles of the back (Fig. 2–31) cause vertebral column extension and rotation of the trunk to the right and left. The quadratus lumborum, located on the right and left sides between the iliac crest on the dorsal and lateral sides, causes lateral flexion to the right and to the left. The muscles of the erector spinae group and other small muscles of the back cause extension, rotation, and lateral flexion of the trunk.

POSTURAL ALIGNMENT OF THE TRUNK

The muscles of the trunk and vertebral column provide the forces necessary to produce and maintain the alignment of the trunk and pelvis in "good posture." Basically, good posture stems from the control

AEROBIC DANCE-EXERCISE INSTRUCTOR MANUAL

Table 2–3

MAJOR MUSCLES OF THE LOWER EXTREMITY AND THEIR MOVEMENTS

MUSCLE	ARTICULATIONS CROSSED	MOVEMENT CAUSED
Iliopsoas	Intervertebral Hip	Flexion Flexion
Gluteus medius Gluteus minimus	Hip	Abduction
Gluteus maximus External rotators	Hip	Extension Lateral rotation Transverse abduction
Tensor fascia lata	Hip	Abduction
Rectus femoris (quadricep)	Hip Knee	Flexion Extension
Pectineus Adductors	Hip	Adduction Transverse adduction
Gracilis	Hip	Adduction Transverse adduction
Sartorius	Hip Knee	Flexion Lateral rotation Flexion
Biceps femoris (hamstring)	Hip Knee	Extension Flexion Lateral rotation
Semitendinosus Semimembranosus (hamstrings)	Hip Knee	Extension Flexion Medial rotation
Popliteus	Knee	Flexion Medial rotation
Gastrocnemius (Achilles)	Knee Ankle	Flexion Plantar flexion
Soleus (Achilles)	Ankle	Plantar flexion
Tibialis posterior Flexor digitorum Flexor hallucis	Ankle Subtalar	Plantar flexion Inversion
Peroneus longus Peroneus brevis	Ankle	Plantar flexion
Tibialis anterior	Ankle Subtalar	Dorsiflexion Inversion
Extensor digitorum	Ankle Subtalar	Dorsiflexion Eversion

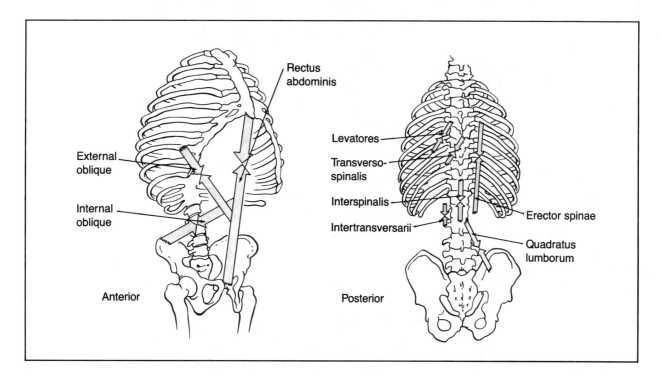

of the lumbar vertebrae and the pelvis. Figure 2–32 illustrates three lumbar postural alignments: (a) ideal (normal), (b) anterior pelvic tilt, and (c) posterior pelvic tilt.

FIGURE 2–30 *(left)* Abdominal muscles (Redrawn from Kreighbaum and Barthels 1985, 264)

FIGURE 2–31 *(right)* Posterior muscles of the vertebral column (Redrawn from Kreighbaum and Barthels 1985, 264)

Ideal Posture

In the ideal postural alignment, the pelvis is resting over the hip joints in a balanced position and the vertebral column displays the "normal" curvatures. The "normal" curvatures in the anteroposterior direction exist as an anterior curve in the cervical area, a posterior curve in the thoracic area, and an anterior curve in the lumbar area, as shown earlier in Figure 2–5.

Anterior and Posterior Pelvic Tilt

Anterior tilt or protraction of the pelvis, shown in Figure 2–32(b), is produced when the pelvis tilts forward on the femur. The pelvis tilting forward causes the lumbar area to accommodate by exaggerating its curvature. Extreme lumbar curvature results in lower back pain due to the "crunching" of the posterior disks located between the vertebrae. This malady is common in women, particularly gymnasts, who have not been coached to tighten the abdominals and maintain the stability of the trunk.

Posterior pelvic tilt, in which the pelvis is tilted backward or retracted relative to the femur, is not as common. This condition, shown in Figure 2–32(c), causes a flattening of the natural lumbar vertebral curve.

These two misalignments (anterior tilt and posterior tilt) can be rectified by proper conditioning of the vertebral column and pelvic musculature. An anterior tilt results from weak abdominals. Strengthening the abdominals and the hip extensor muscles and stretching the lower back and hip flexor muscles will pull the pelvis back into balanced alignment. Posterior tilt can be caused by weak lower back and hip flexor muscles and overpowering abdominal and hip extensor muscles. If not congenital, posterior tilt can be rectified by stretching the

AEROBIC DANCE-EXERCISE INSTRUCTOR MANUAL

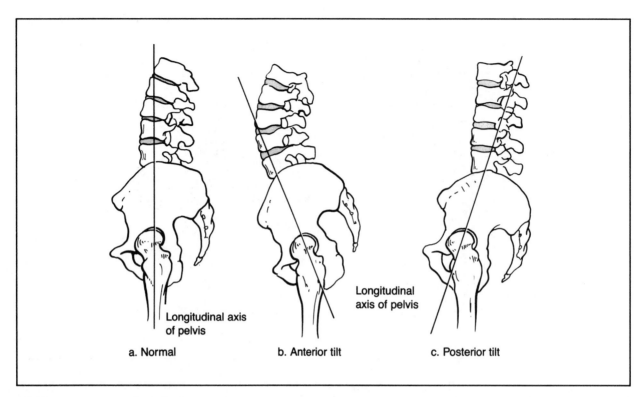

Longitudinal axis
of pelvis

a. Normal

Longitudinal
axis of pelvis

b. Anterior tilt

c. Posterior tilt

FIGURE 2-32 Three lumbosacral
alignments (Redrawn from Kreighbaum and Barthels 1985, 265)

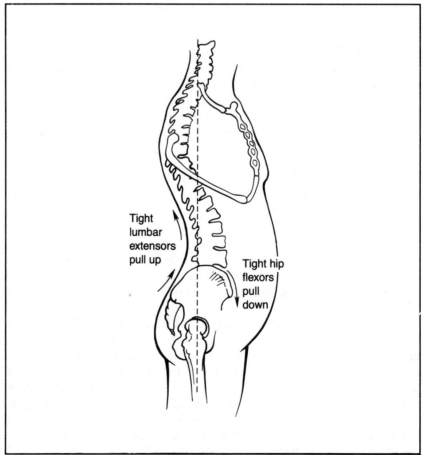

Tight
lumbar
extensors
pull up

Tight hip
flexors
pull
down

FIGURE 2-33 Lordosis

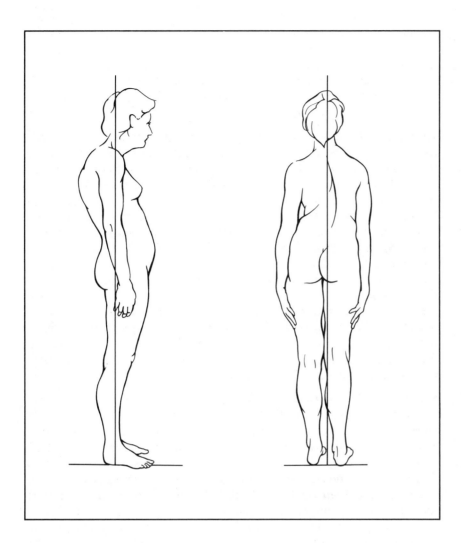

FIGURE 2–34 (*left*) Kyphosis

FIGURE 2–35 (*right*) Scoliosis

abdominals and the hip extensors and strengthening the lower back and hip flexor muscles to pull the pelvis back over the femur and into a balanced position over the hip.

Pathological Postures

Three vertebral column misalignments are considered pathological, or diseased: lordosis, kyphosis, and scoliosis. Lordosis is an extreme anteroposterior curvature in the lumbar area. Kyphosis is an exaggerated thoracic curvature in the anteroposterior plane. Scoliosis is an extreme mediolateral curvature in the thoracic area.

LORDOSIS.   **Lordosis,** often called "swayback," is an exaggerated sagittal curvature of the lumbar area. Associated with anterior tilt or protraction of the pelvis, lordosis (if not congenital) is caused by weak hip extensors and vertebral column flexors and shortened, inflexible vertebral column extensors and hip flexors. Figure 2–33 presents a side view of a person with lordosis.

Willfully placing or forcing the lumbar vertebrae into excess hyperextension will create a predisposition to lordosis. Persons at risk include female gymnasts, pregnant women, middle-aged men with large paunches, and people with weak abdominals. The low-back pain encountered in middle age is often caused by compression of the posterior vertebral disks and stretching of the anterior vertebral ligaments. Strengthening and stretching those muscles that will retract the pelvis into a balanced position over the hip joints alleviates this condition. The muscles that need strengthening are the abominals and the hamstrings; the back extensor muscles and the hip flexors need stretching.

KYPHOSIS. **Kyphosis** is an exaggerated sagittal curvature of the thoracic area. The resulting reduction in the curvature of the lumbar vertebrae gave rise to another name for this condition—"flat back." Figure 2–34 shows a person with kyphosis. If not congenital, kyphosis is frequently seen in older women and therefore has been associated with osteoporosis and osteoarthritis. In gravity-induced cases of kyphosis, it is advisable to strengthen the vertebral column extensors and stretch the vertebral column flexors, particularly in the thoracic area. With kyphosis a forward bending of the thoracic area places the shoulder girdles under the influence of gravitational force that pulls the shoulder girdle into protraction or abduction. Thus, kyphosis has also been associated with "rounded" shoulders. The shoulder girdle retraction muscles must continually work to overcome the shoulder's tendency to sag forward. As the shoulder girdle is pulled into vertical alignment, the shoulder girdle protractors (e.g., the pectoralis major and the anterior deltoid) will need to be stretched.

SCOLIOSIS. **Scoliosis** is a lateral curvature of the vertebral column, usually occurring in the thoracic area. Figure 2–35 presents the vertebral column of a person with scoliosis. Functional, or noncongenital, scoliosis is caused by some imbalance in the structure or the musculature between the right and left sides of the body. For example, a person having one short leg or stronger vertebral column extensors on the right side than on the left side would be prone to scoliosis. If identified early enough, functional scoliosis can be partially or entirely corrected by exercise or bracing. The easiest method of identifying scoliosis is to drop a plumb line from the seventh cervical vertebra and notice the right to left alignment of the vertebral column relative to the sacrum. If the condition is caused by a short leg, a lift in the heel of one shoe often solves the problem. Congenital and severe cases of scoliosis are difficult to manage and should be corrected only by a physician or qualified paramedic.

Low-Back Pain

Low-back pain can occur between the lumbar vertebrae, usually between L3 and L4, or at the sacroiliac joint. Most frequently the pain occurs at the intralumbar joints. Recall that the lumbar vertebrae display a natural curvature. Whenever the pelvis is tilted forward and this natural curvature is exaggerated, the lumbar vertebral area is hyperextended and problems may develop.

Some low-back pain may be alleviated by strengthening the vertebral column flexors, stretching the vertebral column extensors, strengthening the hip extensors, and stretching the hip joint flexors. This exercise program will pull the pelvis from an anterior tilt position back into a neutrally aligned position over the femurs.

The sit-up exercise is frequently used to strengthen the abdominals; however, this exercise can actually cause low-back pain if per-

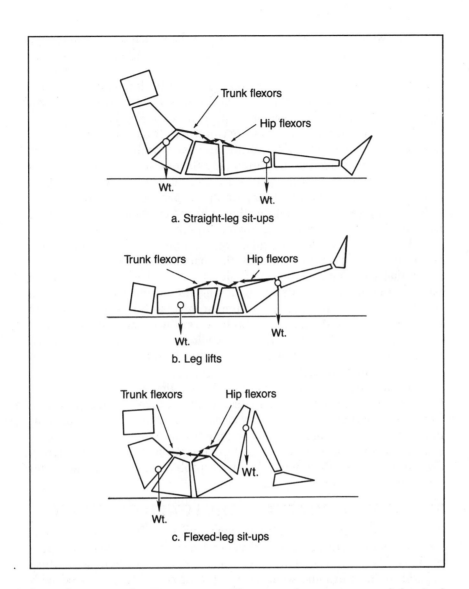

a. Straight-leg sit-ups

b. Leg lifts

c. Flexed-leg sit-ups

FIGURE 2-36 Abdominal strengthening exercises (Redrawn from Kreighbaum and Barthels 1985, 268)

formed improperly. Figure 2-36 illustrates three common abdominal strengthening exercises: the straight-leg sit-up, the flexed-leg sit-up, and leg lifts. Two groups of muscles must be kept in mind here—the abdominals, which are attached to the base of the sternum and the pubic bone at the base of the pelvis, and the hip flexors, several of which are attached to the top of the pelvis and the femur or tibia. Contracting the abdominals brings the base of the sternum toward the middle and the base of the pelvis toward the middle. Thus, the abdominals flex the vertebral column and tend to rock or tilt the pelvis back. The hip flexor muscles, which are attached to the top of the pelvis, tend to rock or tilt the pelvis anteriorly or forward while they flex the hip joint. Because low-back pain can develop when the pelvis is tilted forward, the abdominal muscles must be strong enough during abdominal exercise to prevent the pelvis from tilting forward when the hip flexor muscles are contracted.

To ensure that the pelvis does not tilt forward, the best exercise is the sit-up with knees and hips flexed. If the hips are already flexed, the hip flexors will not have to contract, and the pelvis will not be pulled forward. Thus, no hyperextension of the vertebral column should take place. In terms of low-back pain, leg lifts are the worst of the three exercises discussed here. When the hip flexors are used to flex the hips (lift the legs), their strong contraction will also tend to pull the pelvis forward into an anteriorly tilted position, which, in turn, will hyperextend the lumbar vertebrae and can cause low-back pain.

If the abdominals are weak, performing straight-leg sit-ups will have a similar negative effect on the lumbar vertebrae. To sit up, the weak abdominals need help from the hip flexor muscles. The hip flexor muscles contract to pull the pelvis up, and the pelvis comes up before the rest of the vertebral column. As the upper trunk lags behind the pelvis in the sitting-up motion, the lumbar vertebrae are forced into hyperextension with resulting low-back pain.

The best exercise for strengthening the abdominals depends on the condition of the participants. If the participants are weak in the abdominal area, then the flexed-leg sit-up is best. The instructor should have participants concentrate on flexing the cervical area first, then the thoracic area, and finally the lumbar area, so the body curls up to the sit-up position. Participants who have very weak abdominals should flex only the cervical and upper thoracic areas. As their abdominal strength increases, they can curl up farther to include the lower thoracic and lumbar areas.

One additional note of caution: When the abdominals become fatigued, they will not function adequately to prevent hyperextension. Thus, a participant should be discouraged from trying to perform as many sit-ups as possible in a given time frame. Slow continuous exercises performed only until the participant can feel the lumbar hyperextension will result in fewer low-back problems. See Chapter 11 for a further discussion of low-back pain.

POSTURAL ALIGNMENT OF THE LOWER EXTREMITY

Postures of the lower extremity are very important for the dance-exercise instructor to understand, for several reasons. First, very few people have ideal lower extremity postures. Second, misalignments cause most of the troublesome soreness and pain frequently associated with exercise. Third, the dance-exercise instructor can be instrumental in helping participants strengthen and stretch the appropriate muscles for alleviating pain and difficulty. Fourth, lower extremity misalignments and biomechanical problems can be associated with selecting the proper footwear. Proper footwear can help correct some misalignments; improper shoes may aggravate or even cause misalignments. See Chapter 11 for guidelines on selecting an aerobics shoe.

Ideal Alignment

Normal alignment should not be confused with ideal alignment. Normal alignment is what occurs on the average in the general population, and it is far from ideal. Ideal alignment of the lower extremity is similar to a column upon which a building contractor places the weight of a roof. The sections should be in vertical alignment without any twisting. One section should be directly over the section below it.

In the lower extremity, the sections in the column are the pelvis, the femur, the tibia, and the rearfoot. The pelvis, balanced over two columns while standing, is often balanced over one column during

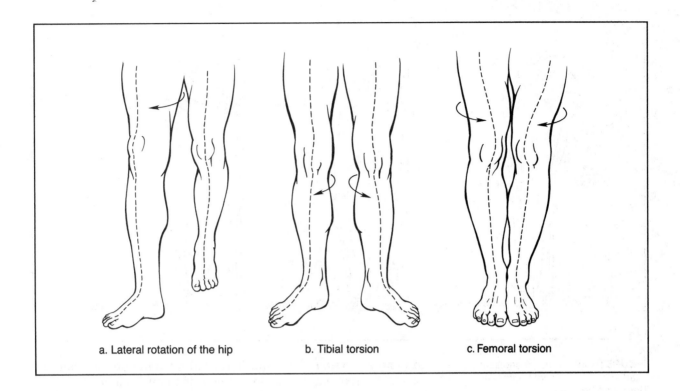

a. Lateral rotation of the hip   b. Tibial torsion   c. Femoral torsion

walking, running, jumping, and exercising in general. Depending on the width of the hips, the femurs are inclined inward as they descend to the knee. Ideally, this inclination should be kept to a minimum. If one segment is out of line, all segments above and below will be affected.

FIGURE 2–37 Rotational misalignments

Rotational Misalignments

Rotational misalignments cause the foot to be directed inward or outward from the midline of the body. Of these two, toeing out is by far the more troublesome. Toeing out can be caused by lateral rotation of the hip joint as seen in ballet dancers (see Fig. 2–37a). Many people walk with their hips rotated laterally. If the hips are rotated outward, the knees and the feet will point outward. Lateral rotation of the hip joint can be corrected by strengthening the medial rotators of the hip and stretching the lateral rotators.

Toeing out can also be caused by lateral rotation at the knees, as illustrated in Figure 2–37(b). Frequently referred to as **tibial torsion,** this condition is seen more frequently in men, because the biceps femoris of the hamstring muscle group is stronger than the two semimuscles (the semitendinosus and the semimembranosus). The biceps is a lateral rotator of the knee and the semimuscles are medial rotators. Tibial torsion can be corrected by strengthening the medial rotators of the knee while stretching the lateral rotators.

Toeing in is not frequently seen and is not associated with painful syndromes of the lower extremity. In some people, toeing in can cause the foot to be inverted. When landing from a jump or landing on the inverted foot while running, the person can "turn" the ankle and sprain the lateral ligaments. People with this problem should stretch the subtalar inversion muscles and strengthen the eversion muscles.

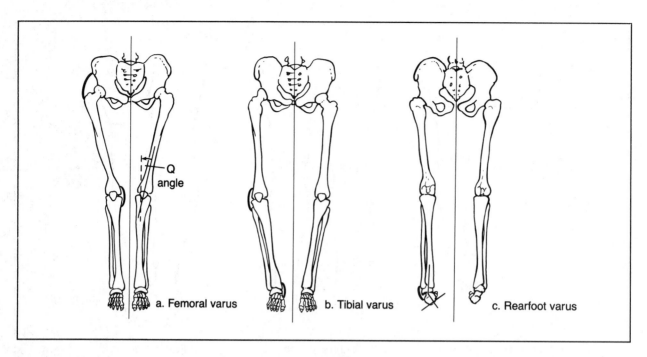

FIGURE 2–38 Varus conditions (Redrawn from Kreighbaum and Barthels 1985, 248)

In **femoral torsion,** the femur is rotated medially on the tibia (see Fig. 2–37c). Frequently seen in women, femoral torsion causes the patella (kneecap) to rotate in with the femur. Thus, when the person is standing with the feet parallel and pointing straight ahead, the knees appear to be inward looking. When the person is standing with the knees pointing straight ahead, the feet are toeing out. People who have this condition may be helped by strengthening the lateral rotators of the hip and stretching the medial rotators, in addition to strengthening the medial rotators of the knee and stretching the lateral rotators. Exercise of the knee extensor muscles is important. However, the exercises should involve only the last 30 degrees of extension of the knee. Extending the knee from a position of further flexion against resistance may result in pain for some people. The exercises for the knee must be done with the hip exercises, or the hip will return to neutral and the leg will be rotated out.

Varus and Valgus Postures

Varus and valgus postures describe whether a segment in the lower extremity is tending inward or outward from its proximal end to its distal end. In a **varus** condition, the femur, the tibia, or the rearfoot follows a line that goes inward from its proximal to its distal end (see Fig. 2–38). Often women are said to suffer from femoral varus because of a wider pelvis. Femoral varus places more stress on the medial side of the knee joint. In a **valgus** condition, the femur, the tibia, or the rearfoot follows a line that goes outward from its proximal to its distal end (see Fig. 2–39). A valgus condition displayed by the tibia is called "knock-knee"; a valgus condition displayed by the femur is called "bowleg."

Maladies of the Lower Extremity

Misalignments of the lower extremity cause several painful conditions associated with exercise and physical stress. The most common maladies are discussed in the following paragraphs.

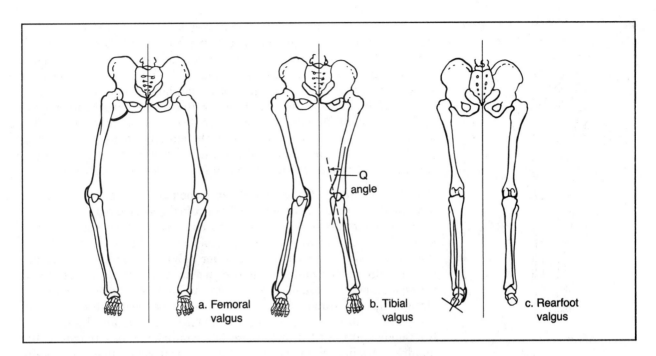

a. Femoral valgus

b. Tibial valgus

Q angle

c. Rearfoot valgus

PRONATED FOOT. The pronated foot is the most common condition associated with lower extremity misalignments. A foot is pronated if the ankle is dorsiflexed, the subtalar joint is everted, and the forefoot is abducted. The ankle falls to the middle (refer to Fig. 2–16). Several maladies are associated with pronated feet, including shin splints and Achilles tendinitis.

Correcting pronation requires strengthening the ankle plantar flexors and the subtalar invertors and stretching the ankle dorsiflexors and the subtalar evertors. Whenever the dorsiflexors are stretched, a position should be assumed in which the ankle is being pushed into plantar flexion with the foot toeing inward, and flexibility exercises should be performed with the knee extended and with the knee flexed. This procedure, as you recall, will stretch both Achilles tendon muscles—the gastrocnemius and the soleus.

UNEQUAL LEG LENGTH. One leg is shorter than the other in approximately 60% of the population. The difference in length between the legs can vary from several millimeters to several centimeters. When viewing a person from the back, look at the crests of the right and left pelvic bones as they come around to the sacrum. If the pelvis is slightly tilted to one side, one leg is shorter than the other. When the person exercises, the abductor muscles of the hip on the long-leg side must work harder to keep the pelvis level. The result is often hip pain on the long-leg side, low back pain, or sacroiliac pain. Putting a lift in the shoe of the shorter leg will usually alleviate the problem.

SHIN SPLINTS. Shin splints refers to pain occurring on the anterior side of the tibia. Developing during long periods of bouncing, jumping, or running, the pain can result from numerous causes including microtears in the muscle tissue where it attaches to the tibia and small fatigue fractures in the tibia itself. Running and jumping on hard surfaces frequently stimulates pain in and around the shin. The tibialis anterior, as you recall, originates on the anterior side of the tibia, crosses the ankle and subtalar joints, and attaches on the anterior and medial

FIGURE 2–39 Valgus conditions (Redrawn from Kreighbaum and Barthels 1985, 250)

AEROBIC DANCE-EXERCISE INSTRUCTOR MANUAL

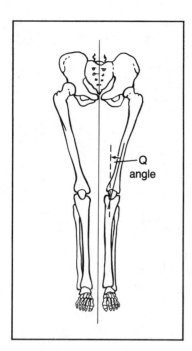

FIGURE 2–40 Quadriceps (Q) angle

side of the foot. This muscle dorsiflexes and inverts the foot. When the foot is everted and plantar flexed, the tibialis anterior is stretched. Stretching occurs each time a person with a toed-out foot pushes against the floor in walking, running, and jumping. Repeating the stretching several thousand times in jogging or in aerobic dancing will probably cause pain on the anterior side of the leg, thus developing "shin splints." The toe-out condition can be seen in people with laterally rotated hips such as ballet dancers, in people with laterally rotated knees as in tibial torsion, and in people with pronated feet. Correcting the misalignment that causes the toeing out often helps shin splint sufferers.

CHONDROMALACIA   **Chondromalacia** is the pain that occurs under and around the patella or kneecap. Chondromalacia is diagnosed by the discomfort and crackling sounds in the knee when flexed and extended. Most often found in women, chondromalacia has been associated with the femoral varus induced by the wider pelvis. As the knee flexes and extends, the patella slides up and down in a groove at the distal end of the femur called the patellar groove. As long as the patella is pulled straight up and down, little friction occurs between the groove and the undersurface of the patella. However, if there is misalignment of the femur and the tibia or if there is an imbalance of strength in the quadriceps muscles on the medial and lateral sides, then the patella is pulled to one side and its undersurface scrapes on the side of the patellar groove. After repeated scraping, the undersurface of the patella begins to wear away. The roughened undersurface causes greater friction and the condition worsens. Eventually, pieces of the patella are scraped off and lodge around the articular capsule causing a catching in the knee as it is flexed or extended.

The **quadriceps angle,** or **Q-angle,** is often measured to determine the misalignment of the femur and tibia associated with chondromalacia. Figure 2–40 illustrates the Q-angle measurement. The line formed by the patellar tendon on the tibia crosses the line formed by the femur and forms an angle. A Q-angle greater than 15 degrees has been associated with misalignment, specifically chondromalacia. A femoral varus or a tibial valgus condition will increase the Q-angle. Femoral or tibial torsion will also cause the patella to ride to one side of the patellar groove resulting in chondromalacia.

Strengthening the quadriceps muscles seems to alleviate the problem somewhat. However, strengthening the knee extensors by extending against a large resistance should only be performed during the last 30 degrees of extension. Using a knee-extension machine in which the exerciser sits on a bench and extends through 90 degrees to 180 degrees is contraindicated. From full flexion to 160 degrees' extension, much of the quadriceps contraction force compresses the patella against the patellar groove, compounding the problem. The knee flexion and extension range of motion used during running or climbing stairs is appropriate.

CENTER OF GRAVITY, BALANCE, AND STABILITY

The **center of gravity** of the body is an imaginary point around which the masses of the body segments are balanced. For example, the body of someone lying supine (face up) on a teeter-totter, is balanced if the center of gravity is directly above the fulcrum. Similarly, someone standing on the teeter-totter is balanced if the center of gravity is directly above the fulcrum. Thus, a body is **balanced** if its center of gravity is above the base of support. When a person stands on one foot, the body balances if the center of gravity is directly over the foot as its base. The body will tip or fall if the center of gravity is outside the base of support.

The location of the body's center of gravity varies from person to person because it depends on which segments are largest and which are smallest. Generally, the center of gravity is located just below the navel. Women with massive thighs and abdomens have lower centers of gravity. Men with massive shoulders and upper bodies have higher centers of gravity.

Stability describes how difficult it is for a body to lose its balance. A more stable body is more difficult to tip than a less stable body. Stability can be increased by widening the base of support, by lowering the center of gravity, or by keeping the center of gravity in the center-most portion of the base. A body is less stable if its center of gravity is close to the edge of the base. This less stable position is seen when athletes assume the "ready position": the knees are flexed and the center of gravity is close to the leading edge of the base, usually the toes. Although less force is needed to topple forward from this position, the athlete intends to move forward quickly and will be aided by less stability.

Generally, less muscle tension is produced in a position of balance and stability. Assuming a balanced posture uses less energy than continually "fighting gravity."

Equilibrium is the state of a system whose motion is not being changed, accelerated or decelerated (Kreighbaum and Barthels 1985). When a body part first starts to move, that part must accelerate from zero motion and that disturbs its equilibrium. When a body part stops moving, as at the end of the range of motion of an exercise, its equilibrium is disturbed by deceleration. If the body is running at a constant velocity, it is in equilibrium. If the body accelerates to run faster or decelerates to run slower, disequilibrium occurs. A balanced body is in *static* equilibrium. A body that is moving at a constant speed is in *dynamic* equilibrium.

BUILDING AN EXERCISE PROGRAM

A dance-exercise instructor will be asked several questions about building an exercise program. Some participants will want to know how to develop specific muscles. Most, however, will be interested in general strength and flexibility gains to enhance their physical fitness level. Therefore, typical questions might focus on such areas as strengthening the muscles surrounding the shoulder or increasing or maintaining the flexibility of the back.

Two-Joint Muscles

Frequently, both one- and two-joint muscles cross an articulation. Many of the body's muscles, particularly those used for locomotion, cross two articulations and thus effect motion and are affected by motion in both articulations. When planning exercises, the nature of two-joint muscles must be kept in mind. Refer back to Tables 2–2 and 2–3 to determine which major muscles of the extremities cross two articulations.

Two-joint muscles should be strengthened or stretched over both joints. To exercise these muscles properly, strengthen the muscle by shortening it over one joint while stretching it over the other, or by shortening the muscle over both articulations simultaneously. Conversely, contract the muscle over the second joint while stretching it over the first joint.

When devising exercises for flexibility, the instructor must remember that a one-joint muscle only needs to be stretched over that one articulation. A two-joint muscle, however, must be stretched *simultaneously* over both articulations. The following three examples illustrate exercises designed to strengthen or stretch two-joint muscles.

STRENGTHENING THE HAMSTRINGS. The hamstring muscles, as a group, extend the hip and flex and rotate the knee. To strengthen the hamstring group, all of these functions should be used. Choose exercises that simultaneously extend the hip, and flex and medially rotate the knee against a resistance. These exercises will tax the semitendinosus and semimembranosus muscles. Next choose exercises that simultaneously extend the hip, and flex and laterally rotate the knee against a resistance. These exercises will tax the biceps femoris. For example, lie on the floor in a prone position. Simultaneously, extend the hip, flex the knee, and medially rotate the knee. Repeat while laterally rotating the knee.

To stretch the hamstring group, select flexibility exercises that simultaneously force the joints into movements that are opposite to the movements caused by the hamstrings. Choose exercises that simultaneously flex the hip and extend the knee.

STRETCHING THE HIP FLEXORS. When preparing to stretch the hip flexors, the rectus femoris and the iliopsoas must be considered. To stretch the rectus femoris, a two-joint muscle causing hip flexion and knee extension, simultaneously extend the hip and flex the knee. This exercise would probably not affect the iliopsoas, however, because the hip would not extend enough to cause this muscle to stretch. Therefore, to stretch the iliopsoas, keep the knee extended (to slacken the rectus femoris) while extending the hip.

PREVENTING PROBLEMS WITH THE ACHILLES TENDON. To prevent Achilles tendon problems, the gastrocnemius and the soleus muscles of the Achilles tendon must be stretched. The gastrocnemius passes over the posterior knee and ankle; to stretch this muscle extend the knee and dorsiflex the ankle simultaneously. Because the gastrocnemius is a two-joint muscle, it tightens before the soleus tightens. To stretch the soleus, slacken the gastrocnemius by flexing the knee and, while the knee is flexed, dorsiflex the ankle. This is an important set of exercises to prevent Achilles tendon problems. Performing only one of these exercises will not stretch the entire Achilles tendon.

Method of Analysis

There are far too many exercises to analyze how each relates to different fitness goals. However, by using the following method, a dance-exercise instructor can select exercises that will have the desired physical fitness effects.

1. *Establish a set of exercise goals* based on physiological parameters such as strength, flexibility, and muscular endurance. These goals may be for general body conditioning or articulation specific. For example, a general goal may be to develop overall muscular endurance, while

Table 2-4

MUSCLES USED TO PRODUCE SPECIFIC MOVEMENTS OF THE JOINTS IN THE UPPER EXTREMITY

MOVEMENT	MUSCLE	ARTICULATION	ACTION
Shoulder flexion	Biceps brachii	Shoulder	Flexion
		Elbow	Flexion
		Radioulnar	Supination
	Anterior deltoid	Shoulder	Flexion
			Transverse flexion
	Coracobrachialis	Shoulder	Flexion
			Transverse flexion
	Pectoralis major (clavicular)	Shoulder	Flexion
			Transverse flexion
Shoulder extension	Posterior deltoid	Shoulder	Extension
	Triceps	Shoulder	Extension
		Elbow	Extension
	Latissimus dorsi	Shoulder	Extension
	Teres major		Medial rotation
Shoulder abduction	Middle deltoid	Shoulder	Abduction
	Supraspinatus		
Shoulder adduction	Pectoralis major	Shoulder	Adduction
		Sternoclavicular	Protraction
	Latissimus dorsi	Shoulder	Adduction
	Teres major		Medial rotation
Shoulder medial rotation	Latissimus dorsi	Shoulder	Medial rotation
	Teres major		
Shoulder lateral rotation	Infraspinatus	Shoulder	Lateral rotation
	Teres minor		
Shoulder transverse adduction	Pectoralis major	Shoulder	Transverse adduction
		Sternoclavicular	Protraction
	Coracobrachialis		Flexion
	Anterior deltoid		
Shoulder transverse abduction	Triceps	Shoulder	Transverse abduction
	Posterior deltoid		Extension
Elbow flexion	Biceps brachii	Elbow	Flexion
		Shoulder	Flexion
		Radioulnar	Supination
	Brachialis	Elbow	Flexion
	Brachioradialis	Elbow	Flexion
		Radioulnar	Supination and pronation to midposition
Elbow extension	Triceps	Elbow	Extension
		Shoulder	Extension

Table 2-5

MUSCLES USED TO PRODUCE SPECIFIC MOVEMENTS OF THE JOINTS IN THE LOWER EXTREMITY

MOVEMENT	MUSCLE	ARTICULATION	ACTION
Hip flexion	Iliopsoas	Hip	Flexion
		Vertebral column	Flexion
	Rectus femoris	Hip	Flexion
		Knee	Extension
	Sartorius	Hip	Flexion
		Knee	Flexion
Hip extension	Gluteus maximus	Hip	Extension
	Biceps femoris	Hip	Extension
		Knee	Flexion
			Lateral rotation
	Semitendinosus	Hip	Extension
	Semimembranosus		Medial rotation
Hip abduction	Tensor fascia lata	Hip	Abduction
	Gluteus medius		
	Gluteus minimus		
Hip adduction	Pectineus	Hip	Adduction
	Adductor longus		
	Adductor magnus		
	Adductor brevis		
	Gracilis		
Hip lateral rotation	Six external rotators		Lateral rotation
	Gluteus maximus		
Hip medial rotation	Iliopsoas	Hip	Medial rotation
		Vertebral column	Flexion
	Tensor fascia lata	Hip	Medial rotation
			Flexion
Knee flexion	Biceps femoris	Knee	Flexion
			Lateral rotation
		Hip	Extension
	Semitendinosus	Knee	Flexion
	Semimembranosus		Medial rotation
		Hip	Extension
	Sartorius	Knee	Flexion
		Hip	Flexion
Knee extension	Rectus femoris	Hip	Flexion
		Knee	Extension
	Vastus lateralis	Knee	Extension
	Vastus medialis		
	Vastus intermedius		
Ankle dorsiflexion	Tibialis anterior	Ankle	Dorsiflexion
		Subtalar	Inversion
	Extensor digitorum longus	Ankle	Dorsiflexion
		Subtalar	Eversion

MUSCLES USED TO PRODUCE SPECIFIC MOVEMENTS OF THE JOINTS IN THE LOWER EXTREMITY (continued)

MOVEMENT	MUSCLE	ARTICULATION	ACTION
Ankle plantar-flexion	Gastrocnemius	Ankle	Plantar flexion
		Knee	Flexion
	Soleus	Ankle	Plantar flexion
	Tibialis posterior	Ankle	Plantar flexion
		Subtalar	Inversion
	Flexor digitorum longus	Ankle	Plantar flexion
		Subtalar	Inversion
	Flexor hallucis longus	Ankle	Plantar flexion
		Subtalar	Inversion
	Peroneus longus and brevis	Ankle	Plantar flexion
		Subtalar	Eversion
	Peroneus tertius		

a specific goal may be to strengthen the shoulder joint or to increase the flexibility of the hip joint.

2. *Select movements that will accomplish the stated objectives.* For strengthening the shoulder, decide if it is important for the participant to be strong specifically in shoulder flexion or shoulder abduction, or whether the person wants to increase general shoulder condition for all movements.

3. *Decide which muscles must be involved to achieve the desired goals.* List those muscles and determine whether they are one-, two-, or multijoint muscles. If a muscle is a one-joint muscle, then only that articulation need be considered when devising an exercise.

4. *Select exercises that strengthen and stretch the entire muscle, considering all of the articulations that it crosses.*

For example, let's analyze the goal of strengthening and stretching the hip joint in the anteroposterior direction. The hamstrings on the posterior side and the rectus femoris and iliopsoas on the anterior side are the major muscles involved. The muscles of the hamstring group are two-joint muscles crossing the hip and the knee. The rectus femoris is a two-joint muscle crossing the hip and the knee; the iliopsoas is a two-joint muscle crossing the lumbar intervertebral joints and the hip. Remember, an exercise to strengthen a two-joint muscle should shorten the muscle across both joints that it crosses. To stretch a two-joint muscle, the exercise should stretch the muscle across both joints at the same time. Muscles only work in a strengthening mode when they are causing a movement or resisting the movement caused by another force such as gravity. (Identifying what the articulation is doing does not necessarily determine which muscles are working; an extensor may be working as the articulation is flexing.)

In a pull-up, for example, during the up phase, the shoulder joint is extending and the elbow is flexing. The muscles being worked are the posterior deltoid, the triceps, the lastissimus dorsi, and the teres major for the shoulder joint and the brachialis, the biceps brachii, and the brachioradialis.

As a second example, in side leg raises the hip joint is being abducted. The muscles being exercised are the tensor fascia lata, the gluteus medius, and the gluteus minimus.

If, on the other hand, the objective is to exercise a particular muscle, such as the triceps, the movement must include the extension of the shoulder and the elbow. Selecting the pull-up only exercises the triceps to extend the shoulder joint. To exercise that part of the triceps that extends the elbow, the participant could extend a dumbbell over the head while keeping the shoulder joint in full flexion.

Until you are familiar with the muscles, the articulations that they cross, and the movements that they cause, refer to Table 2–4 for the upper extremity muscles and to Table 2–5 for the lower extremity muscles.

SUMMARY

To tailor an exercise program to meet the needs of participants, a dance-exercise instructor must understand how the body moves. Body movements used in dance exercise are produced through the interaction of five systems—cardiovascular, pulmonary, nervous, skeletal, and muscular. The structure, function and interrelationship of these systems was the focus of this chapter.

A familiarity with how and why the body segments or links move and how muscles and outside forces such as gravity effect movements is a prerequisite for analyzing an exercise to determine its muscular components and its impact on the person performing the exercise. This information, along with a discussion of postural alignment, balance, and stability, was presented to help the instructor identify the movements that will satisfy the participants' exercise goals, determine which muscles are involved in those movements, and select those exercises that will satisfy those goals without causing injury.

REFERENCES

Kreighbaum, E. and K. Barthels. *Biomechanics: A Qualitative Approach for Studying Human Movement.* 2nd ed. Minneapolis: Burgess Publishing Co., 1985.

Langley, J. B. *Structure and Function of the Human Body.* Minneapolis: Burgess Publishing Co., 1978.

SUGGESTED READING

Hollinshead, W. H. *Functional Anatomy of the Limbs and Back.* Philadelphia: W. B. Saunders, 1976.

Kreighbaum, E. and K. Barthels. *Biomechanics: A Qualitative Approach for Studying Human Movement.* 2nd ed. Minneapolis: Burgess Publishing Co., 1985.

Langley, J. B. *Structure and Function of the Human Body.* Minneapolis: Burgess Publishing Co., 1978.

Ricci, B., M. Marchetti, and F. Figura. "Biomechanics of the Sit-up Exercises." *Medicine and Science in Sports and Exercise* 13 (1981):54–59.

Rogers, C. C. "Upper Body Exercise: 'Jarming Instead of Jogging.'" *The Physician and Sportsmedicine* (April 1986): 181–186.

Vincent, W. J., and S. D. Britten. "Evaluation of the Curl-up—A Substitute for the Bent Knee Sit-up." *Journal of Physical Education, Recreation and Dance* 51 (1980):74–75.

Nutrition and Weight Control

Ellen Coleman

Ellen Coleman, M.A., M.P.H.R.D., is the program director of the Riverside Cardiac Fitness Center, a cardiac rehabilitation program in Riverside, California. She is the author of *Eating for Endurance* and numerous magazine articles, and she lectures extensively on nutrition and fitness. A competitive athlete since 1974, Ms. Coleman has completed eleven 200-mile bicycle races, nine marathons, and two Ironman triathlons in Hawaii.

3

IN THIS CHAPTER:

- Nutrition basics: the six classes of nutrients, the well-balanced diet, special nutritional needs of women.

- Nutrition and exercise: preventing cardio-vascular disease and osteoporosis, enhancing athletic performance.

- Weight control: overweight versus overfat, the diet/exercise combination, dangerous and ineffective weight-loss techniques.

- Eating disorders: anorexia nervosa and bulimia.

A proper diet is necessary for health and optimum athletic performance. It is important for instructors to have a basic knowledge of good nutrition because health-conscious people, including those in a dance-exercise class, are often willing to try any dietary regimen or nutritional supplement in their quest for improved health, athletic performance, or weight loss. Many will go beyond common sense and sound nutrition practices in search of a magic formula. Unfortunately, many popular dietary practices are ineffective and contribute nothing to the physically active person's goals for fitness and health, and some dietary fads are actually harmful.

In addition to being a positive role model, the instructor should be able to offer information on good nutrition, guidance on the intensity and duration of exercise most effective for weight control, and moral support and encouragement for everyone in the class. However, instructors should never attempt to counsel participants on their personal nutrition needs or prescribe diets. Participants with special questions or medical problems should be referred to a qualified professional.*

---

*The American Dietetic Association has a list of registered dietitians qualified to provide nutrition counseling: 1-800-621-6469.

NUTRITION BASICS

A basic principle of applied **nutrition** is balance. The key to positive health and physical fitness cannot be found in any one food or nutrient, but in a proper combination of foods that provides the nutrients we need. This section describes how to meet the body's need for nutrients through a well-balanced diet. By communicating these nutrition basics, either verbally or as handouts or wall posters, an instructor can help steer participants away from gimmicks and fads and toward sound dietary practices.

Nutrients

In physiological terms, food satisfies three fundamental body needs: (a) the need for energy, (b) the need for new tissue growth and tissue repair, and (c) the need to regulate the metabolic functions constantly taking place in the body. These three needs are met by components of foods called **nutrients.** There are six classes of nutrients; each class has unique chemical characteristics suited to meet specific body needs.

WATER.   The most essential of all nutrients, water is second only to oxygen as a substance necessary to sustain life. Because water is readily available and has no caloric value, its importance during exercise is often overlooked. An adequate supply of water is necessary for all energy production in the body, for temperature control (particularly during vigorous exercise), and for elimination of waste products from metabolism. **Dehydration,** or the excessive loss of body fluids, reduces endurance and increases the risk of heat exhaustion and heat stroke.

MINERALS.   **Minerals** are inorganic compounds that serve a variety of functions in the body. Some minerals, such as calcium and phosphorus, are used to build bones and teeth. Others are important components of hormones, such as the mineral zinc in insulin. Iron is crucial in the formation of hemoglobin, the oxygen-carrying pigment within red blood cells. Minerals also contribute to a number of the body's regulatory functions, including the regulation of muscle contraction, conduction of nerve impulses, clotting of blood, and regulation of normal heart rhythm.

Minerals are classified into two groups based on the body's need. *Major* minerals are needed in amounts greater than 100 mg per day. Calcium, phosphorus, magnesium, sodium, and chloride fall into this category. *Minor* minerals, or trace elements, are needed in amounts less than 100 mg per day. Iron, zinc, selenium, copper, and iodine are minor minerals.

VITAMINS.   **Vitamins** are organic compounds that the body requires in small amounts but cannot manufacture. Vitamins provide no calories and cannot be used as fuel. Instead, they function as metabolic regulators that govern the processes of energy production, growth, maintenance, and repair. Thirteen vitamins have been identified. Each has a special function in the body and also works in complicated ways with other nutrients.

Vitamins are divided into two groups: water soluble and fat soluble. The solubility characteristic is important in determining whether the body can store the vitamin. Fat-soluble vitamins include A, D, E, and K, which are stored in the body fat, principally in the liver. Taking a greater amount of fat-soluble vitamins than the body needs over a significant period can produce serious toxic effects. Vitamin C and the B complex vitamins are soluble in water. Excess water-soluble vitamins are excreted, mainly in the urine, and have to be replaced on a regular basis. However, excessive consumption of such water-soluble vitamins as niacin, B_6 and C also can produce serious toxic effects.

PROTEIN.   **Protein,** a major structural component of all body tissue, is needed for growth and repair. Proteins are also necessary components of hormones, enzymes, and blood-plasma transport systems. Normally protein is not used as fuel to any significant degree, either at rest or during exercise. Only when caloric intake is inadequate, as during fasting or semistarvation, or when the amount of dietary carbohydrate is inadequate, as in a high-protein, high-fat diet, does the body use protein for energy.

The proteins in both plant and animal sources are composed of the same basic structural units—**amino acids.** Of more than 20 amino acids that have been identified, 9 are essential to health. Meat, fish, and poultry contain all 9 essential amino acids and are, therefore, termed **complete proteins.** Vegetables and grains, eaten alone, are incomplete proteins, because they do not supply all of the amino acids. However, a well-balanced vegetarian diet can supply the body's protein needs, because amino acids from different plant foods work together, or complement each other, to provide the complete protein needed for growth and repair. For example, beans eaten with rice, or peanut butter smeared on wheat bread provide proteins as complete as those from meat sources.

FATS.   Fats also called lipids, are the most concentrated source of food energy. One gram of fat supplies about 9 kilocalories,* compared to the 4 kilocalories supplied by carbohydrates and protein. As essential to health as the other nutrients, fats are the only source of linoleic acid, needed for growth and skin maintenance. Fats insulate and protect the body's organs against trauma and exposure to cold and are also involved in the absorption and transport of the fat-soluble vitamins.

In addition, fats are the source of fatty acids, which are divided into two categories: saturated and unsaturated (including monounsaturated and polyunsaturated fatty acids). The distinction is based on the bonding between carbon and hydrogen atoms. In more useful terms, **saturated fat** is solid at room temperature and is derived mainly from animal sources; **unsaturated fat** is liquid at room temperature and is found mainly in plant sources. A diet rich in polyunsaturated fats is the most healthful, for it tends to lower the blood cholesterol level. Saturated fats tend to raise the level of blood cholesterol, while monounsaturates seem to have no effect at all. The relationship between dietary fats and cholesterol is important, because high cholesterol is associated with increased risk of coronary heart disease. This issue will be discussed later in this chapter.

CARBOHYDRATES.   **Carbohydrates** are the most readily available source of food energy. During digestion and metabolism, all carbohydrates are broken down to the simple sugar **glucose** for use as the body's principal

---

*Kilocalories (kcal) are the units by which the energy in food is measured. In referring to diet and exercise, a kilocalorie is often mistakenly called a calorie. Actually one kilocalorie equals 1,000 calories. For example, a plain potato contains 100 kcal and one hour of jogging would expend approximately 500–600 kcal.

energy source. Glucose is stored in the liver and muscle tissue as **glycogen.** A carbohydrate-rich diet is necessary to maintain muscle glycogen, the preferred fuel during aerobic exercise.

There are two types of carbohydrates: complex and simple. Complex carbohydrates provide both nutrients and fiber with their calories, and are found in fruits, vegetables, breads and cereals, and beans. Simple, or refined carbohydrates, found in sugar and sweets, represent an energy source but have no other nutritional value. Therefore, a healthful diet is rich in complex carbohydrates and sparing in simple carbohydrates.

The Well-Balanced Diet

The optimum diet contains adequate amounts of each of the six essential nutrients. In the early 1940s the National Research Council of the National Academy of Sciences defined the daily nutrient requirements for Americans. Their findings were published in the form of **Recommended Dietary Allowances (RDAs),** which were revised in 1980. The RDA represents the daily amount of a nutrient recommended for practically all healthy persons to maintain optimal health. The recommendations include a large margin of safety. For example, although the body needs only 10 mg of vitamin C to prevent the deficiency disease scurvy, the RDA for vitamin C is 60 mg. Tables 3–1 and 3–2 outline the RDAs for essential vitamins and minerals.

As valuable as RDAs may be, it is difficult for the average person to translate them into practical terms. To aid in meal planning, the Daily Food Guide, commonly referred to as the **Basic Four Food Groups,** was published by the US Department of Agriculture in 1957. This guide provides a framework for making dietary selections by grouping together foods with similar nutrients, and then recommending the number of servings that should be eaten daily from each group (Table 3–3).

The four food groups are milk, meat, fruit and vegetable, and grain and cereals. Foods not included in these four categories, labeled "other," supply few nutrients. These "others" include the fats and oils used in cooking, sweets and condiments, and beverages such as coffee, alcohol, and soft drinks. The average person who eats a variety of foods from each of the four groups will meet basic vitamin and mineral requirements and will not need vitamin and mineral supplements.

In addition to the RDAs and the Four Food Groups, there is another guide to sound dietary practices. In 1977 the Senate Select Committee on Nutrition and Human Needs, chaired by Senator George McGovern, evaluated the American diet and found it to be too high in total calories, sugar, and fat—particularly saturated fat. As a result, the committee set forth new nutritional guidelines intended to reduce the incidence of major diseases such as cancer and heart disease. If followed, these guidelines, known as the Dietary Goals of the United States, would increase the consumption of complex carbohydrates and decrease fat consumption. Figure 3–1 compares current eating trends with those set forth by the guidelines. As seen in the figure, at least 48% of the total number of calories consumed should be in the form of complex carbohydrates; no more than 30% in fat; about 12% in protein; and no more than 10% in refined and processed sugars.

Table 3–1

VITAMINS: SOURCES AND ADULT RDAs

VITAMIN	SOURCES	ADULT RDAs
	FAT SOLUBLE	
A	Liver, fortified milk and margarine, butter, egg yolk, leafy green and yellow vegetables, dried apricots, cantaloupe, peaches	4,000–5,000 I.U.*
D	Fortified milk, egg yolk, fish, and sunlight (absorbed through the skin)	400 I.U.
E	Vegetable oils, wheat germ and whole grains, nuts	30 I.U.
K	Leafy green vegetables, cabbage and cauliflower, tomatoes, wheat bran (adults also produce vitamin K in their intestines), milk	70–140 mcg†
	WATER SOLUBLE	
C	Citrus fruits, tomatoes, strawberries, melons, potatoes, broccoli, green peppers	50–60 mg°
B_1 (Thiamine)	Pork, organ meats, legumes, whole-grain and enriched cereals and breads, wheat germ	1.0–1.5 mg
B_2 (Riboflavin)	Organ meats, milk and dairy products, whole-grain and enriched cereals and breads, eggs, fish, leafy green vegetables	1.2–1.7 mg
Niacin	Fish, liver, meat, poultry, eggs, peanuts, grains, legumes	13–19 mg
B_6 (Pyridoxine)	Meat, cereal bran and germ, egg yolk, legumes	1.8–2.2 mg
B_{12}	Liver, kidney, meat, fish, milk, cheese (only in foods of animal origin)	3.0 mcg
Folic Acid (Folacin)	Green vegetables, organ meats, lean beef, eggs, fish, dry beans, lentils, asparagus, yeast	400 mcg
Pantothenic Acid	Whole-grain cereals, organ meats, eggs, vegetables (found in most plant and vegetable foods)	4–7 mg
Biotin	Liver, egg yolk, peanuts, yeast, milk, legumes, bananas, cereal	100–200 mcg

*International Units
†micrograms
°milligrams

AEROBIC DANCE-EXERCISE INSTRUCTOR MANUAL

Table 3-2

MINERALS: SOURCES AND ADULT RDAs

MINERAL	SOURCES	ADULT RDAs
	MAJOR MINERALS	
Calcium	Milk and milk products, dark green leafy vegetables, broccoli, sardines, clams, oysters	800 mg°
Phosphorus	Meat, fish, poultry, legumes, milk, dairy products, whole-grain cereals, soft drinks	800 mg
Magnesium	Whole grains, nuts, dark leafy vegetables, grains, legumes	300-400 mg
Potassium	Citrus juices, bananas	*
Sodium	Table salt, seafood, milk, eggs (abundant in most foods, except fruit)	*
	TRACE MINERALS	
Iron	Liver, meat, fish, poultry, egg yolks, legumes, whole grains, dried fruit, dark green leafy vegetables	10-18 mg
Copper	Liver, kidney, shellfish, oysters, whole grains, nuts, legumes, chocolate	2-3 mg
Zinc	Liver, shellfish, eggs, meat	15 mg
Iodine	Iodized table salt, seafood, water	150 mcg†
Fluoride	Fluoridated water, coffee, tea, soybeans, spinach, gelatin, onion, lettuce	*

°milligrams
†micrograms
*U.S. RDA has not been established.

Special Needs of Women

Two minerals, calcium and iron, are of special concern to women. Nutritional deficiencies of either mineral can impair a woman's ability to exercise and possibly lead to health problems.

Calcium, the most abundant mineral in the body, is critical for the conduction of nerve impulses, heart function, muscle contraction, and the operation of certain enzymes. The bones and teeth contain 99% of the body's calcium; the remaining 1% circulates in the bloodstream. When the supply of calcium in the blood is too low, the body withdraws calcium from the bones.

An inadequate supply of calcium is one of the major contributing factors to **osteoporosis,** an age-related disorder in which bone mass

Table 3-3

BASIC FOUR FOOD GROUP PLAN

FOOD GROUPS	DAILY SERVINGS FOR ADULTS	MAIN NUTRIENTS
MILK		

1 cup milk or yogurt
or calcium equivalent:
  1½ ounces cheese
  1 cup pudding
  1¾ cup ice cream
  2 cups cottage cheese
	2 or more	Vitamin D
		Calcium
		Riboflavin
		Protein

MEAT		

2-3 ounces cooked lean meat,
fish, poultry or protein equivalent:
  2 eggs
  2 ounces cheese
  1 cup dried beans, peas
  4 tablespoons peanut butter
	2 or more	Protein
		Calcium
		Iron
		Thiamine
		Riboflavin

FRUIT AND VEGETABLE		
½ cup cooked or juice 1 cup or 1 piece raw	4 or more	Vitamin A Vitamin C Carbohydrate
GRAIN AND CEREAL		
1 slice bread 1 cup cold cereal ½-¾ cup cooked cereal	4 or more	Carbohydrate Thiamine Iron Niacin

decreases and susceptibility to fracture increases. Osteoporosis is a major public-health problem in the United States, affecting an estimated 15-30 million people and 25%-35% of the women past menopause. Because of their lower bone mass, women are more susceptible to osteoporosis. Also, after menopause women produce less estrogen, which further accelerates bone loss. Osteoporosis is called the "silent disease" because it usually is not detected until a fracture occurs, often in the hip, wrist, or spine.

The amount of bone mass a woman has at age 35 will strongly influence her susceptibility to fractures in later years. Therefore, calcium is as important to adults, especially adult women, as it is to children. The RDA for calcium is 800 mg per day for adult men and women. According to a recent survey, 50% of all females age 15 and over consume less than 800 mg and 75% of women over 35 have inadequate calcium intake (*Dairy Council Digest* 1982). The prevalence of calcium deficiency among women becomes even more serious in

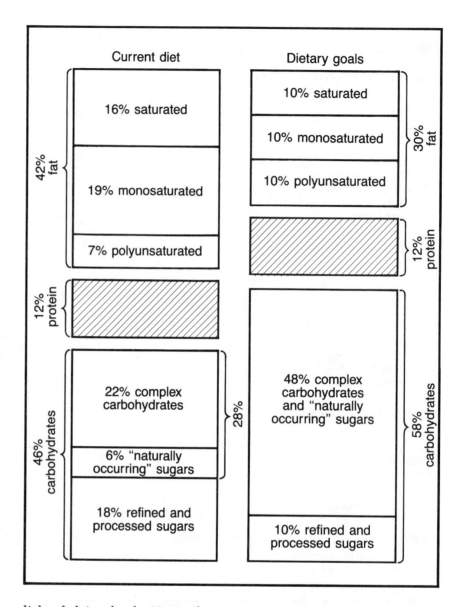

FIGURE 3-1 Dietary Goals of the U.S.

light of claims by the National Institutes of Health (NIH) and nutrition experts that the calcium needs of women actually are well above the recommended 800 mg level. These experts recommend that adolescent women consume 1,200 mg of calcium per day, premenopausal women consume 1,000 mg, and postmenopausal women (not on estrogen replacement therapy) consume 1,500 mg.

Dairy products represent the best sources of calcium (Table 3-4). Many factors determine how much calcium is absorbed by the body. For example, a high consumption of protein interferes with calcium absorption by increasing the amount excreted in the urine. Too much phosphorus (phosphates in soft drinks are a rich source of phosphorus) increases the need for calcium and may create a deficiency even if consumption meets recommended levels. Inactivity, common among the elderly, also speeds calcium loss.

Today more and more women are becoming aware of their calcium needs and turning to supplements. Dance-exercise participants may ask their instructors for advice on this matter. It is important to remem-

Table 3—4

CALCIUM SOURCES

FOOD	SERVINGS	AMOUNT OF CALCIUM (mg)
Whole Milk	1 cup	290
Skim Milk	1 cup	300
Low-fat (2%) milk	1 cup	298
Low-fat plain yogurt	1 cup	415
Frozen yogurt (2%)	1 cup	200
Ricotta cheese	¼ cup	167
Cottage cheese	1 cup	160
Cheddar cheese	1 ounce	210
Canned sardines with bones, packed in oil and drained	3½ ounces	370
Canned salmon with bones, packed in own juice	3½ ounces	200
Shrimp	1 cup	147
Oysters	1 cup	226
Broccoli, cooked	1 cup	140
Kale, cooked	1 cup	210
Blackstrap molasses	1 tablespoon	140
Spinach, cooked	½ cup	106

Source: US Department of Agriculture

ber that the role of the dance-exercise instructor is to make students aware of basic nutrition needs and sound dietary practices. An instructor who does not have the proper qualifications should not recommend supplements or prescribe nutrition therapy. The safest approach is still a well-balanced diet containing calcium-rich foods. Before taking a supplement, a woman should consult a registered dietitian or physician to make sure that her calcium intake does not exceed recommended levels. Too much calcium can also be detrimental. In some people, excessive calcium intake increases the risk of urinary-tract stones.

AEROBIC DANCE-EXERCISE INSTRUCTOR MANUAL

Iron deserves special attention because **iron-deficiency anemia** is the nation's most common nutritional deficiency, affecting approximately 40% of women between the ages of 20 and 50 (Aftergood and Alfin-Slater 1980). Iron is needed to form hemoglobin, an iron-containing protein that carries oxygen in the blood and releases it to the tissues. When the total hemoglobin concentration drops, the muscles do not receive as much oxygen. A hemoglobin level below 12 mg/dl for women and below 14 mg/dl for men is considered anemic. An anemic person has less endurance and cannot exercise as strenuously because the maximum oxygen uptake, or aerobic capacity, is reduced due to the decreased oxygen-carrying capacity of the blood caused by low hemoglobin levels.

Iron deficiency in women is usually the result of menstrual blood loss and inadequate dietary iron intake. There is also evidence that strenuous training accelerates the destruction of red blood cells, increases iron loss in sweat, and decreases iron absorption. The RDA for iron is 18 mg for women, but the average woman consumes only 10 mg per day. There are many ways to increase iron intake and correct this deficiency.

1. Increase consumption of animal products, such as lean red meats and the dark meat of chicken and turkey. Animal protein provides the best and most readily absorbed source of iron.

2. Combine animal and vegetable products (a meat-and-bean burrito, for example) to increase the iron absorbed from the vegetable product.

3. Eat foods rich in vitamin C with each meal. Vitamin C enhances iron absorption from the intestine. A glass of orange juice with breakfast can increase iron absorption nearly 300%.

4. Use cast-iron cookware as often as possible. The more acidic the food and the longer it is cooked in a cast-iron container, the higher the iron content of the food. For example, the iron content of ½ cup of spaghetti sauce increases from 3 mg to 88 mg when simmered in a cast-iron pot for 3 hours.

5. Do not drink tea and coffee with meals. Studies have found that both beverages greatly reduce iron absorption.

6. Increase consumption of iron-rich fruits and vegetables, such as dark leafy green vegetables, legumes, strawberries, watermelon, raisins, dried apricots, and prunes.

Because obtaining 18 mg of iron each day is a difficult task, and because many women are concerned about anemia, the supplement question again arises. Self-supplementation of iron is particularly dangerous. That "tired, listless feeling" can be caused by numerous conditions, and an iron deficiency can only be determined by measuring serum ferritin (storage iron) and checking the hemoglobin level. Iron supplementation will not improve the health or performance of a woman with normal iron stores. On the other hand, excessive intake can produce an iron overload and cause deficiencies of the trace minerals copper and zinc. The best advice to give a woman who believes that her iron intake is inadequate is to see her physician for a check-up. A registered dietitian can provide personalized dietary recommendations to increase the iron content of the diet.

NUTRITION AND EXERCISE

Nutrition and exercise are two essential components of the fitness equation. Good nutrition combined with exercise plays a large role in the prevention of such debilitating diseases as osteoporosis and coronary heart disease. Even in well-trained athletes, good nutrition is necessary if they are to perform to their full potential. This section will explore the complementary roles played by nutrition and exercise in preventing disease and enhancing athletic performance.

Preventing Disease

According to the American Heart Association (1982), cardiovascular diseases claim more American lives than all other causes of death combined. **Coronary heart disease (CHD)** accounts for over half the deaths from cardiovascular disease, making it the number one killer in the United States. CHD is almost always the result of **atherosclerosis,** a gradual buildup of fatty deposits, called **plaques,** in the arterial walls. As the plaques enlarge, the artery loses its elasticity and the passages become narrower, decreasing the blood flow. If a blood clot develops, the flow can be stopped entirely.

Atherosclerosis may involve the arteries to many areas of the body. When the disease affects the arteries leading to the heart, a heart attack can result. When the arteries leading to the brain are affected, a stroke is the result.

One of the major culprits in CHD is a fatty substance called **cholesterol,** which is found in foods and also produced in the body. Cholesterol is an essential component of cell structures and hormones. However, a diet that is too high in saturated fat may produce too much serum (blood) cholesterol, which ends up as plaque that clogs arteries. In an early and now well-known study of 12,000 middle-aged men in seven countries, Ancel Keys and his colleagues (1957) found that the people of eastern Finland had the highest death rate from coronary disease. They also had the highest percentage of saturated fat in their diets and the highest blood cholesterol levels. On the other hand, in Greece, where most fat is unsaturated, death from CHD was far less common, and in Japan, where only 10% of the diet is fat and most fat is polyunsaturated, the cholesterol levels were very low and the death rate from CHD was more than 10 times lower than in Finland.

As a result of research in recent years, physicians no longer consider only a person's **total cholesterol** level when predicting the risk of heart disease. Instead, they look at the relative proportion of two different types of cholesterol, identified according to the molecules, called **lipoproteins,** that distribute cholesterol throughout the body. **Low-density lipoproteins (LDLs),** carry cholesterol into the system, leaving a residue in the arterial walls. Most cholesterol in the body is carried by LDLs. **High-density lipoproteins (HDLs)** remove cholesterol from the system, including the arterial walls, and transport it to the liver where it is reprocessed or eliminated. Therefore, the cholesterol carried by low-density lipoproteins (LDL-C) is "bad" cholesterol because it contributes to plaque buildup in arterial walls. The cholesterol carried by high-density lipoproteins (HDL-C) is "good" cholesterol because it removes the fatty deposits from arterial walls. Premenopausal women have higher HDL-C levels than men of the same age, which may account, in part, for their lower rate of CHD.

The ratio between HDL-C and total cholesterol is the single most important factor in determining risk for heart disease. This ratio is called the **coronary heart disease risk ratio.** The lower the ratio, the lower the risk. For men, a total cholesterol/HDL-C ratio of 5.0 is associated with an average risk of developing heart disease. A ratio of 3.5 corresponds to a 50% reduction in risk. For women, a ratio of 4.4 is associated with average risk, and 3.4 represents a 50% reduction in risk. Another way of representing the same concept is to say that HDL-C should represent at least 20% of total cholesterol and, preferably, 25% or more.

A low total cholesterol in itself is no guarantee of a low risk for heart disease. For example, a man with a total cholesterol of 150 (very low) and an HDL-C of 20 has a ratio of 7.5, definitely in the high-risk zone. On the other hand, a person with HDL-C of 60 (a high figure) is not necessarily at a lower risk unless the total cholesterol is relatively low. A man with a HDL-C of 60 and a total cholesterol of 400 is still at extremely high risk for heart disease. Therefore, to lower the risk for heart disease, the HDL-C should be increased and the total cholesterol decreased by lowering the LDL-C.

Research has shown that diet and exercise are the keys to lowering total cholesterol and raising HDL-C. Arntzenius et al. (1985) studied the relationship between diet, lipoproteins, and the progression of coronary lesions in 39 patients who had angina pectoris (severe cardiac pain caused by inadequate blood supply to the heart) and obstruction of at least one coronary vessel. For 2 years, the patients followed a low-cholesterol, vegetarian diet that had a 2:1 ratio of polyunsaturated to saturated fats. The researchers found that the dietary changes were associated with weight loss, lower systolic blood pressure, and, most significant for this discussion, lower total cholesterol and a lower ratio of total cholesterol to HDL-C. Patients who initially had a high total cholesterol/HDL-C ratio, and who lowered that ratio by dietary intervention, showed no further lesion growth in the coronary arteries. However, coronary heart disease continued to progress significantly in those patients whose ratios remained high.

For the dance-exercise instructor, these findings mean that participants can change their health status by changing their diet. However, while change is possible, it will not be quick and easy. Taking vitamin and mineral supplements will not lower a person's total cholesterol/HDL-C ratio, nor will a crash diet or an eating program that lasts only a month or two. The instructor should encourage participants to make gradual, healthful changes in dietary habits (as outlined earlier in this chapter), so that a well-balanced diet becomes part of their lifestyle.

To reduce the amount of saturated fat in the diet, keep meat portions small and emphasize chicken, turkey, and fish over beef and pork. Trim all visible fat and broil or roast meat instead of frying it. Dairy products made from whole milk or cream, especially butter and hard and processed cheeses, are also high in saturated fat. Therefore, it is best to substitute low-fat or skim milk and low-fat cheese for whole-milk products and polyunsaturated oils (safflower, soybean, sunflower, or corn oil) for saturated fat in cooking. Since egg yolks are very high in cholesterol—a single yolk provides 250 mg of cholesterol, nearly the total daily allowance—limit them to 3 or fewer per week.

In addition to consuming less saturated fat, there are other dietary measures that may reduce the risk of atherosclerosis. Research has shown that fiber from fruits and vegetables, legumes, and whole oats may be effective in lowering serum cholesterol levels. There is also evidence that the type of polyunsaturated fat found in coldwater fish, such as salmon, mackerel, sardines, and trout, may lower serum cholesterol. Therefore, eating more fish and high-fiber vegetable products may improve one's coronary heart disease risk ratio.

Diet, however, is only one part of the fitness equation. Numerous studies have shown that although exercise does not decrease total cholesterol, it does favorably alter the total cholesterol/HDL-C ratio. For example, Williams et al. (1982) identified 81 healthy, sedentary men aged 30–55 and randomly assigned them to one of two groups, a supervised running group or a sedentary control group. The researchers then measured the plasma lipoproteins, fitness, and percent body fat of the two groups at 3-month intervals. Two findings are important for dance-exercise instructors:

1. The total cholesterol/HDL-C ratio did not begin to change until a threshold exercise level of 10 miles per week was maintained for 9 months or more.

2. Fitness increased and percent body fat decreased sooner and at lower exercise levels than required for changes in the concentration of LDL-C and HDL-C.

In other words, while some benefits of aerobic exercise will be seen fairly quickly, other important health-related changes will occur only over an extended period. Another recent study (Wood, Terry, and Haskell 1985) had similar findings: Fourteen sedentary, middle-aged men who engaged in a progressive running program over 2 years showed an increase in HDL-C, a decrease in LDL-C, and a decrease in percent body fat. However, while the total cholesterol was significantly reduced at 6 months, an increase in HDL-C was not seen until 12 months. As with diet, an instructor should stress the benefits of gradually integrating a regular program of exercise, such as 3 one-hour aerobics classes per week (enough to expend 1,000 kcals per week), into the lifestyle, and, at the same time, warn participants against plunging into a frenzied period of exercise with the expectation of immediate health benefits.

The message is clear: a high-carbohydrate, low-fat diet and aerobic exercise can favorably influence a person's total cholesterol/HDL-C ratio and, therefore, lower the risk of coronary heart disease. Other studies have shown that smoking lowers HDL-C and raises LDL-C, and that the ratio is related to the number of cigarettes smoked per day. People who stop smoking can achieve HDL-C levels similar to nonsmokers. Fortunately, an aerobic exercise program often helps smokers to cut back on the number of cigarettes they smoke or to stop smoking completely.

Good nutrition and aerobic exercise can also reduce the risk of osteoporosis. There is strong evidence that weight-bearing exercise, as seen in an aerobics class, increases bone mass. Like muscle, bone responds to stress by becoming stronger. Several studies of tennis players have shown that the bone mass of the playing arm is much greater than that of the nonplaying arm. Studies of the elderly have found that bone mineral loss is not always a function of age and that mineralization can increase with activity. In reviewing the role of exercise in preventing osteoporosis, Smith (1982) concludes that bone atrophy occurs in sedentary people and bone hypertrophy occurs with sufficient physical activity. Therefore, weight-bearing aerobic exercise, plus an adequate calcium intake (as explained earlier in this chapter), is the best approach for preventing osteoporosis in later years.

Athletic Performance

Nutrition is an important complement to physical training for both the beginning exerciser and the accomplished athlete. There is no evidence, however, that the nutritional needs of the active person are any different from those of the sedentary population. Physically active people will burn more calories and, therefore, may consume more food without gaining weight, but do not require a special diet. A dance-exercise instructor should be prepared to answer questions about nutrition as it relates to exercise and to counter the many popular misconceptions about diet and performance.

MAINTENANCE OF GLYCOGEN STORES.   Because carbohydrates are the source of glycogen, the most efficient fuel for aerobic exercise, the high-carbohydrate, low-fat diet recommended in the Senate Guidelines is the best regimen for both overall health and aerobic exercise. When muscle glycogen stores are reduced to low levels, a dance-exercise participant will become exhausted and will either have to stop exercising or reduce exercise intensity.

Muscle glycogen decreases progressively during high-intensity exercise exceeding 90 minutes, such as running a marathon. However, glycogen stores can also be depleted gradually over several days of heavy exercise. As the glycogen stores decrease, aerobic exercise becomes more difficult and less enjoyable. Instructors with a heavy teaching load may experience this phenomenon, and all instructors should be alert to the problem in beginning exercisers who attempt too ambitious a program or advanced participants who make take 3–4 classes per week and engage in other physical activities such as jogging or cycling. Over several days, the participant becomes increasingly tired and cannot maintain a normal exercise pattern.

This chronic state of fatigue and staleness can be prevented by periodic rest days and a diet rich in carbohydrates. Complex carbohydrates promote glycogen storage better than refined carbohydrates. Refined sugars can give fast energy because they enter the bloodstream quickly but that energy does not last. Complex carbohydrates, on the other hand, are absorbed more slowly, providing energy over a longer time. Complex carbohydrates also supply fiber and nutrients with their calories. Bread, cereal, pasta, potatoes, rice, vegetables, and fruit are good sources of complex carbohydrates. The high-protein, high-fat diet typical of many Americans will not replace the glycogen lost during heavy training.

EATING BEFORE EXERCISING.   There are several good reasons for not eating just before exercising. During exercise, the body relies on existing stores of muscle glycogen and body fat. A meal just before exercise will not increase muscle glycogen stores, and when blood is diverted to the working muscles, food remaining in the stomach can cause nausea. A large meal will distend the stomach and may restrict breathing.

Although a preexercise meal will not contribute energy for the workout, it may help ward off feelings of weakness and fatigue. The best solution is to eat a light, high-carbohydrate meal several hours before prolonged exercise so the stomach and upper bowel are empty before exercise begins. The meal should be low in protein, which takes 24 hours to move through the digestive system as compared to approximately 3 hours for carbohydrates. The meal should also be low in fat, which slows food transit time. A breakfast that meets these guidelines consists of cooked or dry cereal (low in sugar) with nonfat or low-fat milk, and fresh fruit. Experiment with different foods to see which provide the best and longest lasting energy.

HYDRATION.   Water is the most commonly overlooked endurance aid. Proper hydration is essential for proper exercise performance. During exercise in a warm environment, the body relies primarily on the evaporation of sweat to dissipate heat. This loss of body fluids gradually compromises the body's ability to circulate blood and regulate body temperature, because the blood transferring oxygen to muscle tissue must be diverted to the skin to transfer heat from the body's core to the environment. This competition for blood between the muscles and the skin places a greater demand on the cardiovascular system. As a person becomes dehydrated, the heart rate increases, the blood flow to the skin decreases, and the body temperature rises steadily. In practical terms, performance begins to decline and exercise becomes labored. If the body temperature continues to rise, the participant may suffer heat exhaustion or heat stroke. (See Chapter 14 for a discussion of heat illnesses.)

An adequate intake of fluids is obviously the best way to prevent dehydration. Normally, a person's water intake is governed by the thirst mechanism, which is regulated by the hypothalamus. However, when exercising in a hot environment, thirst is not an accurate indicator of the body's need for water. A person who is exercising vigorously and losing a large quantity of water through sweat may become dehydrated before feeling thirsty. Therefore, fluids should be taken according to a schedule.

Instructors who are teaching in hot weather should inform their class of the importance of fluid intake and remind participants to stop periodically to drink water. A person planning to exercise in hot weather should drink 2–3 cups of water about 2–3 hours before exercising, and another 1–2 cups about 15 minutes before exercising (some experts suggest 1-½ hours before). This technique, known as **hyperhydration,** helps to lower the body's core temperature and to reduce the added stress heat placed on the cardiovascular system. During exercise, the participant should drink 4–8 ounces of fluid every 10–20 minutes to replace sweat losses and to maintain blood volume.

Cold water is the best fluid for exercisers. Cold drinks empty more rapidly from the stomach than warm drinks and also help to lower the body's core temperature. Drinks containing too much sugar are absorbed into the system more slowly and, therefore, function less effectively as a fluid replacement. Commercial sport drinks with a high sugar content (glucose, fructose, or sucrose) may actually harm exercise performance. Fifteen minutes after drinking 1 cup of water, 60%–70% of the water has been absorbed into the system. However, if the 1 cup of fluid is a beverage containing 10% sugar (the sugar content of soft drinks), 95% of the fluid will still be in the stomach 15 minutes later. Commercial sport drinks containing more than 2.5% sugar should be diluted to 2.5% before being consumed. These drinks also supply electrolytes, which the average dance-exercise participant does not need. Water is a much more effective, and much less expensive, fluid for aerobic exercise.

MYTHS AND MISCONCEPTIONS.   There are many popular myths and misconceptions about how to enhance exercise performance. Even experienced exercisers can be misinformed. An exercise instructor will most likely hear the following myths in class.

Myth: Protein supplements can help meet the demands of a heavy exercise schedule.

Protein requirements increase only slightly with activity, and the amount of protein athletes typically consume more than meets the requirement. There is no evidence that protein powders improve either strength or endurance.

Most Americans already eat 2–3 times more protein than they need. The RDA for protein is calculated according to the ideal body weight and, as all RDAs, provides a generous allowance to meet the needs of nearly all healthy people. The average adult requires 0.36 grams of protein per pound of body weight. For a 125-lb woman, the daily protein requirement is 45 grams. By consuming 3 servings of foods high in protein—such as 2 cups of skim milk (17.6 grams), 1 egg (5.7 grams), and 3 ounces of cooked beef (24 grams)—a woman can more than meet her protein requirement. The requirement for a 160-lb man, which is 57.6 grams, can be met by adding ½ cup of cottage cheese (15 grams). Vegetarians can satisfy their protein requirements through a balanced diet as well, because many foods besides meat contain protein. For example, ½ cup of cooked kidney beans contains 7.2 grams, 1 cup of cooked spaghetti contains 6.5 grams, and 1 banana contain 1.3 grams of protein.

Protein supplements are not only unnecessary, they may be harmful. Excess protein calories, like excess calories from any nutrient, are stored as fat. Too much protein, whether ingested through foods or supplements, produces extra nitrogen in the body; and the kidneys and liver must work harder to eliminate this excess. The kidneys require more water to dilute the nitrogen for excretion; this increased water requirement may contribute to dehydration.

Myth: Eating sugar before exercising will provide an extra boost of energy.

A high-sugar snack consumed just before exercising will not improve performance, and a growing body of evidence indicates that it may impair performance. Sugar enters the blood a few minutes after ingestion, producing a rapid increase in blood sugar and causing the body to overreact and produce more insulin. The insulin inhibits the metabolism of fatty acids by the muscles, forcing the muscles to rely more heavily on glycogen stores. The insulin also lowers the blood sugar level, which is already being lowered as the muscles draw on glycogen for energy. As the blood sugar level falls, the exerciser may experience weakness and fatigue. One study (Keller and Schwarzkopf 1984) found that college distance runners could ride a bicycle ergometer 25% longer after drinking a caffeine-free, sugar-free drink than after drinking a glucose drink. In other words, ingestion of sugar before prolonged exercise can reduce the time a participant is able to exercise before becoming exhausted.

Myth: Caffeine should be used to enhance endurance.

Caffeine is a drug, a stimulant to the central nervous system, found in coffee, chocolate, colas, and aspirin medications. Some athletes ingest caffeine before a competitive event to enhance their endurance during continuous high-intensity aerobic exercise lasting 90 minutes or longer. Some researchers believe caffeine increases the availability of free fatty acids early in exercise, thus depleting glycogen at a slower rate and increasing endurance. Other studies have failed to substantiate that claim.

However, the amount of caffeine necessary to produce this effect is 4–5 mg per kilogram of body weight. This amount of caffeine represents a pharmacological dose. As a drug, caffeine is not sanctioned for use by the US Olympic Committee or the American College of Sports Medicine. Associated side effects include nausea, muscle tremors, and headache. Caffeine is also a diuretic and may contribute to dehydration by increasing water loss through urination.

Myth: Athletes should take salt tablets to replace the salt lost through sweat.

The American diet provides more than enough sodium for physically active people. Salt tablets are potentially dangerous because the excess sodium draws water out of the body's cells, dehydrating them and impairing their performance. Concentrated doses of salt also can irritate the stomach lining and cause nausea. The best way to replace lost sweat is with plain water and the salt provided through a balanced diet.

Myth: A physically active person needs vitamin and mineral supplements to maintain a high energy level.

Current evidence suggests that the dietary requirements of the athlete are the same as those of the nonathlete, so even the most avid dance-exerciser should not need to head for the vitamin bottle. In some cases, the use of supplements can actually do more harm than good, because it fosters the illusion of proper self-care while obscuring the fact the proper eating is the basis of good health and athletic performance.

Neither vitamins nor minerals are a direct source of energy. Unless a person has a shortage of a particular vitamin or mineral, supplements will not improve performance, strength, or endurance.

Exceptions to this rule should be mentioned, even though they do not apply to a typical dance-exercise setting. Regular use of certain drugs and illnesses such as chronic infections or chronic intestinal disorders can produce vitamin deficiencies. Heavy smokers may be deficient in vitamin C, and heavy drinkers may require more thiamine, niacin, B_6, and folacin than nondrinkers. People who fail to consume a variety of foods, a common problem among dieters and the elderly, may also benefit from supplementation, under the guidance of a physician or a registered dietitian.

Megadoses of vitamins and minerals (amounts 10 times the RDA or more) are usually worthless and potentially dangerous. At this level, vitamins no longer function as vitamins; they function as drugs, often producing serious side effects. An instructor should never encourage megavitamin self-therapy. The best approach to health and performance is a balanced diet. A participant interested in supplementation should seek guidance from a professional who is qualified to assess the needs and risks as well as the benefits.

Myth: A beer or two improves psychological well-being and aids proper hydration during aerobic exercise.

Alcohol is the most abused drug in our country and a major contributor to accidents and disease. Drinking alcohol before aerobic exercise may harm performance, because alcohol is a central nervous system depressant that impairs balance and coordination. Because alcohol redirects blood flow away from the heart and toward the periphery, a person with heart disease who has not yet shown symptoms of the disease may be at risk during exercise. Alcohol also may decrease the liver's output of glucose, leading to low blood sugar (hypoglycemia) after several hours of exercise.

Both the American College of Sports Medicine (1982) and the American Dietetic Association (1980) have concluded that alcohol does not contribute to performance and in most cases appears to be detrimental. A person who wants to drink a beer or any other form of alcohol should wait until after exercising. An instructor who suspects that a participant has been drinking should advise the person of the potentially harmful effects and recommend that the person not drink before coming to class.

WEIGHT CONTROL

Weight loss is a big business in this country. The bestseller list usually contains at least one diet book, and billions of dollars are invested each year in diet aids, special foods, exercise gimmicks, and special weight-loss programs. More than any other aspect of fitness, weight loss is replete with misinformation and potential hazards. While some weight-loss gimmicks merely slim down the wallets of those who try them, others endanger the health of their victims. Almost all fail to produce permanent weight loss.

Many participants come to a dance-exercise class for the purpose of controlling or reducing their weight. An uninformed instructor can perpetuate an already negative and repetitive cycle of weight loss followed by weight gain. On the other hand, a knowledgeable instructor can steer participants away from unrealistic goals and ineffective, often dangerous practices and toward sensible, safe, long-range approaches to maintaining desirable weight and body composition.

Overweight versus Overfat

In our society, the bathroom scale has a following worthy of a political party or religion. In the rush to shed pounds, however, most people overlook an important question: How fat am I?

The term **overweight** means that a person weighs more than the average for his or her weight, height, and frame size, as defined by standard scales. Most diet-conscious people assume that a gain in weight means a gain in fat, and that weight loss equals fat loss. The scale, however, cannot differentiate between fat pounds and muscle pounds. An extremely fit person with a high muscular density may be classified as overweight because muscle is denser than fat, while a person of normal weight can be at risk for health problems because a high percentage of that weight is fat.

A more accurate indicator of fitness is body composition, or the percentage of total body weight that is fat mass and the percentage that is lean body mass (everything that is not fat, including muscle, bones, skin, and organs). The most accurate and practical ways to measure body composition are hydrostatic (underwater) weighing and measuring the thickness of skinfolds at various sites (see Chapter 6). Both techniques must be performed by trained personnel to insure accuracy. For men, 15% body fat is the upper limit for general health, and over 23% is considered obese. For women, the upper limit is 25%, and over 30% is considered obese.

Obesity, a condition characterized by excessive, generalized storage of fat, is the nation's most serious nutritional problem. An estimated one out of four Americans is obese. Adults have 30–40 billion fat cells that shrink or swell as fat is stored or burned. Part of the physiological mechanism that protects humans from starvation, fat cells never disappear even in someone who is starving. In 1985, the National Institutes of Health Consensus Panel in Obesity told the nation that obesity is not just a matter of appearance: It is a disease that increases a person's risk of heart disease and cancer and is highly associated with diabetes.

While a low percentage of body fat is associated with increased fitness and higher HDL-C levels, some fat is needed to maintain health. A body fat percentage of 3%–6% for men and 8%–12% for women is considered essential, or the amount needed for normal physiological functioning. Attempts to reach a very low percentage, like attempts to reach a very low weight, can be physiologically and psychologically devastating. Physically active persons should stay below the upper limits of body fat established for general health. Within that range, each person should try to achieve the percentage of body fat at which he or she feels and performs best.

The Diet/Exercise Question

What is the best approach to weight loss: diet, reducing the number of kilocalories consumed, or exercise, increasing the number of kilocalories burned? The answer, of course, is both, but to understand why requires an understanding of the concept of energy balance.

The energy content of food is constantly being transformed into other forms of energy, including the energy used for muscular contractions. **Energy balance** means that the body weight will stay the same when caloric intake equals caloric expenditure. An imbalance between expenditure and intake will cause a change in body weight. For example, when a person expends more energy (kilocalories) than provided by the food he or she consumes, the body draws on its fat reserves to meet the extra demand. Conversely, when more kilocalories are consumed than he or she expended, the extra energy is stored in body fat.

To lose weight a negative caloric balance, or a caloric deficit, must be achieved. A deficit of 3,500 kcal is required to lose a pound of stored fat. Therefore, a woman who consumes an average of 2,500 kcal per day and reduces her daily consumption by 500 kcal would lose one pound per week. However, research has shown that lean body tissue as well as fat is lost by dieting. With extreme caloric restrictions, much of the weight loss (estimated between 25% and 45%) may come from the lean body mass. Even a sensible, well-balanced diet that produces a loss of one or two pounds per week may also result in some loss of lean body weight.

A further drawback to dieting alone is suggested by the **setpoint theory,** which contradicts the traditional theory of weight control based on energy balance. According to the setpoint theory, the body strives to maintain a certain level of body fat, or setpoint. When a person diets to drop below that level, the body thinks it is starving and lowers its metabolism to become more energy efficient.

For example, in one study (Bray 1969) 6 obese subjects on a diet restricted to 450 calories for 3½ weeks experienced only a 3% drop in body weight, but a 17% drop in normal energy expenditure (including basal metabolic rate). On the other hand, when normal-weight college students ingested 2–3 times their normal intake of kilocalories over 3–5 months, they increased their weight by only 16–20 pounds instead of the expected 75 pounds (Sims et al. 1968). The body attempted to maintain its setpoint by using calories less efficiently and increasing its energy expenditure. It also appears that a high-fat diet increases the setpoint and that repeated bouts of dieting make the setpoint mechanism more efficient. In other words, it becomes harder to lose weight and easier to regain it. In light of this information, the challenge is to lower the setpoint.

Fortunately, aerobic exercise appears to lower the body's setpoint by increasing the metabolic rate. Research has shown that after exercise, the metabolic rate remains elevated for hours, increasing the energy expenditure beyond the energy cost of the exercise itself. Losing weight by increasing energy expenditure also greatly reduces the loss of lean muscle mass (even with dietary restrictions) and increases the loss of fat. It is important to note that not all exercise is conducive to weight loss. Weight lifting, while better than nothing at all, will not burn calories like jogging or bicycling. The two keys to exercise for weight loss are moderate intensity and long duration. The body does not begin burning fat for fuel until exercise has continued for 20 minutes or more.

The best approach to weight loss is a combination of diet and exercise, or a moderate decrease in kilocalories consumed and a moderate, regular increase in physical activity. Exercise enables a person to burn more fat and improve muscle tone and develop the cardiovascular system. During the first few months of an exercise program, there may be little, if any, weight change because the lean weight initially increases at about the same rate as fat weight is lost. What the scales do not show is the change in appearance. As lean body mass increases in proportion to body fat, the body will appear trimmer and clothing will be looser even if the weight remains the same.

The American College of Sports Medicine (1983) has provided sound guidelines for healthful weight loss. The guidelines recommend a caloric intake not lower than 1,200 kcal for normal adults, combined with an endurance exercise program of 20–30 minutes at least 3 days per week. The caloric deficit may range from 500 to 1,000 kcal, depending on individual caloric requirements. The rate of sustained weight loss should not exceed 2 pounds per week. Long-term weight control, the guidelines state, "requires a lifelong commitment, an understanding of our eating habits and a willingness to change them. Frequent exercise is necessary, and accomplishment must be reinforced to sustain motivation." The instructor can play an instrumental role by providing the motivation and reinforcement for exercise.

Dangerous and Ineffective Weight-Loss Techniques

Weight loss is big business, and the American public is bombarded with appetite suppressants, fad diets, and exercise gimmicks that claim to make the process "quick and easy." At best, these techniques are ineffective; at worst, they are potentially harmful. The dance-exercise instructor can provide a valuable service by offering accurate, scientifically based information to counter false advertising claims.

Spot reduction is often promoted to eliminate the so-called cellulite in specific areas of the body. Cellulite is just another name for subcutaneous fat that has a dimpled appearance. The only way to get rid of fat deposits is through diet and exercise. Exercise, even when localized, draws from all the fat stores of the body and not just from selected fat depots. Sit-ups will increase the muscle tone for the abdomen, for example, but will not burn off the "tummy roll."

Vibrating belts, elastic belts, and electric muscle stimulators are equally ineffective methods of reducing body fat. The claim that vibrating belts "break up" fat has no basis in fact. While the vibration may relax the muscles, such passive exercise does not increase a person's caloric expenditure and, therefore, cannot decrease body fat. Similarly, elastic belts cannot "melt away" fat because, again, no caloric deficit is created. The belts may cause temporary water loss from the area or compress the tissues, so the waistline looks thinner for a time. However, the figure soon returns to normal. Electric muscle stimulators, placed on specific muscle groups, discharge a small electric current, causing the muscles to contract. While these devices may help rehabilitate injured muscles, they do not increase caloric expenditure enough to result in the loss of body fat.

Rubber or plastic suits worn during exercise are more dangerous and equally ineffective. A person wearing one of these suits will lose weight, but it will be primarily water, not fat. Furthermore, these suits prevent the evaporation of sweat, which is crucial to regulating body temperature during exercise. A rubber suit will not "sweat off" fat, but it may lead to dehydration and heat stroke, especially if worn in hot, humid weather. Sitting in a sauna also results in water loss, and therefore weight loss, which is quickly replaced when fluids are consumed.

Diet pills should be avoided entirely. Diet pills usually contain a stimulant, such as amphetamines, to suppress the appetite. However, the appetite suppressant effect is temporary, so the rate of weight reduction tapers off with time. More important, amphetamines can be addictive and cause insomnia, high blood pressure, headaches, and dizziness. Phenylpropanolamine, another hunger-controlling ingredient, can cause high blood pressure as well as irregular heart rhythm and liver damage.

Fad diets, which radically alter a person's intake of nutrients, can also be extremely dangerous. Diets that severely restrict carbohydrate calories cause glycogen depletion, which induces an obligatory water loss, since about 3 parts of water are stored with 1 part of glycogen. Dieters love the rapid weight loss and assume they are losing fat. Actually their body fat stores remain virtually untouched. Exercisers will perform poorly due to reduced glycogen levels. Complications associated with low-carbohydrate fad diets include ketosis (increased blood acids), potassium depletion, calcium depletion, dehydration, weakness, and possible kidney problems. Prolonged, unbalanced diets consisting of only one or two foods, such as grapefruit and eggs, can lead to vitamin and mineral deficiencies.

Fad diets are faulty from a behavioral standpoint as well; they fail to stress the need for a permanent change in a person's eating habits and thus perpetuate the myth that weight loss can be achieved quickly and easily. The dieter is not encouraged to learn about and practice good nutrition, but instead told to follow rigid rules for a short time. When the dieter abandons the diet, the weight is regained.

So consumer beware! Instructors should advise their participants to avoid any weight-loss plans with unrealistic claims. It is impossible to lose 10 pounds of fat in 10 days. Even on a total fast, a large part of the weight lost will be lean body mass and not fat, and much of the lost weight will be quickly regained when the person resumes normal eating patterns. Moderate caloric restriction combined with a regular program of aerobic exercise is the best way to lose weight and keep it off and, ultimately, to make weight control a permanent part of a healthful lifestyle.

EATING DISORDERS

Anorexia nervosa and bulimia are serious, widespread problems in our society, and ones that instructors are likely to encounter in their classes. Both are most common among women, especially athletes striving for a low body fat percentage or a performance edge and dancers who must be thin; but men may suffer from these disorders as well. An instructor cannot cure someone with an eating disorder. However, by providing sound nutritional advice and setting realistic time frames for weight loss, the instructor can play a role in the prevention of eating disorders.

Anorexia nervosa is self-imposed starvation to the point of emaciation. Anorexics often lose up to 25% of their body weight; because of an extremely distorted body image, however, they still feel heavy. Research has shown that most anorexics are intelligent, high achievers who are encouraged to lose weight as children or adolescents, either for the sake of appearance alone or for the purpose of athletic competition. They lose the weight and feel in control, but the need to stay in control remains long after the weight-loss goal has been achieved. Anorexics' ability to resist food remains an obsession, unrelated to the basic nutritional and exercise requirements for health and fitness.

Bulimia literally means "ox hunger." Bulimia is characterized by a binge/purge cycle in which huge amounts of food are eaten over a short period and then vomiting is induced or laxatives or diuretics are used to control weight. These episodes of binging, followed by feelings of shame and guilt and then purging, are usually carried out secretly, and even family and close friends often remain unaware of the problem. Like the anorexic, the bulimic is trapped by an obsession with thinness. Unlike the anorexic, the bulimic is usually of normal weight.

In a recent study (Rosen et al. 1986) of 182 female collegiate athletes, 32% reported that they practiced one or more weight-control behaviors defined as pathogenic (producing disease), including binging, self-induced vomiting, and using laxatives, diet pills, or diuretics. Unfortunately, these practices only impair health and performance. The complications of eating disorders can be serious, and sometimes lethal: malnutrition, electrolyte imbalances (caused by diet pills, laxatives, and other drugs to control weight), dehydration, irregularities in heartbeat, fatigue, fainting, and seizures. Some anorexics have literally starved themselves to death.

On the surface, it may not be easy to tell the difference between a participant's healthy concern for ideal body composition and athletic performance and an obsessive, destructive concern for being thin. A highly motivated exerciser may exhibit some of the compulsive behaviors common among persons with eating disorders. Both share the drive to excel and to control mind and body. Both set goals just beyond reach and experience depression or anxiety when their personal rituals cannot be maintained. However, an instructor who observes the following symptoms in a participant should suspect an eating disorder:

1. Repeated complaints about feeling fat, even when the person is of normal weight or underweight.
2. A drive to exercise excessively, beyond the requirements of health and fitness.
3. Wide fluctuations in weight over short periods.
4. Edema or bloating of the face, hands, or ankles, not related to menstrual periods.
5. Complaints of light-headedness, fatigue, and muscle cramps.
6. Questions about the use of laxatives, diuretics, or diet pills for weight loss.
7. More than average dental problems (caused by erosion and decay from repeated vomiting of highly acidic stomach contents).

An alert instructor can help a participant overcome an eating disorder. First, instructors should be good role models, with positive and realistic self-images. An instructor who is always complaining about his or her weight will only feed the obsession of a participant with anorexia or bulimia. Second, instructors should openly address the general problem of eating disorders in class, stressing the importance of realistic time frames for weight loss and the importance of good nutrition, and providing a list of professional resources for anyone who has, or knows someone who has, the problem.

Finally, an instructor who suspects a participant is anorexic or bulimic should speak privately to that person in a supportive, non-judgmental way. Ask if binging or laxatives or diuretics are used and express concern as a fitness professional and a caring person. If the participant is willing to talk, listen, offer encouragement, and provide the names of physicians, psychologists, or dietitians who specialize in eating disorders. If the participant denies the problem, keep the channels of communication open and let him or her know that help is available if needed. Although it is normal to feel hesitant about approaching someone, ignoring the problem increases the danger to the participant. An eating disorder that remains undiagnosed and untreated may lead to permanent physical injury.

SUMMARY

Fitness-oriented persons often seek the secret ingredient that will improve their health and physical performance. Thus, nutritional faddism is more prevalent in the fitness world than anywhere else. Expensive vitamin and mineral supplements, fad diets, and exercise gimmicks are promoted to boost performance and reduce body fat. The fact remains, however, that there is no quick and easy way to lose weight or to enhance performance, and many products that make such advertising claims are potentially dangerous to the consumer.

The instructor can greatly contribute to the health and fitness of dance-exercise participants by serving as a positive role model and providing them with sound, basic information on nutrition and weight control. A diet high in complex carbohydrates and low in fat, especially saturated fat, is the best regimen for both endurance athletes and armchair athletes. There is no dietary supplement or special food that will enhance a good diet or redeem a poor one. Excess body fat increases a person's risk for heart disease and cancer and is highly associated with diabetes and a host of other health problems. The best way to lose weight is to combine a modest reduction in calories with low to moderate aerobic exercise of 20 minutes or more at least 3 times per week. The instructor's role is to promote a healthful lifestyle, counter the many myths and misconceptions about diet and exercise, and discourage the use of short-term and unrealistic diet and exercise plans.

REFERENCES

Aftergood, L., and P. B. Alfin-Slater. "Women and Nutrition." *Contemporary Nutrition* (General Mills, Inc.) 5 (1980):n.p.

American Dietetic Association. "Position Statement on Nutrition and Physical Fitness." *Journal of the American Dietetic Association* 76 (1980):437–43.

American College of Sports Medicine. "Position Statement: Proper and Improper Weight Loss Programs." *Medicine and Science in Sports and Exercise* 15 (1983):ix–xiii.

American College of Sports Medicine. "Position Statement: The Use of Alcohol in Sports." *Medicine and Science in Sports and Exercise* 14 (1982):ix–xi.

American Heart Association. *Heart Facts 1983*. Dallas: American Heart Association, 1982.

Arntzenius, A. C., et al. "Diet, Lipoproteins, and the Progress of Coronary Atherosclerosis." *New England Journal of Medicine* 312 (1985):805–11.

Bray, G. A. "Effect of Caloric Restriction on Energy Expenditure in Obese Patients." *Lancet* 32 (1969):397.

"Diet and Bone Health." *Dairy Council Digest* 55 (1982):25–30.

Keller, K., and R. Schwarzkopf. "Preexercise Snacks May Decrease Exercise Performance." *The Physician and Sportsmedicine* (April 1984):89–91.

Keys, A., J. Anderson, and F. Grande. "Serum Cholesterol Response to Dietary Fat." *Lancet* 1 (1957):787.

Rosen, L. W., D. B. McKegg, D. O. Hough, and V. Curley. "Pathogenic Weight-Control Behavior in Female Athletes." *The Physician and Sportsmedicine* (January 1986):79–86.

Sims, E. A., and E. S. Horton, "Endocrine and Metabolic Adaptation of Obesity and Starvation." *American Journal of Clinical Nutrition* 21 (1968):1455–70.

Smith, E. L. "Exercise for Prevention of Osteoporosis: A Review." *The Physician and Sportsmedicine* (March 1982):72–83.

US Senate Select Committee on Nutrition and Human Needs. *Dietary Goals for the United States.* 2nd ed. Washington, D.C.: US Government Printing Office, 1977.

Williams, P. T., P. D. Wood, W. L. Haskell, and K. Vranizan. "The Effects of Running Mileage and Duration on Plasma Lipoprotein Levels." *Journal of the American Medical Association* 247 (1982):2674–79.

Wood, P. D., R. B. Terry, and W. L. Haskell. "Metabolism of Substrates: Diet, Lipoprotein Metabolism, and Exercise." *Federation Proceedings* 44 (1985):358–63.

SUGGESTED READING

Brody, J. *Jane Brody's Nutrition Book.* New York: W. W. Norton, 1981.

Clark, N. *The Athlete's Kitchen.* New York: Bantam Books, 1983.

Coleman, E. *Eating for Endurance.* Riverside: Rubidoux Printing, 1982.

Cummings, C., and V. Newman. *Eater's Guide: Nutrition Basics for Busy People.* Englewood Cliffs, New Jersey: Prentice-Hall, 1981.

Kahn, M. *The 200 Calorie Solution.* New York: W. W. Norton, 1982.

Katch, F., and W. McArdle. *Nutrition, Weight Control and Exercise.* Philadelphia: Lea and Febiger, 1983.

Pollock, M., J. Wilmore, and S. Fox. *Exercise in Health and Disease.* Philadelphia: W. B. Saunders, 1984.

Tufts University Diet and Nutrition Letter, 475 Park Avenue South, New York, New York 10016.

SCREENING, TESTING AND PROGRAMMING

PART II

Instructors are more than just exercise experts; they are teachers. Anyone who thinks teaching is easy probably hasn't stood in front of a class of twenty eager beginning exercisers. This largest section of *The Aerobic Dance-Exercise Instructor Manual* takes the instructor through every major aspect of teaching a dance-exercise class. Five chapters cover the topics of initial health screening and fitness testing, designing and modifying routines, monitoring exercise intensity, and employing a variety of teaching styles. Because more and more women are continuing to exercise during pregnancy, two special chapters examine the factors instructors should consider when incorporating pregnant women into traditional dance-exercise classes. The information in this section will be a valuable resource for instructors who seek out further training, and provide food for thought for more experienced instructors.

Health Screening

Steven Van Camp

Steven P. Van Camp, M.D., is a cardiologist in private practice in San Diego. He is a professor in the College of Professional Studies at San Diego State University, as well as medical director of the exercise physiology laboratory and the Adult Fitness Program. Dr. Van Camp is a fellow of the American College of Cardiology and the American College of Sports Medicine. He also serves on the IDEA Board of Advisors and the IDEA Foundation's Board of Directors.

4

IN THIS CHAPTER:

- Medical disorders and conditions that may make exercise unsafe.

- How to screen participants; when to refer someone for medical evaluation and clearance.

- The effects of medications on the heart-rate response to exercise.

Dance exercise can be a beneficial and enjoyable form of exercise. If instructors screen participants properly, conduct exercise sessions safely, and learn to respond to emergencies, dance exercise can also be a safe form of exercise. This chapter will discuss the important role health screening plays in a dance-exercise program and offer practical screening procedures. These procedures are appropriate for traditional, general classes in an environment where elaborate fitness testing is not the norm.

This chapter cannot teach instructors to be knowledgeable health-care deliverers. Nor can it prepare instructors for all possible health contingencies for participants in a dance-exercise class. However, the screening process presented here will help instructors identify persons who need special attention or who should be exercising in special classes, as well as persons who should not be exercising at all until they obtain medical clearance from their physicians.

The health-screening process has other positive features as well: (a) it can help instructors become more familiar with the physical abilities of their students, (b) it can enhance the credibility of the instructor as a concerned professional, (c) it can help protect instructors against potential legal problems, and (d) it can open lines of communication between physicians and dance-exercise instructors, thus helping instructors gain exposure in their communities as concerned professionals.

MEDICAL DISORDERS THAT AFFECT EXERCISE

While it appears that appropriate exercise will add to the quality and, probably, to the length of life, exercise does carry a health risk for persons with certain medical disorders of the cardiovascular, pulmonary, and musculoskeletal systems. The most significant condition that may make exercise unsafe is coronary heart disease.

Coronary heart disease is the result of **atherosclerosis,** a thickening and hardening of the walls of the arteries by deposits of cholesterol. Atherosclerosis may result in narrowing of the arteries, including the coronary arteries that supply the heart with blood and, therefore, oxygen. Other names for coronary heart disease are coronary artery disease and atherosclerotic heart disease. During exercise the heart beats faster and more forcefully (the heart rate and systolic blood pressure are elevated), which means that the myocardium (heart muscle) needs more oxygen. If the arteries that supply the myocardium with oxygen are significantly narrowed by the cholesterol and calcium deposits of atherosclerosis, the flow of blood is restricted. When the myocardium's demand for oxygen exceeds the supply available through the coronary arteries, **myocardial ischemia** (deficiency of blood supply to the heart muscle) occurs. Myocardial ischemia, in turn, may lead to **angina pectoris** (a feeling of pressure, usually in the center of the chest), cardiac arrhythmias (abnormal heart rhythms), or even a **cardiac arrest** (the heart stops). In addition, people with atherosclerotic narrowings of coronary arteries are at risk for **myocardial infarctions** (heart attacks). Clearly, vigorous exercise is potentially unsafe for people with coronary heart disease, and they should exercise only in accordance with their physician's recommendations. In most cases, participants with diagnosed (known) coronary heart disease should not exercise in dance-exercise programs designed for the general population.

Unfortunately, coronary heart disease is not always obvious to those who have it. Some people either have no symptoms (i.e., they are asymptomatic), or they may misinterpret or not appreciate the significance of their symptoms. Therefore, not only do persons with known heart disease need medical clearance before exercising, persons who are at significant risk for coronary heart disease should also be evaluated by their physicians. Medical research has identified certain **risk factors** that are associated with increased likelihood of disease. Risk factors can be hereditary or the product of lifestyle, or a combination of the two. The more risk factors one possesses and the more severe they are, the greater the chance of having or developing the disease with which they are associated.

The most significant risk factors for a particular disease are termed **primary risk factors.** Less important risk factors are **secondary risk factors.** Generally accepted as primary risk factors for coronary heart disease are cigarette smoking, hypertension, and abnormal blood cholesterol levels (either high total cholesterol or low high-density lipoprotein [HDL] cholesterol). Secondary risk factors are obesity, age over 65, being male, family history of coronary heart disease in relatives younger than 65 years old, sedentary lifestyle, diabetes mellitus, and, possibly, psychosocial stress. A person with a risk-factor profile that indicates a significant possibility of coronary heart disease should, therefore, be evaluated by a physician before beginning an exercise program.

Name_____Date_____

Sex_____Age_____

What is the present state of your general health?

_____

Physician's Name_____

Physician's Telephone Number_____

Person to contact in case of an emergency?

Name_____Phone Number_____

Are you presently taking any medication?_____

Are you now or have you been pregnant within the past
three months?_____

Does your physician know you are participating in a dance-
exercise program?_____

Do you have now or have you
had within the past year: YES   NO

 1. A history of heart problems?   _____   _____

 2. High blood pressure?   _____   _____

 3. Difficulty with physical exercise?   _____   _____

 4. A chronic illness?   _____   _____

 5. Advice from a physician not
     to exercise?   _____   _____

 6. Muscle, joint, or back disorder
     that could be aggravated by
     physical activity?   _____   _____

 7. Recent surgery (within the
     past three months)?   _____   _____

 8. History of lung problems?   _____   _____

 9. Diabetes?   _____   _____

10. Cigarette-smoking habit?   _____   _____

11. Obesity (more than 20 pounds
     overweight)?   _____   _____

12. High blood cholesterol?   _____   _____

13. History of heart problems
     in immediate family?   _____   _____

What regular physical activity do you presently do?

_____

FIGURE 4-1 Sample Health History Form

Exercise may also present a health risk for persons with disorders of the lung, or pulmonary system, such as asthma, emphysema, or chronic bronchitis. Each of these conditions may result in dyspnea (difficult or labored breathing), making exercise difficult. Exercise may aggravate the condition for some people and improve the condition for others. The important point is that anyone with a disorder of the pulmonary system should have a medical evaluation before beginning or continuing an exercise program.

Similarly, people with disorders of the musculoskeletal system can experience difficulty with exercise, and exercise may aggravate their disorder. These disorders—involving any problem with muscles, joints, or the back—include arthritis, bursitis, and tendinitis. After proper medical evaluation, people with these conditions can usually participate in some type of exercise class, although a typical aerobics program may aggravate an existing condition. Some participants may be able to exercise in a standard class by modifying their activities in accordance with their physician's recommendations.

HEALTH SCREENING PROCESS

A health history form (see Fig. 4–1) contains information that should be obtained from participants before they begin an exercise class. Ideal forms are brief enough to be practical and simple enough that participants can complete them without referring to their medical records. The sample included here is only a model; it may be modified according to the needs of each program and the recommendations of that program's medical and legal advisers. The information on the form should be updated on a regular basis, for example, every 6–12 months, and whenever a participant has problems during an exercise program.

Information gathered by this process will help instructors become familiar with new participants. Information about current activity patterns, although not crucial to the health-screening process, will help instructors understand the participant's present fitness level and identify the most appropriate type of exercise program. It will also help instructors in deciding an appropriate rate of progression for each participant.

When a participant's health history or medical symptoms indicate a condition that would make exercise unsafe, referral to a physician for evaluation and clearance is appropriate. To facilitate communication between the instructor, the participant, and the physician, the instructor can submit a medical clearance form (see Fig. 4–2) to the physician that describes the class, including the mode and intensity of exercise, the duration of the class, and how often it meets. This approach helps the physician accurately assess the risks of a particular class for a certain participant. The instructor should keep the medical clearance in a file along with the health history records.

When an instructor notices any of the following risk factors, it is appropriate to refer the participant to a physician and to require a written medical clearance before the person begins or continues an exercise program:

Date_____

Dear Doctor:

   Your patient_____wishes to

exercise with_____exercise program. The

activity will involve the following:

   (type, frequency, duration and intensity of_____

   activities)_____

   If your patient is taking medications that will affect

his or her heart rate response to exercise, please indicate

the manner of the effect (raises, lowers or has no effect on

heart rate response): Type of medication_____

Effect_____

   Please identify any recommendations or restrictions that

are appropriate for your patient in this exercise program:

_____

_____

Thank you.
Sincerely,

Jane Jones
Super-Duper Aerobics
Address
Phone
- -

_____has my approval to exercise in

the_____program with the recommendations or

restrictions stated above.

   Signed_____Date_____

FIGURE 4-2 Sample Medical
Clearance Form

1. *Age over 40 years for men and over 45 for women.* Older participants will have increased risk of conditions that would make exercise hazardous or difficult.

2. *Pregnancy or childbirth within the previous 3 months.* It is important to obtain a written clearance from the participant's physician before allowing a pregnant or recently pregnant woman into a dance-exercise program (see Chapter 8).

3. *History of heart disease.* The eligibility of a participant with a history of heart problems depends on the type and severity of the condition. Heart conditions may range from inconsequential to severe, but any such history requires evaluation and clearance by the participant's physician.

4. *Hypertension (high blood pressure).* In general, participants with medically controlled high blood pressure will be allowed to exercise by their physicians. However, these participants should avoid exercises with significant isometric components. Such exercises may produce a potentially dangerous rise in blood pressure. Medications used to treat high blood pressure will be discussed later in this chapter.

5. *Past difficulty with physical exercise.* If the difficulty was mild, or if it is explainable by factors no longer present (e.g., pregnancy, anemia, or an infectious disease), referral to a physician may be appropriate, but it is not absolutely necessary.

6. *A chronic illness.*

7. *Advice from a physician not to exercise.*

8. *Musculoskeletal problems, including muscle, joint, or back disorders, that could be aggravated by physical activity.*

9. *Recent surgery (within the past 3 months).* The extensiveness of the surgical procedure, the patient's recovery, and the time since the surgery will be important in a physician's decision to allow or encourage exercise.

The presence of any of the following indicate that referral to a physician is appropriate, but not absolutely necessary.

1. *Age of 35–40 years old for men, 40–45 for women.* These people are in an age range in which medical referral is not absolutely necessary, but in which there begins to be a possibility (usually small) of problems with exercise.

2. *History of lung problems, including chronic bronchitis, emphysema, or asthma.*

3. *Diabetes mellitus.* Referral is especially important if the participant is receiving insulin. Diabetes mellitus, an abnormality of glucose metabolism, may be significantly benefited by regular exercise. However, each person's situation and exercise program should be discussed carefully with his or her physician to maximize the program's benefits and minimize the problems.

4. *Cigarette-smoking habit.*

5. *Obesity (over 20% above ideal weight, or over 30% body fat for women and over 23% body fat for men.)*

6. *High blood cholesterol.*

7. *History of heart problems in the immediate family.*

Persons with the last four characteristics have increased risk of heart disease, even if they have no symptoms. The risk increases with the severity of the factors. In other words, a person who smokes four packs of cigarettes per day is at greater risk than someone who smokes half a pack. In most cases referral to a physician may not be crucial, but in all cases it benefits the person, and so it is recommended.

In summary, medical clearance should be required for men over 40 years old, women over 45 years old or pregnant, and anyone answering yes to one of the first 7 questions on the health history form (Fig. 4–1). Medical referral should be carefully considered for men 35–40, women 40–45, and anyone answering yes to one of the questions 8 through 13 on the form.

The health screening process should also note any medications that class participants are taking. An instructor who knows which participants are taking medications can observe them carefully for exercise-related difficulties or unusual heart-rate responses. Certain situations may require further assessment. Instructors and studio owners should discuss their approach to medication-related issues with their program's medical consultants.

Once the health-history information has been collected, it should be used and not just filed away and forgotten. The information can be helpful in designing the dance-exercise class and providing support and guidance for participants. The information obtained from a health history form should be supplemented by observation of participants.

MEDICATIONS

Many participants in dance-exercise classes take prescription and non-prescription (over-the-counter) medications that affect their heart-rate response to exercise. These medications may be identified by the participant directly or by the health-screening process, or they may be brought to the instructor's attention when a participant has an unusual heart-rate response to exercise (15 or more beats per minute higher or lower than would be expected).

It is important to understand the effects of these medications on heart-rate response to assist participants in their exercise programs. A medication may be referred to by its manufacturer's brand name or by its scientific generic name. For example, Inderal is a brand name for the beta blocker propranolol. Lasix is a brand name for the diuretic furosemide. To understand the probable effects of a specific medication, an instructor needs to identify the general category to which it belongs. Table 4–1 shows the general effects of several categories of medications on heart-rate response. These are the typical effects that may be seen in most persons. To use the table, consult the participant, participant's physician, or a medical reference to find the correct category for a participant's medication.

When evaluating a participant's response to medications and exercise, it is important to remember that individual responses will vary. For example, the effects of many medications are dose related, which means that greater effects occur with larger doses. An important factor in this dose-related response is the time the medication was administered in relation to the exercise session. For instance, if a small dose of medication is taken a long time before an exercise session, the effect will probably be small. On the other hand, if a large dose is taken shortly before exercise, the effect will probably be larger. In addition,

AEROBIC DANCE-EXERCISE INSTRUCTOR MANUAL

Table 4-1

EFFECTS OF MEDICATIONS ON HEART-RATE (HR) RESPONSE

MEDICATIONS	RESTING HR	EXERCISE HR	MAXIMAL EXERCISING HR	COMMENTS
Beta-adrenergic blocking agents	↓	↓	↓	Dose-related response
Beta-adrenergic blocking agents with intrinsic sympathomimetic activity (ISA)	↔ or ↓	↓	↓	Dose-related response; decrease in resting HR is smaller than in beta blockers without ISA
Diuretics	↔	↔	↔	
Antihypertensives	↑, ↔ or ↓	↑, ↔ or ↓	usually ↔	Many antihypertensive medications are used. Some may decrease, a few may increase, and others do not affect heart rates. Some exhibit dose-related response.
Calcium-channel blockers	↑, ↔ or ↓	↑, ↔ or ↓	↓ or ↔	Variable & dose-related responses
Antihistamines	↔	↔	↔	
Cold medications: without SA / with SA	↔ / ↔ or ↑	↔ / ↔ or ↑	↔ / ↔	
Tranquilizers	↔, or if anxiety reduced may ↓	↔	↔	
Antidepressants and some antipsychotic medication	↔ or ↑	↔	↔	
Alcohol	↔ or ↑	↔ or ↑	↔	Exercise prohibited while under the influence; effects of alcohol on coordination increase possibility of injuries

EFFECTS OF MEDICATIONS ON HEART-RATE (HR) RESPONSE (continued)

MEDICATIONS	RESTING HR	EXERCISE HR	MAXIMAL EXERCISING HR	COMMENTS
Diet pills: With sympathomimetic activity (SA)	↑ or ↔	↑ or ↔	↔	Discourage as a poor approach to weight loss; acceptable only with physician's written approval
Containing amphetamines	↑	↑	↔	
Without sympathomimetic activity or amphetamines	↔	↔	↔	
Caffeine	↔ or ↑	usually ↔	↔	
Nicotine	↔ or ↑	↔ or ↑	↔	Discourage smoking; suggest lower target heart rate & exercise intensity for smokers

↑ = increase   ↔ = no significant change   ↓ = decrease

Note: Many medications are prescribed for conditions that do not require clearance. Don't forget other indicators of exercise intensity, e.g., participant's appearance, ratings of perceived exertion.

some classes of medications have variable effects. For instance, as shown in the table, **calcium-channel blocking drugs** may either increase, decrease, or have no effect on the heart rate. Therefore, while it is important to understand the general effects of different types of medications, it is equally important to remember that individual responses can vary widely.

BETA BLOCKERS   Among the most commonly administered medications are **beta-adrenergic blocking agents** or **beta blockers,** which may be used to treat a variety of cardiovascular and other disorders. These medications exert their effects by blocking beta-adrenergic receptors and, thus, limiting adrenergic (sympathetic) stimulation. In simpler terms, they block the effects of catecholamines (adrenalin or epinephrine and norepinephrine) throughout the body and reduce the resting, exercise, and maximal heart rates.

Patients have similar general responses to beta blockers. However, the size of the response may vary from patient to patient because beta blockers are competitive, reversible blockers of sympathetic activity.

Therefore, the effects are dose related (greater effects with higher doses of medication), temporary (usually lasting for hours), and dependent on a person's own catecholamine levels.

If an exerciser is taking a beta blocker as treatment for angina pectoris, high blood pressure, a previous heart attack, or abnormal heart rhythm, then medical clearance must be obtained before exercising. It is important to understand the effects of beta blockers because some exercise participants taking beta blockers will be appropriately cleared by their physicians. These medications are also used for conditions that do not require medical clearance, such as migraines and familial tremors. (See Chapter 9 for a discussion of appropriate ways to monitor heart rates for participants on beta blockers.)

DIURETICS **Diuretic** medications have no effect on the heart rate. However, because they produce excretion of water and electrolytes (including sodium) from the kidney, diuretics may decrease blood volume and, thus, predispose an exerciser to dehydration. Therefore, participants taking diuretics should be especially careful to maintain adequate fluid intake before, after, and sometimes during an exercise session. Fluid intake is especially important when exercise is prolonged or done in a warm, humid environment.

ANTIHYPERTENSIVES Several medications are available for treating hypertension, including beta-adrenergic blocking agents and calcium-channel blockers. As shown in Table 4–1, those medications can vary widely in their effects on heart-rate response. Any medication affecting the resting or exercising heart rate may require adjustment in desired target heart-rate range.

COLD MEDICATIONS Cold medications may contain an antihistamine or a medication with sympathomimetic activity or both. Those with antihistamines alone generally have no significant effect on heart rates. Those with sympathomimetic activity may increase heart rates at rest and possibly during exercise.

SUMMARY

Health screening is a crucial first step in maintaining the safety of a dance-exercise program. Health screening also enhances an instructor's credibility and opens lines of communication with physicians. After initial screening at the beginning of an exercise program, periodic reassessment is important. Instructors should use screening information when designing and conducting classes and should back up this information by careful observation. Any participant who is identified as at risk, either during the initial screening or as a result of symptoms exhibited during an exercise program, should be referred to a physician.

Components of an Aerobic Dance-Exercise Class

Karen Clippinger-Robertson

5

Karen Clippinger-Robertson, M.S.P.E., is a kinesiologist for Seattle Sports Medicine and a consultant to Pacific Northwest Ballet, the US Weightlifting Federation, and various fitness facilities. She has lectured nationally for such organizations as the Olympic Training Center and The International Symposium of Biomechanics in Sports, and she conducts fitness-instructor training programs for Seattle Sports Medicine and the Washington State Recreation and Parks Association.

IN THIS CHAPTER:

- Sequencing a dance-exercise class: AER-CAL versus CAL-AER.
- Warm-up: selecting exercises, progression.
- Aerobics: duration, intensity, content, progression.
- First cool-down: lowering the heart rate, preventing pooling of blood in extremities.

- Calisthenics: strength versus endurance, alignment and technique, selecting exercises, modifying intensity, sequence.
- Final cool-down: selecting flexibility exercises, modifying stretches, and progressing to include more muscle groups and more complex positions.

A dance-exercise class is intended to enhance physical fitness—to increase physical capacity so that overall health and quality of life improve. But to realize the potential gains from an aerobic dance-exercise class, which include improved cardiovascular endurance, body composition, flexibility, muscular endurance, and muscular strength, it is essential to design the class appropriately. Table 5–1 outlines a sample design for a dance-exercise class. This design, based on principles discussed in this chapter, serves as a guide that may be varied to meet specific class objectives or the needs of a particular group of participants.

CLASS FORMAT

Typically, a dance-exercise class begins with a warm-up, which generally uses movements with a low-to-moderate speed and range of motion. These movements are designed to promote body awareness and to increase blood flow to the muscles. An aerobics or calisthenics component follows the warm-up. The aerobics component, which is aimed at improving cardiovascular endurance and body composition,

AEROBIC DANCE-EXERCISE INSTRUCTOR MANUAL

Table 5–1

SAMPLE DANCE-EXERCISE CLASS DESIGN

COMPONENTS		EXAMPLES OF CONTENT
Warm-Up (5–10 minutes)	Isolation exercises	Neck flexion, neck rotation side-side, shoulder rotations, trunk flexion with pelvic tilts, hip isolations, knee flexion and extension, ankle circles, foot push-releases.
	Full body movements	Pliés, step-touches, step-touches with arm movements, side-reaches, small lunges, small lunges with increasing range arm movements.
	Flexibility exercises	Calf, hamstring, and low-back standing stretches.
Aerobics (20–30 minutes)	Aerobic warm-up	Step-touches, touch-backs, heel-touches, knee lifts and light jogging with arms increasing in range of motion.
	Peak aerobics	Jogging with full arm movements, side leg-kicks, lunges with full arm movement, knee lifts with hops, 3-step kick with traveling.
	Aerobic cool-down	Same as aerobic warm-up, (i.e., movements with less traveling, less range in leg and arm movements, less impact, slower tempo).
Cool-Down I (5–20 minutes)	Large, rhythmical movements	Rhythmical movements, such as walking or pliés, to aid in returning blood to the heart, but at a low enough intensity to allow heart rate to gradually decrease toward a resting level.
Calisthenics (15–20 minutes)	Trunk exercise	Abdominal curl-ups.
	Upper extremity exercises	Push-ups, posterior shoulder exercise.
	Lower extremity exercises	Hip flexor and quadriceps strengthening (front leg-lift), hip abductor exercise (side leg-lift), hip adductor exercise (side leg-pull), hip extensor exercise (back leg-lift), tibialis anterior exercise, tibialis posterior exercise, and peroneal exercise.
Cool-Down II (7–10 minutes)	Flexibility exercises	Flexibility routine shown in Figure 5–35 including stretches for the hamstrings, hip adductors, shoulder extensors, hip abductors, low back, quadriceps femoris, hip flexors, gastrocnemius and soleus.

uses large body movements performed continuously so that the heart rate stays elevated. Following the aerobic workout, a cool-down gradually reduces the heart-rate toward resting levels and prevents excessive pooling of blood in the lower extremities. A calisthenics component generally includes exercises designed to increase muscular endurance or strength in specific muscles. Some exercises, such as the biceps curl, may isolate and exercise a single muscle group, while others, such as the push-up, involve several muscle groups. The class ends with a further cool-down, which include stretching and relaxation exercises designed to lower the heart rate further, help prevent muscle soreness, enhance flexibility, and reestablish the body's equilibrium.

Emphasis

Although the four components—warm-up, aerobics, calisthenics, and cool-down—are common to most dance-exercise classes, the emphasis given to each will vary depending on the objective of a particular class, as well as the fitness level, age, health, and physical skill of its participants. For example, a class for previously sedentary people may emphasize the calisthenics portion while reducing the duration and intensity of the aerobics section. This approach could decrease the possibility of injury by increasing flexibility and muscular strength to prepare the body for the stresses of aerobics. Another class with a primary objective of changing body composition might emphasize the aerobics segment because the longer duration of aerobic exercise helps to metabolize fat (Pollock, Wilmore, and Fox 1984). The young or extremely fit may benefit from a 1½-hour class that includes a 30–45 minute aerobics segment as well as a rigorous calisthenics section that uses resistance to enhance overload. With elderly or obese people, a long, slow cool-down is advisable.

Sequence

An area of continuing controversy in dance exercise, about which we have little evidence at present, is whether it is better to place the calisthenics segment before or after the aerobics segment. The two sequences are outlined in Table 5–2. Proponents of calisthenics first (CAL-AER) argue that calisthenics extend the warm-up, thus allowing the body to accommodate gradually to the increased workload of the aerobics segment (Gerson 1985). They also argue that this sequence can alleviate the potential problem of postural hypotension. During exercise, there is a tremendous increase in blood flow to the working muscles. A change in position, especially raising the head above the heart by standing up after floor exercises, can result in hypotension (a drop in blood pressure). The decreased blood flow to the brain can cause dizziness or faintness. Some proponents of CAL-AER also argue that fatigue after the aerobics segment could lead to poor technique and greater risk of injury during calisthenics. Others feel that because glycogen stores are used during calisthenics, the body will begin metabolizing fat sooner during aerobics. At this time, there is insufficient data to substantiate these arguments and more research is needed.

Proponents of aerobics first (AER-CAL) argue that calisthenics may fatigue the large muscles enough to increase the risk of injury during the faster pace of aerobics. In the author's experience, most dance-exercise injuries result from overuse during aerobics rather than during

AEROBIC DANCE-EXERCISE INSTRUCTOR MANUAL

Table 5-2

CLASS SEQUENCING

CAL-AER CLASS	AER-CAL CLASS
Warm-up	Warm-up
Calisthenics	Aerobics
Aerobics	Warm-up
Warm-up	Peak
Peak	Cool-down*
Cool-down*	Cool-Down I**
Cool-Down I**	Calisthenics
Cool-Down II***	Cool-Down II***

*Reduce intensity to lower heart rate to low end of target heart-rate zone.

**Rhythmic movements to lower heart rate to 120 beats per minute or less.

***Stretching and relaxation.

calisthenics. Some proponents of AER-CAL (Jones 1985) believe that this sequence produces a slightly greater cardiovascular benefit and use of calories. When the heart rate has been elevated to the target zone by aerobic exercise, it may remain sufficiently elevated during part of the calisthenics to provide a greater aerobic benefit and caloric expenditure than would occur if the calisthenics were performed first. Individual class design might make the difference in this respect. For example, a calisthenics section that began by using large muscle groups (such as hip, thigh, or trunk) and emphasizing muscular endurance might be more likely to provide these benefits than one that began with smaller muscle groups (ankles, arms) or one that emphasized slow repetitions with holds that would allow the heart rate to fall rapidly. Further investigation is needed to see if these hypothesized benefits actually occur, and if so, if the gains they offer are large enough to have any practical significance.

Because so little scientific evidence is available to decide this issue of sequencing aerobics and calisthenics, instructors should stay abreast of the issue as further information accumulates, and in the meantime, carefully evaluate the alternatives for their own programs and participants. For purposes of illustration, this chapter will follow the AER-CAL sequence.

In addition to appropriate sequencing of class components, it is important to design the movements within each component for safe and effective class development. An instructor who understands the purpose of each component and the physiological stress needed to produce desired changes can design movements that effectively produce these changes instead of simply increasing repetitions. The reader may want to refer to Chapter 2 for illustrations and descriptions of the muscles and joints referred to in the following discussion.

WARM-UP

The purpose of the **warm-up** is to prepare the body for the more rigorous demands of the aerobics and calisthenics segments by raising the internal temperature. For each degree of temperature elevation, the metabolic rate of the cells increases by about 13% (Astrand and Rodahl 1977). In addition, at higher body temperatures, blood flow to the working muscles increases, as does the release of oxygen to the muscles. Because these effects allow more efficient energy production to fuel muscle contraction, the goal of an effective warm-up should be to elevate internal temperatures one or two degrees, so that sweating occurs.

Increase in temperature has other effects that are beneficial for exercisers, as well. The physiological benefits of warm-up include

- higher metabolic rate
- increased blood flow to muscles
- higher rate of oxygen exchange between blood and muscles
- more oxygen released within muscles
- faster nerve impulse transmission
- decreased muscle relaxation time following contraction
- increased speed and force of muscle contraction
- increased muscle elasticity
- rehearsal effect (the body practices muscular patterns to be used later)
- reduced risk of abnormal electrocardiogram
- increased flexibility of tendons and ligaments

Many of these physiological effects may reduce the risk of injury because they have the potential to increase neuromuscular coordination, delay fatigue, or make the tissues less susceptible to damage (Astrand and Rodahl 1977, Shellock 1983).

Selecting Exercises

Practically speaking, in a typical 1-hour class, the warm-up will last 5–10 minutes. Initial movements should use a small range of motion that can gradually increase as the body warms. For example, the early part of the warm-up might use small knee-lifts but not high kicks with the knee extended.

SPECIFICITY. Movements in the warm-up should specifically prepare the body for movements used in the aerobics routines. Specificity not only insures that the appropriate muscles are warmed up, but it also provides a **rehearsal effect.** That is, the neuromuscular system has a chance to practice or rehearse muscular patterns similar to those used in later parts of the class. This rehearsal effect may enhance performance and reduce injury (DeVries 1966). For example, the warm-up for a low-impact class that uses a lot of arm exercises would include movements to prepare the shoulders and arms. In contrast, a high-impact class would include exercises for the ankles and feet, such as push-releases, which replicate the movements needed for jumping and landing. The push-release (see Fig. 5–1) begins with the weight of the body forward, supported mostly by the foot in front. The exerciser

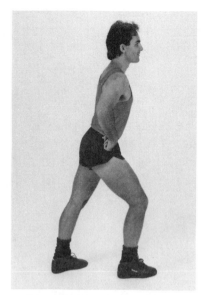 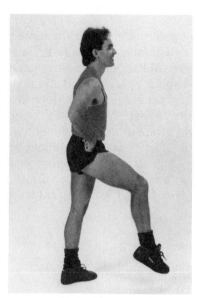 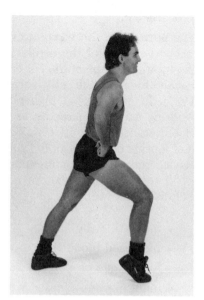

a. Start with foot flat and body weight forward.

b. Push off the floor, raising the foot slightly.

c. Land gently on toe and roll back onto ball and then heel of foot. Repeat.

FIGURE 5-1 Push-releases

forcefully pushes away from the floor while pointing the toe (ankle plantar flexion), so that the foot rises slightly off the floor. The exerciser then gradually lowers the body weight, using controlled movement, emphasizing eccentric use of the ankle plantar flexors and the intrinsic foot muscles.

BODY ISOLATION. Although specificity is important, a common error in the warm-up is to overemphasize body isolation and flexibility exercises. Many classes begin with a series of isolation movements, such as forward head rolls (without rolling the head back into hyperextension), shrugs, shoulder rolls, and torso twists. Although these exercises are useful to begin with and to increase kinesthetic awareness, they should progress to movements that use more muscle mass so that internal body temperature rises.

STRETCHES. Like body isolations, stretches are insufficient to elevate internal temperature. There is also less discomfort, less risk of injury, and probably greater gain in flexibility when stretching is performed after the muscles have warmed up. Hence, stretches are probably most effective after an initial warm-up and/or after the aerobics or calisthenics segments. One approach using the AER-CAL format is to include stretches at the end of the warm-up for the muscle groups that will be most challenged by the aerobics section. For example, most dance-exercise classes challenge the calf, hamstring, and low-back muscles, and so stretches for these three areas can be done before the aerobics, leaving the rest of the stretching for the end of class when the muscles are thoroughly warmed. Classes using a lot of lunges or other movements challenging hip flexor extensibility can include stretches for the hip flexors, including the quadriceps femoris.

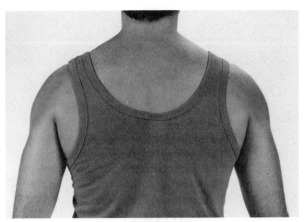

a. Begin with shoulders relaxed and arms hanging.

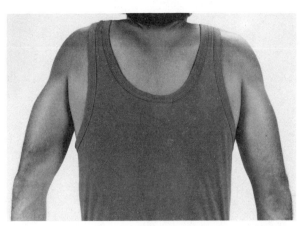

b. Shoulder shrugs: Bring shoulders up, elevating shoulder blades, and then lower.

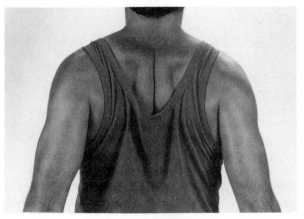

c. Shoulder rolls: Bring shoulders up, pull the shoulders back and down.

FIGURE 5–2 Shoulder shrugs and shoulder rolls

Progression

One way to meet the various criteria for the warm-up is to organize it into three phases. The first phase uses small, isolated movements intended primarily to increase kinesthetic awareness, or help participants shift from their previous activities and focus on their bodies. These movements, which begin to increase blood flow to the contracting muscles, include side-to-side neck rotations, shoulder shrugs (Fig. 5–2a, b), shoulder rolls (Fig. 5–2c), hip isolations, ankle circles, and pelvic tilts (Fig. 5–3). Pelvic tilts can provide practice for correct postural alignment throughout the rest of the class. It is usually easier for participants to follow movements that flow in sequence, either from head to toe or from toe to head.

From the first phase, movements should progress to include more muscle groups simultaneously and, thus, elevate internal body temperature. During the second phase, movements can include pliés (knee bends), side reaches, step-touches, and heel-touches. The second phase,

AEROBIC DANCE-EXERCISE INSTRUCTOR MANUAL

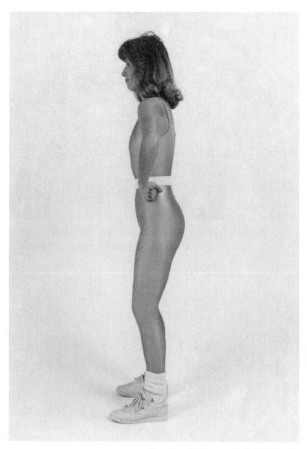

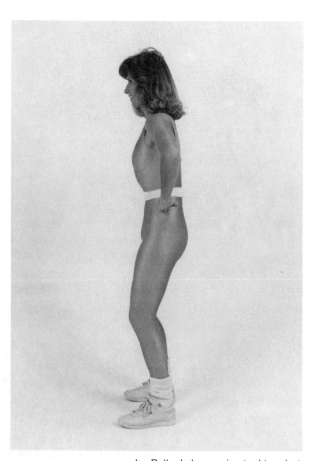

a. Begin with knees slightly bent, hands on waist.

b. Pull abdomen in, tucking buttocks under.

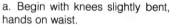

FIGURE 5–3 Pelvic tilt

with movements that are slower and simpler than during peak aerobics, is a perfect time to emphasize correct alignment and technique. Because the body is not yet prepared to generate or absorb large forces, movements should be limited in impact and range of motion. Exercises such as deep lunges, jumping jacks, or single-leg jumps are inappropriate. As the warm-up proceeds, movements can build both in range of motion and complexity, always being carefully selected to prepare the body for the specific challenges of the particular class.

A short series of stretches compose the last phase of the warm-up. In the AER-CAL format, many instructors prefer standing stretches (see Fig. 5–4) so that the class can move easily into aerobics. Stretches for the low back, hamstrings, and calf muscles are especially important. With any standing stretch, the hands may be used to help support the upper body by placing them on the thighs or on a wall, chair, or barre. To perform the low-back stretch (Fig. 5–4a), round the low back by using the abdominal muscles to produce an extreme posterior pelvic tilt. To perform the hamstring stretch (Fig. 5–4b), lean forward at the waist over the front leg, which is extended. Be sure to use the hands for support so that the low back bears less stress. To perform the gastrocnemius stretch (Fig. 5–4c), keep the rear foot straight and the heel on the ground as the body weight shifts forward over the front foot. Shifting the weight slightly to the back and bending the back knee will modify this stretch to stretch the soleus muscle (Fig. 5–4d).

FIGURE 5–4 Standing stretches

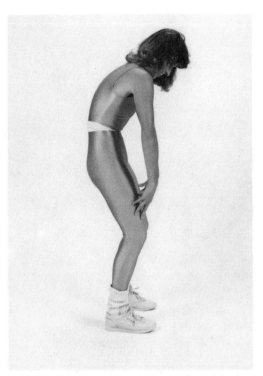

a. Low-back stretch: Round the low back by using the abdominal muscles to produce an extreme posterior pelvic tilt.

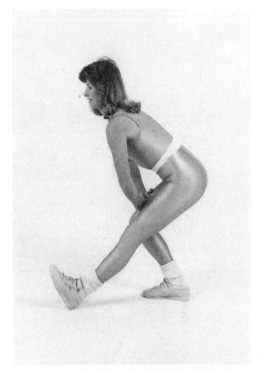

b. Hamstring stretch: Extend one leg and lean forward at the waist, using the hands for support.

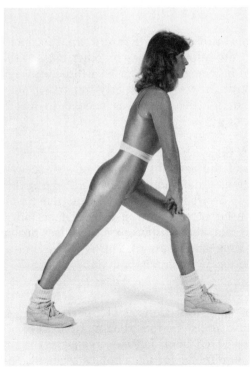

c. Gastrocnemius stretch: Keep the rear foot straight and the heel on the ground. Shift the body weight forward over the front foot.

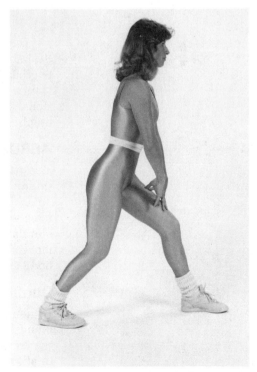

d. Soleus stretch: Shift the weight slightly to the back and bend the back knee.

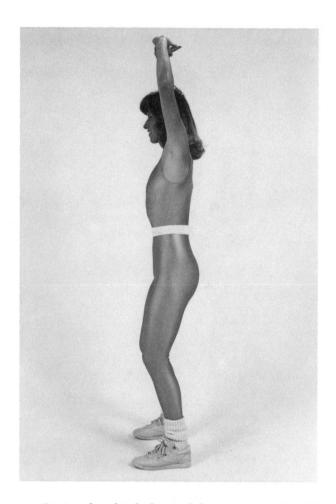

FIGURE 5–5 Shoulder extensor stretch: Flex the knees slightly and bring arms overhead with palms up. Pull arms back behind head, being careful not to arch the back or drop the head.

During this third phase of the warm-up, shoulder stretches are also desirable for low-impact classes or other classes that use many full overhead arm movements. Figure 5–5 illustrates a shoulder extensor stretch, effective for this particularly important muscle group. Additional stretches may be added as needed to meet specific choreographic demands.

AEROBICS

The purpose of the aerobics segment of a dance-exercise class is to improve cardiovascular endurance by challenging the heart and lungs. To achieve this desired effect, participants must maintain their heart rates within a target zone for an extended period. To maintain this elevated heart rate, **aerobic dance-exercise** uses prolonged, continuous movement of large muscle groups. This type of exercise can also improve body composition by reducing body fat.

Duration

Although the American College of Sports Medicine (1978) recommends aerobic-exercise periods ranging from 15 to 60 minutes, within the constraints of a 1-hour dance-exercise class it usually works well to allow 20–30 minutes for the aerobics segment. At least 20 minutes is needed to burn enough calories and apply sufficient stimulus to improve body composition and cardiovascular fitness while working at a safe intensity. Usually a maximum of 30 minutes is recommended for the basic dance-exercise class. In that time, participants achieve cardiovascular benefits (assuming they are working at appropriate intensities) and reduce their risk for musculoskeletal injury.

For some specialized classes the duration of the aerobics segment may be extended. For example, a longer duration—approximately 40 minutes—at a lower intensity would be appropriate for a class with a primary goal of improving body composition. Some studios offer a 90-minute class for persons who are very healthy and fit, and in these cases, a longer aerobics segment of 40–50 minutes may be appropriate. However, with these longer durations, careful medical screening, meticulous class design, and gradual increase in intensity are essential to avoid musculoskeletal injury. One study found that musculoskeletal injuries to the lower body doubled when a 30-minute aerobics segment was increased to 45 minutes in walk-jog-run programs for beginners (Pollock et al. 1977).

Intensity

For safe and effective cardiovascular gains, most experts recommend exercising at an intensity of 60%–80% of maximum heart-rate reserve (see Chapter 9 for a detailed discussion of target ranges and heart-rate monitoring techniques). Although 60%, the threshold necessary for cardiovascular improvement, is a helpful guide, it is important to understand that fitness gains will be affected by the initial fitness of each participant. Cardiovascular gains occur in unfit persons at exercise intensities lower than 60%, while the fit exerciser often has to work at higher intensities to show significant improvement (Pollock, Wilmore, and Fox 1984). As the upper range of the recommended intensities is approached or surpassed, risk increases for musculo-skeletal injury and cardiovascular symptoms, while participant compliance decreases. Therefore, in a recreational dance-exercise class it is best to avoid the higher intensities. Pollock, Wilmore, and Fox (1984) recommend an intensity in the lower to middle range for beginning, asymptomatic adults, and Neiman (1986) recommends that only people in excellent physical condition work at an intensity in the upper portion of the range.

It is total workload (energy expenditure) that determines cardiovascular improvement. Thus, positive gains can accumulate from either long duration at low intensity or shorter duration at higher intensity. It is the combination of exercise intensity and duration that counts. Considering that medical histories are often incomplete and that it is difficult to individualize classes adequately, it seems prudent for an instructor to aim for a moderate combination of exercise duration and intensity in the dance-exercise class. Encouragingly, recent studies have found that exercise sessions of 30 minutes duration, at a moderate intensity, 3–5 times per week, can increase aerobic fitness and provide significant protection from heart disease (Cooper 1982).

Participants need to know what their target zones are and how to alter their heart-rate response, or intensity. For example, to lower intensity, they can limit the range of motion of their movements or eliminate the arm motions of an exercise. As shown in Figure 5–6, the intensity of an exercise can be reduced by lifting the knee less (sequence a) or by reducing or eliminating the arm movements (sequence b). Intensity can be further reduced by traveling less and removing the hop.

FIGURE 5–6 Decreasing movement intensity

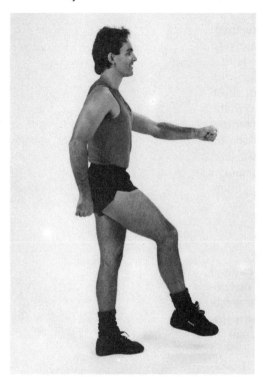

a. Low intensity: Use low kicks instead of high kicks.

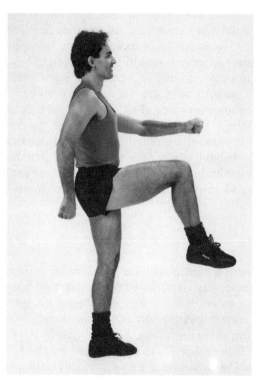

High-intensity.

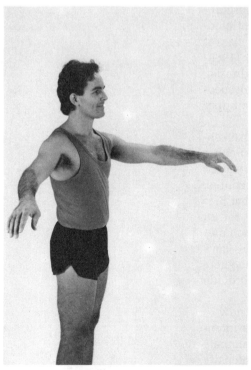

b. Low intensity: Lower the arms from shoulder height instead of from overhead.

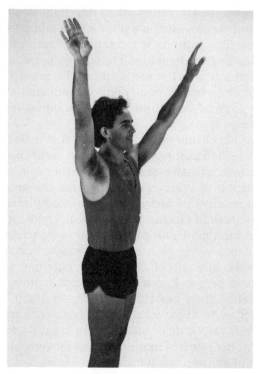

High-intensity.

FIGURE 5–7 Aerobic routine using varied arm movements while jogging

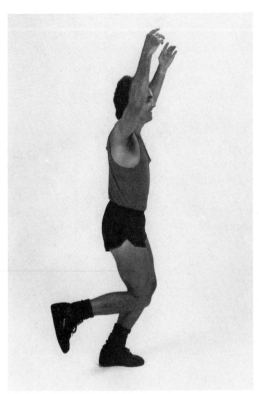

a. Shoulder flexion/extension

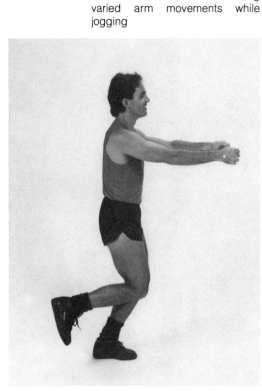

b. Shoulder transverse abduction/ adduction

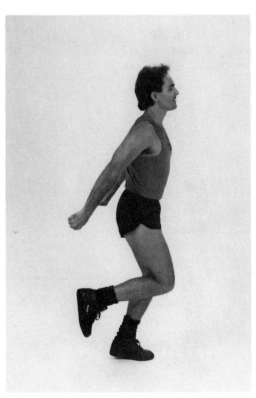

c. Shoulder hyperextension/flexion

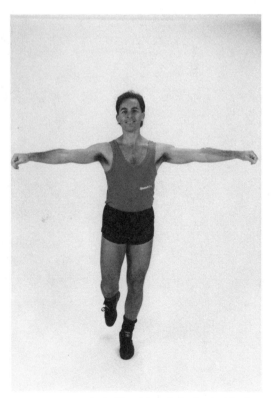

d. Shoulder abduction/adduction

AEROBIC DANCE-EXERCISE INSTRUCTOR MANUAL

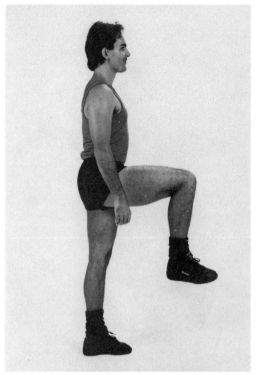

FIGURE 5–8 Front knee-lifts work the hip flexors.

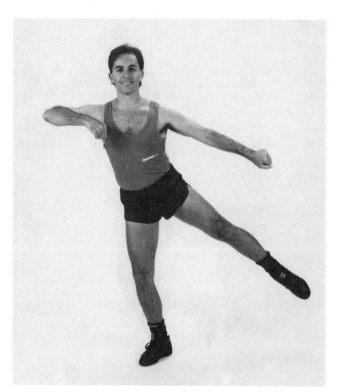

FIGURE 5–9 Side kicks work the hip abductors.

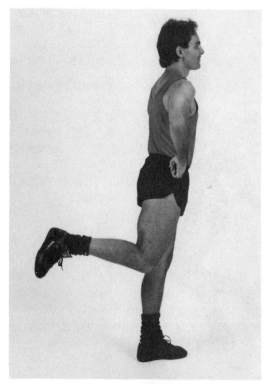

FIGURE 5–10 Back knee-curls work the hamstring muscles.

Content

Many aerobics routines are built from basic movements such as walks, runs (jogs), skips, hops, and jumps. Figure 5–7 presents variations of arm movements combined with jogging in place: in (a) the arms rise overhead and then lower to the sides (shoulder flexion, extension); in (b) the arms cross in front at shoulder level (transverse adduction, abduction); in (c) the arms press back and then return to the front (shoulder hyperextension, flexion); and in (d) the arms rise sideways to shoulder height and then lower again to the sides (shoulder abduction, adduction). Additional variety can come from adding traditional dance steps, such as the Charleston, hustle, swing, polka, or pony.

When building such routines, the instructor should use a balance of muscle groups, including movements to the front, back, sides, and on various diagonals. Arms and legs should work all actions possible at the involved joints; for example, flexion, extension, abduction, adduction, circumduction, and rotation at the hip and shoulder. In designing hip movements, most instructors have a tendency to emphasize the hip flexors with exercises such as front knee-lifts (Fig. 5–8), and to forget the importance of movements such as side kicks (Fig. 5–9) that work the hip abductors and back knee curls (Fig. 5–10) that work the hamstrings. With the arms there is a similar tendency to use front and overhead movements excessively. It is important to work the arms backward (hyperextension, shown in Fig. 5–7c) and rotate them, as well. Including movements on diagonal planes will also incorporate varied muscle groups.

In designing the content of the aerobics segment, movement sequence is another important consideration. Certain movements, such as lunges or jumps that take off and land from the same leg, place large stresses on the joints. Although athletes sometimes use such movements in extreme forms to develop power, as, for example, when they jump for height or distance, or when they lunge with weights, these movements require great strength and they place the inadequately conditioned person at great risk for injury. With the wide range of fitness, age, injury history, and skill among participants in most fitness classes, it is best to leave the development of power to the closely supervised athletic arena. In dance-exercise classes, such movements should be modified. For example, lunges should be limited to 90 degrees and the height of jumps should be reduced. These movements can also be performed with limited repetitions or alternated with exercises that are less rigorous or that challenge different muscle groups. When the fitness routine alternates stresses (Fig. 5–11), it allows muscles enough recovery time to avoid the failure point where injury occurs.

Progression

The intensity of the aerobics section should vary. Like the warm-up, it may be thought of in three phases: the aerobic warm-up, peak aerobics, and the aerobic cool-down.

AEROBIC WARM-UP.   The aerobic warm-up allows the cardiovascular system to adjust gradually to the increasing exercise demands; it also prepares the musculoskeletal system. In contrast with the earlier warm-up at the beginning of class, the aerobic warm-up avoids isolation movements and instead emphasizes continuous movements that involve large muscle mass and that increase internal temperatures along with

AEROBIC DANCE-EXERCISE INSTRUCTOR MANUAL

FIGURE 5–11 Alternate stresses by choosing exercises that challenge different muscle groups.

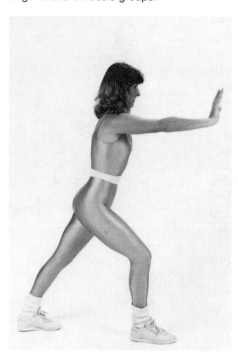

a. Lunges (knee stresses)

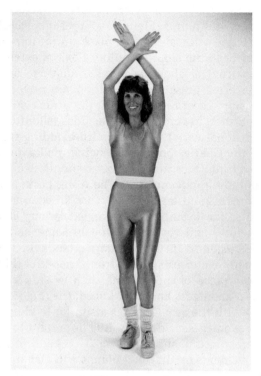

b. Rigorous overhead movements (shoulder stresses)

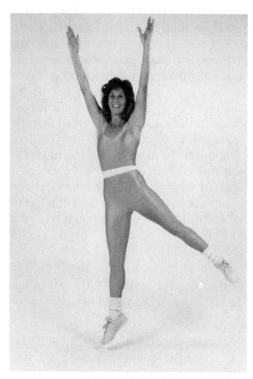

c. Jumps (lower-leg stresses) to each side

Components of an Aerobic Dance-Exercise Class

FIGURE 5-12 Aerobic warm-up movements

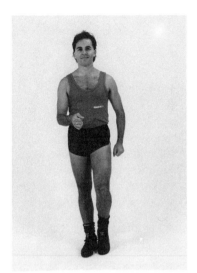

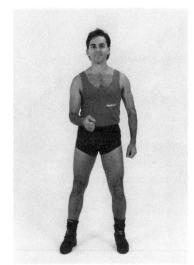

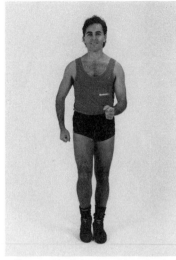

a. Step-touches: Begin with weight on right foot.

Step to side with left foot.

Close with right, touching the ball of the foot to the floor. Reverse.

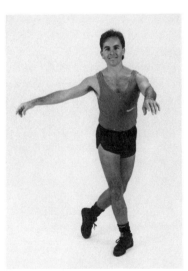

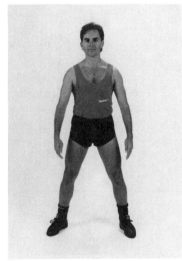

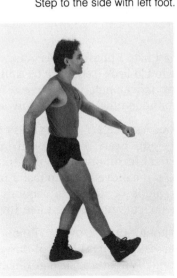

Step to the side with left foot.

Bring the right foot back. Repeat.

b. Touch-backs: Begin with weight on the right foot and the left foot touching back.

c. Heel-touches: Alternate heel touches in front of the body.

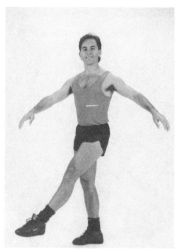

a. Low intensity: Low kick

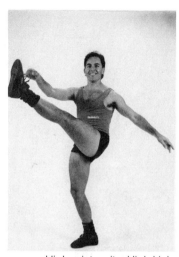

Higher intensity: High kick

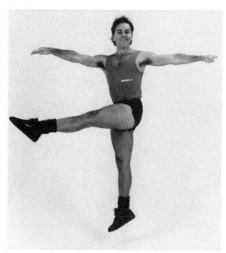

Highest intensity: Kick with a jump

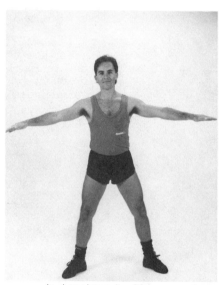

b. Low intensity: Move arms from shoulder height in jumping jacks.

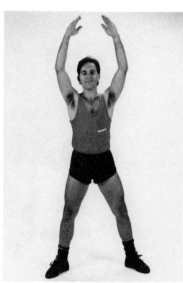

High intensity: Move arms from overhead.

FIGURE 5–13 Increasing movement intensity

heart rate. Appropriate exercises (Fig. 5–12) include step-touch (sequence a), touch-back (sequence b), and heel-touch (sequence c)—all with small arm movements. In all these foot-touches, one foot is always on the ground, so that impact is low and range of motion is low to moderate.

PEAK AEROBICS. As the class moves into the aerobics segment, intensity and heart rates should build gradually. The instructor can use several techniques to build intensity (Fig. 5–13), such as performing the same movements to faster music, adding more traveling steps, adding hops or jumps (a sequence), or using larger arm movements (b sequence) and deeper knee flexion.

AEROBIC COOL-DOWN. Frequently shortchanged in dance-exercise classes, the **aerobic cool-down** allows the cardiovascular system to gradually reestablish equilibrium at a lower intensity. The instructor

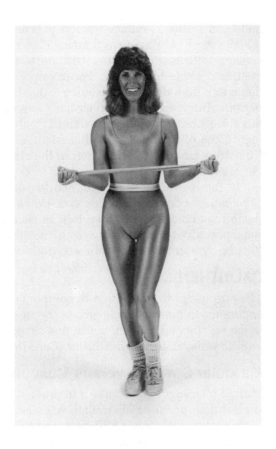

FIGURE 5–14 A Cool-Down I exercise: The legs make small side-to-side step-touches, while the arms perform external rotation using surgical tubing for resistance.

can reduce intensity gradually by progressively reducing range of motion, traveling, impact, and amount of muscle masses used. By the end of the aerobic cool-down, heart rate should be lowered to the low end of the target heart-rate range. The aerobic cool-down provides a smooth transition into the class cool-down, which, for the purpose of clarity, this chapter refers to as Cool-Down I.

COOL-DOWN I

In the AER-CAL sequence, the **cool-down** following the aerobics component is often incorporated into the beginning of the calisthenics component (see Table 5–2). However, because cardiac complications most often occur with the cessation of exercise, this part of the workout is being addressed separately to emphasize its importance. Appropriately designed, the cool-down will continue to lower the heart rate to 120 beats per minute or below and help to prevent excessive pooling of blood in the lower extremities, reduce muscle soreness, and promote faster removal of metabolic wastes (Astrand and Rodahl 1977; Pollock, Wilmore, and Fox 1984).

The music is slower and the range of motion is smaller than in the aerobics component. Movements in which the head is lowered below the heart and then raised again should be avoided because these movements may cause dizziness. The cool-down is an appropriate time for upper-body strengthening, using surgical tubing or weights, while the legs make simple and small movements such as demi-pliés or step-touches (Fig. 5–14). The rhythmic contractions of the legs act as an important muscle pump to help return blood from the lower extremities to the heart. Without such activity, blood pooling in the lower body can result in reduced blood pressure, dizziness, and (in exceptional cases) cardiac arrhythmias. This pooling can be of particular concern with sustained isometric contractions of the legs, because isometrics occlude blood flow. For example, some instructors direct students to hold a deep plié (isometric quadriceps work) for an extended period while performing upper-body exercises. Instead of maintaining this fixed position, exercisers should rhythmically flex and extend their legs in the plié or else use other small, simple, rhythmic movements. Isometrics are better placed later in the class after sufficient cool-down has been achieved.

In the AER-CAL sequence, another cool-down period follows the calisthenics component. This cool-down (Cool-Down II) emphasizes flexibility and relaxation exercises. In classes that follow the CAL-AER sequence, Cool-Down I (lowering the heart rate) and Cool-Down II (flexibility and relaxation) directly follow each other.

CALISTHENICS

The purpose of the **calisthenics** component is to improve strength and endurance in major muscle groups. Some instructors include stretches in the calisthenics section, but in this chapter, stretches will be included with the discussion of flexibility (Cool-Down II).

Muscular Strength versus Muscular Endurance

Muscular strength is important to prevent injuries, and several studies suggest that increases in strength will also produce moderate increases in muscular endurance (Anderson and Kearney 1982; Fox 1984). However, exercise regimes designed to increase muscular endurance do not seem as effective for improving strength. With the information presently available, it seems more efficient and effective to design the calisthenics routine for increasing strength (fewer repetitions at higher resistance) instead of for increasing endurance (more repetitions at lower resistance). For example, it now appears that performing many consecutive abdominal curls does not produce adequate gains in strength. Many athletes and aerobics instructors who perform hundreds of abdominal crunches daily still test out weak in their abdominal muscles (Clippinger-Robertson 1986). Of 88 aerobics instructors recently tested, 89% scored inadequately on standard physical-therapy strength tests (Kendall, Kendall, and Wadsworth 1971) for the abdominals.

The challenge is to design class exercises with enough overload that muscle fatigue can be reached and strength gains achieved within less than about 15 repetitions. In traditional strength training, athletes achieve adequate overload by adding external resistance, such as free weights, wall pulleys, or weight apparatus. Dance-exercisers can usually increase overload adequately by using slower repetitions, greater range of motion, more difficult exercise variations, holds, or external resistance such as light weights, surgical tubing, or elastic bands.

Abdominal curls can illustrate several ways of increasing overload by making an exercise more difficult. Many people who routinely perform 100 curls can achieve better results with fewer repetitions. These people can often achieve muscle fatigue in about 10 repetitions when they perform the curls slowly and increase the height, perhaps to 20 degrees. The waist should remain on the floor for safety (Fig. 5-15a). Another way of increasing difficulty is to add holds at one or more arcs (Fig. 5-15b). The exerciser can curl up to 10 degrees, hold for 5

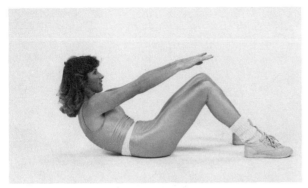

a. Increase the range of motion.

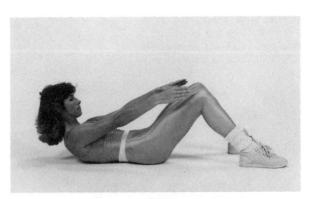

b. Add a 5-count hold at 10–20 degrees of trunk flexion.

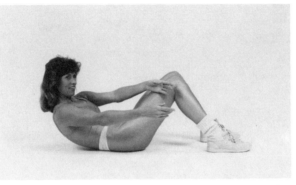

c. Add rotation.

FIGURE 5–15 Increasing overload in curl-ups

counts, curl up farther to about 20 degrees, hold for another 5 counts, gradually curl back down to the floor, and immediately curl up again, repeating the whole exercise 5–10 times. Adding rotation also increases difficulty (Fig. 5–15c). The exerciser curls up to about 20 degrees and rotates to the side, keeping the pelvis stationary as the torso rotates. The opposite shoulder should come up and around to encourage use of abdominal instead of back muscles for rotation. After holding this rotated position for several counts, the exerciser rotates to the other side, rotates back to the center, and then lowers the trunk carefully to the floor.

In making the decision to emphasize muscular strength over muscular endurance, the safety and the specific needs of the class must be considered. For example, adding holds, with the associated elevation of blood pressure, may cause problems for seniors, pregnant women, or exercisers with heart disease. Adding weights may endanger pregnant women or students with arthritis. One approach is to use exercise at higher resistance only in intermediate or advanced, unrestricted classes. Another approach is to add higher resistance to exercises after a 6–10 week conditioning period that uses lower resistance. A third approach is to combine higher and lower resistance in exercises. For example, abdominal strengthening might consist of two sets of 10 repetitions of a difficult version, emphasizing muscular strength, followed by a third set of 30 repetitions of an easier version, emphasizing muscular endurance. With any approach, exercises using high resistance must be appropriate for the participants in the specific class. Instructors should encourage participants to work carefully at their individual fitness levels and with proper technique.

FIGURE 5–16 Maintaining correct alignment: Use the adominals to stabilize the trunk and pelvis to avoid distortions such as arching the low back.

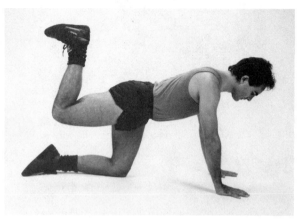

a. Back leg-lifts with correct alignment.

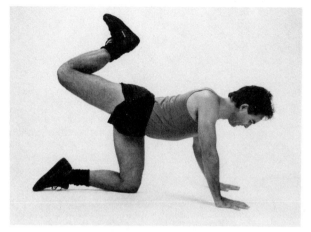

Incorrect alignment.

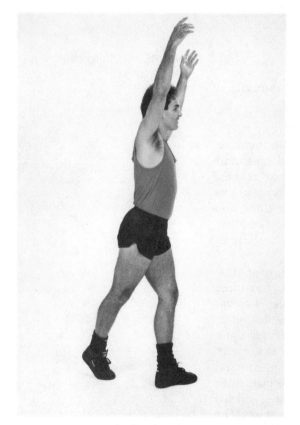

b. Overhead arm movements with correct alignment.

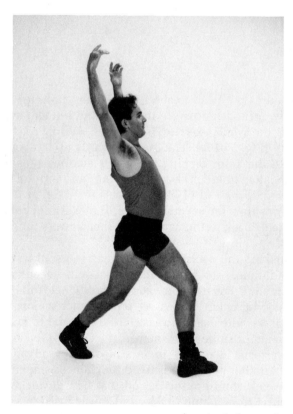

Incorrect alignment.

Components of an Aerobic Dance-Exercise Class

FIGURE 5–17 Side leg-lifts

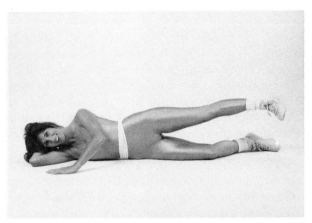

a. Correct: Proper pelvic-spinal alignment.

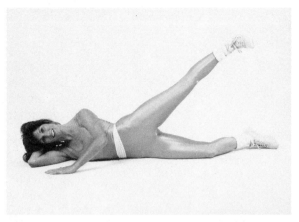

b. Incorrect: Tilting the hip laterally, a common compensation.

FIGURE 5–18 Donkey kick

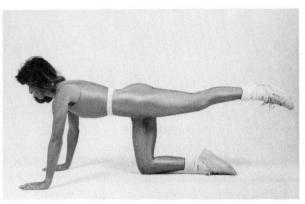

a. Correct alignment: A small range (about 15 degrees of hip extension) and adequate abdominal stabilization.

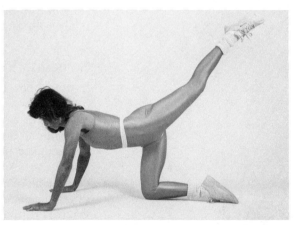

b. Incorrect alignment: Excessive hyperextension of the spine.

Alignment and Technique

Although certain exercises—the plough, the windmill, double-leg raises, the hurdler's stretch—are inherently too risky for a dance-exercise class, almost any exercise can be potentially dangerous if performed with poor alignment and technique. With most exercises, the manner in which they are performed is the critical issue. If instructors understand the correct execution of exercises, anticipate common errors, and cue effectively so that participants can achieve correct form, they reduce considerably the risk of injury in their classes.

One common source of error is the tendency to "cheat" by substituting other muscles as fatigue increases. The resulting musculoskeletal compensation can both cause injury and interfere with desired gains in muscular strength or endurance. To avoid this error, the exerciser must maintain trunk and pelvic stability as well as the movement pattern that uses the correct muscles. Trunk and pelvic stability can generally be achieved through contraction of the abdominal muscles or, in some cases, co-contraction of both the abdominals and the back extensors. After attaining this pelvic and spinal alignment, the goal is to maintain it throughout the exercise without letting the pelvis tilt forward (arching the low back) or allowing excessive lateral pelvic tilt in exercises such as back leg lifts (Fig. 5–16a) and exercises using overhead arm movements (Fig. 5–16b). A subtle change in position can have a dramatic effect on muscle use and body stresses. For example, a common error in performing side leg lifts (Fig. 5–17a) is to allow lateral tilting of the pelvis (Fig. 5–17b), which permits the lateral trunk flexors to assist with the movement, thus reducing the desired load to the hip abductors. This lateral tilt also produces large stresses in the low-back region. Correct technique often requires reducing the range of motion, the repetitions, and the speed, so that the appropriate muscles can stabilize the pelvis and spine, preventing undesired movement. For example, with the donkey kick (Fig. 5–18a), only about 15 degrees of hip hyperextension is possible before the spine must arch and the pelvis tilt forward (Fig. 5–18b). Thus the hip extension movement should use a small range and adequate abdominal stabilization to maintain correct alignment and prevent hyperextension of the spine (Fig. 5–18b). Performing fewer repetitions or using a lower resistance is far safer and more effective than compromising correct technique.

Selecting Exercises

It would be ideal to develop a balance of the muscles that carry out the movement (prime movers) by strengthening both the muscles that assist with a movement (synergists) and the muscles that have the opposite action (antagonists). Overdevelopment of one muscle group can actually be counterproductive, as evidenced in studies that find hamstring strains resulting from strength imbalances between the quadriceps and hamstrings (Burkett 1970; Liemohn 1978). However, in a dance-exercise class with 10–20 minutes available for calisthenics, it is difficult to design routines that develop such a balance. One approach is to select exercises, such as the push-up, that work several muscle groups at once. Another approach is to emphasize muscle groups that are weak in most people and that are important for posture and for injury prevention.

ABDOMINAL STRENGTH.   Abdominal strengthening (see Fig. 5–15 for exercises) is important both to correct the common postural problem of lumbar lordosis and to prevent low-back injury. The oblique and transverse abdominal groups are particularly important in these functions because they generate intra-abdominal pressure (Clippinger-Robertson 1986). Adding rotation to abdominal curls will emphasize the obliques. For effective overload when performing rotated exercises, such as opposite elbow to knee, exercisers should be certain to curl the trunk up to meet the knee (Fig. 5–19a), rather than bring the knee to the elbow (Fig. 5–19b).

To emphasize the transverse abdominals, exercisers should pull the abdomen inward instead of letting it bulge out during the strengthening routine. Pelvic tilts and isometric curl-ups are effective for teaching this isolation technique. The goal of the pelvic tilt is to pull the abdominal wall in toward the low spine at the same time that the pelvis and rib cage are drawn closer together (Fig. 5–20). The top of the pelvis should be tilted backward so that the low-back curve diminishes

FIGURE 5–19 Opposite elbow to knee

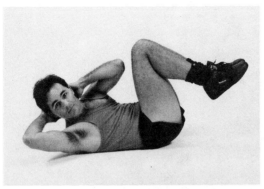

a. Correct: Bring the trunk and elbow up toward the knee.

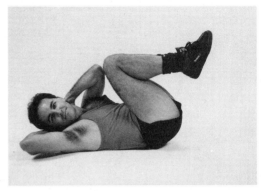

b. Incorrect: The knee is brought up to meet the elbow.

FIGURE 5–20 Transverse abdom-abdominus function in pelvic tilts

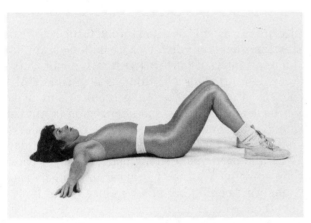

a. Starting position: Knees bent, back relaxed.

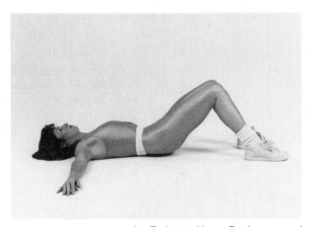

b. End position: Back pressed against floor and buttocks slightly lifted.

and the pubic bone comes forward and up into a tucked position. Isometric curl-ups begin with a basic curl (Fig. 5–15a). At the top of the curl, the hands are placed on the outside of the legs and used to pull the trunk a few inches higher. At this higher arc, the exerciser alternately pushes out and pulls in the abdominal wall to develop better awareness of the muscles involved. Then the exerciser pulls the abdominal wall firmly inward, releases the hands, and holds the position isometrically for 5 seconds. The isometric curl-up may be repeated 5–10 times, depending on the fitness of the participants. As the participants develop better control, they can omit the section in which they alternately push out and pull in the abdominal wall.

SHOULDER STRENGTH. Most people use their arms in front of them to lift, carry, and reach, thus developing stronger and shorter shoulder muscles in front (anterior) than in the back (posterior). Hours of sitting in sedentary jobs, often with slumping posture, further aggravate this tendency by weakening and stretching posterior shoulder and upper-back muscles. This common imbalance between posterior and anterior

AEROBIC DANCE-EXERCISE INSTRUCTOR MANUAL

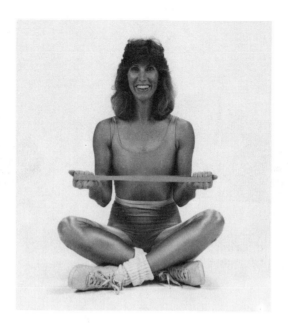

FIGURE 5–21 A strengthening exercise to correct rolled shoulders: Grasp tubing with palms up and elbows close to body and pull hands away from each other.

shoulder muscles easily produces the postural problem of rounded shoulders. Rounded shoulders generally involves weak, long scapular adductors, with tight humeral internal rotators (pectoralis major, latissimus dorsi, and anterior deltoid). This condition is also commonly accompanied by kyphosis. Correction of this problem involves strengthening the upper back and posterior shoulder region (scapular adductors, thoracic spinal extensors, and humeral external rotators) and stretching the shoulder horizontal adductors and the shoulder extensors. In Figure 5–21, the participant strengthens the upper-back and shoulder muscles by grasping a piece of surgical tubing between her hands with her palms up, keeping her elbows close to her body. She then rotates her shoulders so that her hands pull away from each other. Toward the end of the motion, she involves her scapular adductors by pulling her shoulder blades together as her hands continue to pull farther away from each other. Figure 5–22 illustrates shoulder flexibility exercises. In Figure 5–22a, the horizontal adductors, particularly the pectoralis major, are stretched; in Figure 5–22(b), the shoulder extensors, particularly the latissimus dorsi and the pectoralis major (sternal portion), are stretched. Any of these shoulder stretches would fit in well after strengthening exercises such as push-ups, either in the calisthenics section or later in the flexibility (Cool-Down II) section. Correction of rounded shoulders is important, not only for aesthetic reasons, but because the condition can cause improper shoulder mechanics that can lead to problems such as tendinitis.

If the class has time for additional shoulder strengthening, a well-rounded program would include shoulder-extension exercises and the more commonly used flexion and abduction exercises. In the shoulder-extension exercise, the arm begins down at the side (Fig. 5–23a) and then pulls back (shoulder hyperextension), with surgical tubing providing resistance (Fig. 5–23b). Exercisers should be sure that the wrist stays in line with the lower arm, and that the elbow does not hyperextend as the arm pulls back. A well-rounded program would also include exercises for strengthening the rotator cuff—the muscles essential for shoulder stability and for proper mechanics when raising the arm.

Components of an Aerobic Dance-Exercise Class

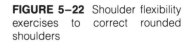
FIGURE 5–22 Shoulder flexibility exercises to correct rounded shoulders

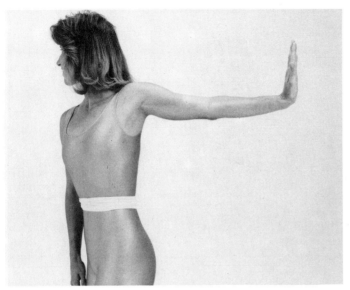

a. Shoulder horizontal adductor stretch: Hand on wall with torso rotating away.

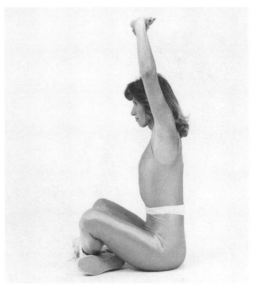

b. Shoulder extensor stretch: Palms up, back straight, pull arms back.

FIGURE 5–23 Shoulder extensor strengthening using surgical tubing

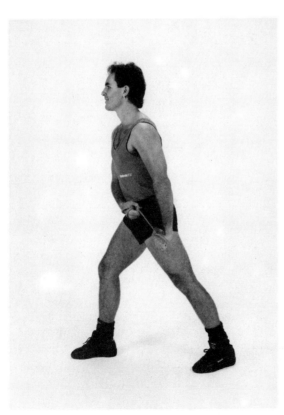

a. Start with arms down at the side.

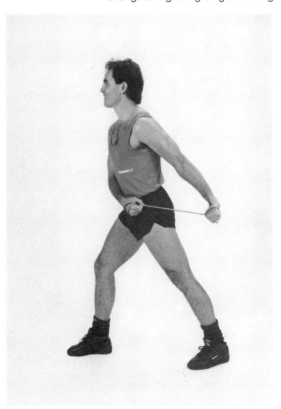

b. Keeping arms straight, pull back as far as possible, and release.

FIGURE 5–24 Strengthening the quadriceps femoris and hamstrings (weight can be added as strength increases.)

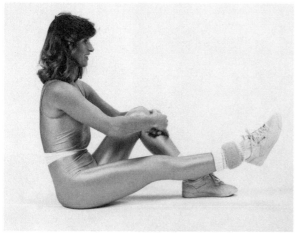

a. Lift the leg with the knee straight.

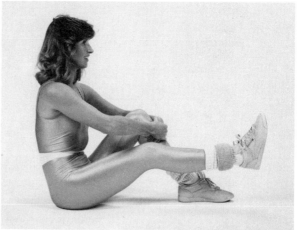

Bend the knee about 20 degrees and raise thigh higher.

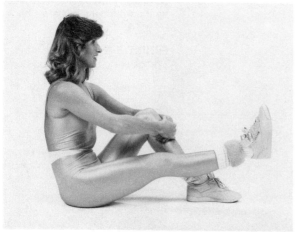

Straighten knee and hold for 3 seconds.

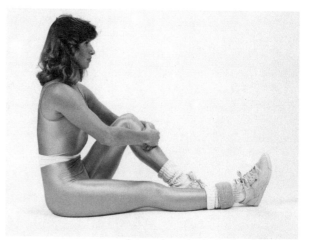

Lower leg slowly to the floor and repeat.

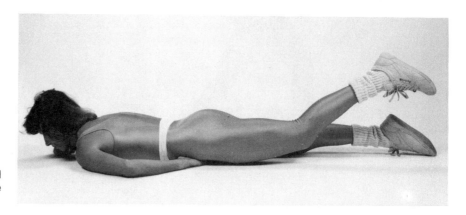

b. Place hands under hips; bend knee 30–40 degrees and lift whole leg.

The exercise illustrated in Figure 5-21 is a good example of movement that strengthens the external rotators of the rotator cuff.

HIP AND KNEE STRENGTH. Strengthening the quadriceps is important to protect the knee and prevent problems with the kneecap, such as chondromalacia patella (Clippinger-Robertson et al. 1986). To prevent muscle strains, however, balanced strength between the quadriceps and hamstrings is necessary; thus, the hamstrings need to be strengthened along with the quadriceps. Remember that the hamstrings and the rectus femoris are biarticulate (cross two joints) and exercises that combine actions at both hip and knee are an effective means of strengthening these muscles.

Figure 5-24 illustrates exercises that combine these actions. To strengthen the quadriceps (Fig. 5-24, sequence a), the seated exerciser first lifts the leg with the knee straight (hip flexion). She then bends the knee about 20 degrees and raises her thigh higher. While holding this new angle of hip flexion, she slowly straightens her knee (knee extension) and holds that position for 3 counts. Then she lowers the leg slowly to the floor and repeats the exercise. As strength increases, resistance may be added by using an ankle weight. For back safety, the abdominal muscles must be used throughout the exercise to prevent the pelvis from tilting forward. A participant who experiences back discomfort may modify the exercise by leaning back on the elbows, by lifting the legs less high, or by performing the exercise without external resistance. To strengthen hamstrings (Fig. 5-24b), the exerciser bends her knee about 30-40 degrees (knee flexion) and then lifts her whole leg (hip extension). It is important to limit the height of the leg lift and to use the abdominals to prevent the low back from arching.

In addition to the hip flexors and extensors, it is desirable to strengthen the hip abductors and adductors, which help to stabilize the gait and assist with other movements such as flexion, extension, and rotation. In the exercise to strengthen the hip abductors illustrated in Figure 5-25a, the top leg is lifted toward the ceiling. A hold may be added here. The leg is then slowly lowered to the floor and the exercise repeated. To strengthen the hip adductors, the lower leg is lifted (Fig. 5-25b), held, if additional difficulty is desired, and slowly lowered. With both exercises, the exerciser should emphasize moving the leg (femur) in relation to the pelvis, avoiding compensations such as laterally tilting the pelvis (Fig. 5-17b), arching the low back, or rocking forward or back on the lower pelvic bone. Using the abdominals can help stabilize the pelvis and the spine.

SHIN STRENGTH. Another area that needs strengthening for injury prevention is the shin and lower leg, the most commonly injured areas in high-impact aerobics classes. Although many people believe that jumping strengthens the shins, actually it primarily strengthens the calf muscles (plantar flexors), which work concentrically on the takeoff and eccentrically on the landing. It is particularly important to strengthen the tibialis—anterior and posterior—and the peroneals. Although some of these muscles aid with plantar flexion, they work more effectively when inversion and eversion, respectively, are added. The shin exercises illustrated in Figure 5-26 use a wide elastic band for resistance. (The band works better than surgical tubing because it does not slide or roll down.) In the strengthening exercise for the tibialis anterior,

AEROBIC DANCE-EXERCISE INSTRUCTOR MANUAL

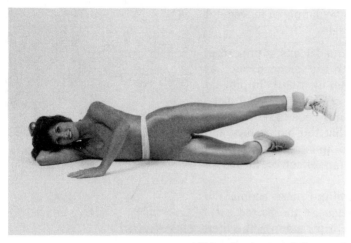

a. Lift top leg toward ceiling and lower slowly to the floor.

FIGURE 5–25 Strengthening the hip abductor and adductor

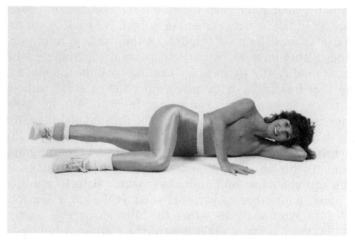

b. Lift lower leg and lower slowly to the floor.

the exerciser pulls the big toes up toward the shin (ankle dorsiflexion, inversion, Fig. 5–26a). In strengthening the tibialis posterior (Fig. 5–26b), the exerciser crosses the feet and points the toes (ankle plantar flexion), then pulls the inner borders of the feet—the big toes—apart and raises them slightly (inversion). In the peroneal-strengthening exercise (Fig. 5–26c), the feet are held parallel and pointed (plantar flexion) as the exerciser pulls the outer borders of the feet—the little toes—apart and slightly up (eversion).

Modifying Intensity

As in the aerobics component, the goal of the calisthenics component is to provide exercises of appropriate intensity, so that muscular strength and endurance improve while injuries are avoided. Because it is common to find wide variation in strength among class members and even among joints and muscles in the same person, the instructor must provide options for modifying exercises. Participants should be warned that if their joints hurt or if they cannot maintain correct form, they

Components of an Aerobic Dance-Exercise Class

FIGURE 5–26 Shin-strengthening exercises with elastic band

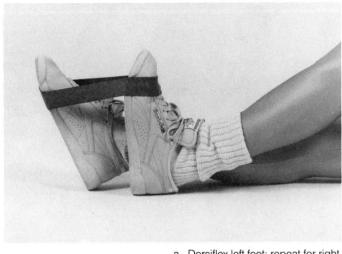

a. Dorsiflex left foot; repeat for right. (Strengthens tibialis anterior.)

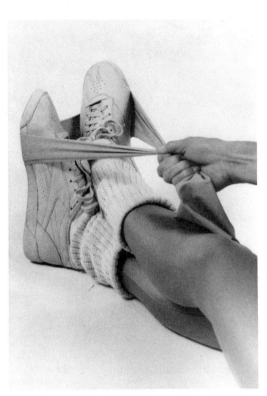

b. Cross legs at ankles. Point toes and pull feet apart, inverting foot. (Strengthens tibialis posterior.)

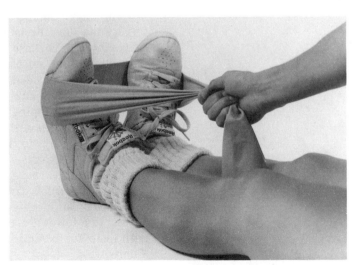

c. Begin with feet parallel and pull feet apart (eversion). (Strengthens peroneal muscles.)

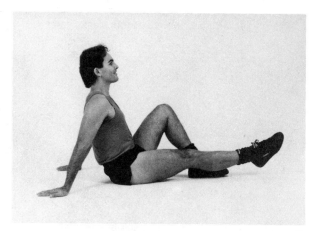

a. Low lift

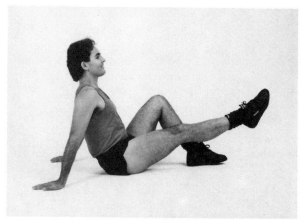

b. High lift

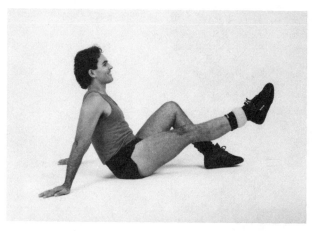

c. High lift with weight

FIGURE 5–27 Increasing intensity of front leg-lifts

are working too hard. They should be encouraged to substitute easier versions of the exercises.

Three convenient ways to modify the difficulty of an exercise are to vary the repetitions, the distance a body part is lifted, or the resistance. Increasing these variables will increase difficulty. For example, with straight-leg raises (Fig. 5–27a), difficulty may be increased by performing 15 instead of 10 repetitions, lifting the leg higher (Fig. 5–27b), or adding ankle weights (Fig. 5–27c). Resistance may also be increased by changing the configuration of body parts, a technique commonly used in curl-ups and push-ups where altering the relationship of body parts to the axis of rotation significantly affects the difficulty of the exercise. Curl-ups, for instance, become progressively more difficult as the arms move farther away from the lumbar spine (Fig. 5–28, a–d). A participant who has difficulty performing a series of curl-ups can modify the exercise by changing the arm position, by curling to a lower arc, or by performing fewer repetitions interspersed with rests: for example, a sequence of 5 curls, brief rest, 5 curls, rest, 5 curls.

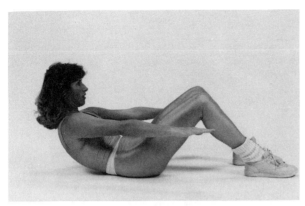

a. Least difficult: Curl-up with arms reaching forward.

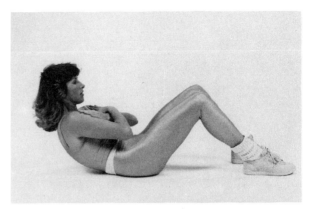

b. More difficult: Curl-up with arms crossed at chest.

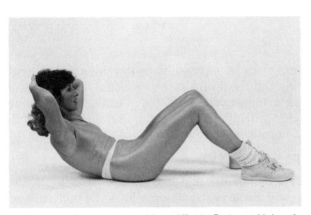

c. More difficult: Curl-up with hands behind head.

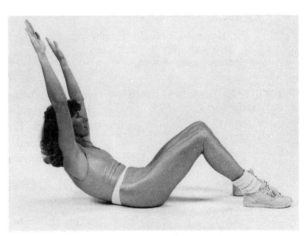

d. Most difficult: Curl-up with arms overhead.

Transitions

The exercise sequence should be designed with smooth transitions between movements. When the routine includes several sets, working alternate muscle groups in a similar body position helps keep a smooth flow. For example, a set of 10 right leg-lifts (Fig. 5—25a) may be followed by a set of 10 left side leg-pulls (Fig. 5—25b). This alternation may be repeated several times with variations in leg position or counts, if desired. An instructor who knows several strengthening exercises for each major muscle group will find it easier to design a sequence that flows well.

Including a few calisthenics in preceding and following segments can sometimes enhance smooth transitions and effective use of limited class time. Shoulder and upper-back exercises can easily fit into the first cool-down while the legs perform simple rhythmic movements (Fig. 5—14). These movements can make a smooth transition into floor work for the abdominals, hip, and knee, or into standing leg work such as front, side, or back leg-lifts, knee extension, and knee flexion.

FIGURE 5—28 Leverage principles applied to curl-ups. By modifying arm positions, curl-ups are made progressively more difficult.

AEROBIC DANCE-EXERCISE INSTRUCTOR MANUAL

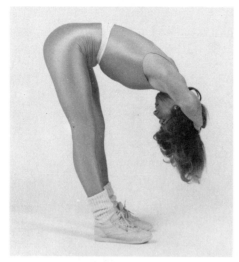

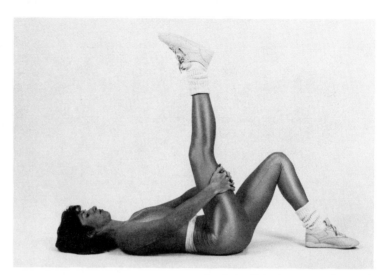

a. Unsafe: Avoid hamstring stretches with extreme unsupported lumbar flexion.

b. Safe: Substitute stretches such as the supine hamstring stretch.

FIGURE 5–29 Back safety while stretching the hamstrings

In a similar manner, exercises for strengthening the shins fit well with simple stretches during the flexibility, or second cool-down, portion of the class. For example, the exercises illustrated in Figure 5–26 may be performed with elastic bands or the hands for resistance while leaning forward for a hamstring stretch.

COOL-DOWN II (FLEXIBILITY)

Because current evidence indicates that it is safer to stretch muscles when they are warm, and because stretching allows the body to cool down, placing most **flexibility** exercises at the end of class during the final cool-down works well, even though some specific stretches may be used after working particular muscle groups during calisthenics. As in other segments of the class, a smooth flow between exercises is necessary. Instructors should group flexibility exercises to avoid awkward transitions and minimize the number of changes in body position. Adequate flexibility is critical for preventing injury; flexibility exercises are designed to maintain or increase the range of motion at key body joints. Correctly performed, a stretch places the muscle in a position of elongation greater than its resting length, such that the exerciser feels the stretch but no pain. The stretch position should be maintained for at least 10 seconds, and preferably 30–60 seconds, with no bouncing.

To select flexibility exercises that yield effective gains without endangering the spine or other joints, the instructor needs a basic understanding of joint biomechanics, and a knowledge of the fitness levels of his or her students. For example, the plough is inappropriate for most dance-exercise participants because it produces large compression forces in the neck. Similarly, stretches using extreme flexion of the lumbar spine should be avoided or used with great caution. For example, in the standing hamstring stretch with unsupported lumbar flexion (Fig. 5–29a), the back muscles relax, leaving the intervertebral discs and ligaments of the spine to support the weight. Other positions, such as the supine hamstring stretch, can stretch the hamstrings without placing the spine in such jeopardy (Fig. 5–29b). Stretches that produce torsion, such as the hurdler's position for stretching the

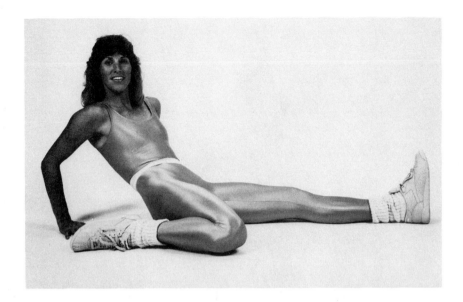

FIGURE 5–30 Avoid the hurdler's position for stretching the quadriceps femoris.

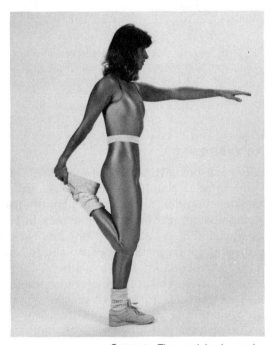

a. Correct: The pelvis is maintained in an upright neutral position as the femur is brought into hyperextension.

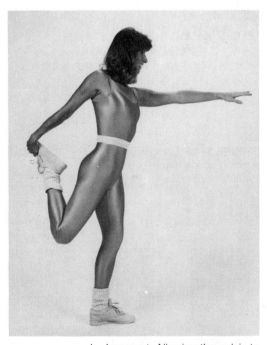

b. Incorrect: Allowing the pelvis to tilt anteriorly slackens the hip flexors.

quadriceps femoris (Fig. 5–30), should be avoided and alternatives substituted that keep the upper leg in line with the lower.

An instructor who understands which muscles are the focus of each stretch and which position of the joints is necessary will be able to help participants stretch more effectively and more safely. For example, in stretching the hip flexors the exerciser should bring the hip into extension while the pelvis maintains a neutral position—straight up and down (Fig. 5–31a). A common error is to allow the pelvis to tilt forward as the hip is brought into extension (Fig. 5–31b). This error slackens the muscles that the exerciser intends to stretch.

FIGURE 5–31 Stretching the hip flexors

AEROBIC DANCE-EXERCISE INSTRUCTOR MANUAL

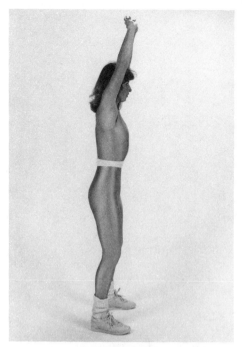

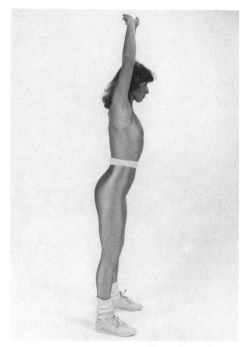

a. Correct: Maintaining proper back alignment with knees slightly bent.

b. Incorrect: Tight shoulder extensors and internal rotators can limit shoulder flexion so that compensatory hyperextension of the lumbar spine is necessary to reach overhead.

FIGURE 5–32 Compensatory arching of low back in overhead stretch

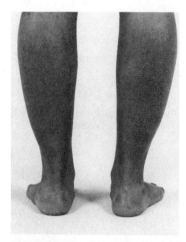

FIGURE 5–33 Compensatory foot pronation. When the calf muscles are tight, compensatory foot pronation often occurs to gain greater ankle dorsiflexion.

Selecting Exercises

Adequate flexibility is especially important to prevent injury in certain areas, such as the anterior shoulder, low back, hamstrings, and calf muscles. Inadequate shoulder flexibility frequently leads to round shoulders and compensatory arching of the low back in positions where the arms are overhead (Fig. 5–32a, b). Tight low-back muscles and hamstrings can disrupt spinal mechanics and lead to low-back injury. Tight calf muscles (gastrocnemius-soleus complex) limit needed dorsiflexion at the ankle during typical locomotor movements (Fig. 5–33). As a result, the foot pronates to achieve greater dorsiflexion at the ankle. Excessive pronation contributes to many lower extremity injuries, including shin splints, Achilles tendinitis, and plantar fascitis. Flexibility exercises for the anterior shoulder, low back, hamstrings, and calf, which should be included in all classes, were described earlier in this chapter as part of the warm-up segment of the class. Alternatives are illustrated in Figure 5–34.

Additional flexibility exercises may be chosen to fit the needs of a specific class. Generally, stretches should be included for the hip flexors, quadriceps femoris, hip abductors, and hip adductors. One standing hip-flexor stretch is illustrated in Figure 5–31. In Figure 5–34a, the exerciser takes a lunge position stretching the hip flexors of the back leg. The exerciser should take care to use the hands for balance, keep the front knee over the foot, and use the abdominal muscles to keep the pelvis from tilting forward. If the front knee hurts during this stretch, a less rigorous stretch, such as the one illustrated

Components of an Aerobic Dance-Exercise Class

FIGURE 5–34 A stretching routine

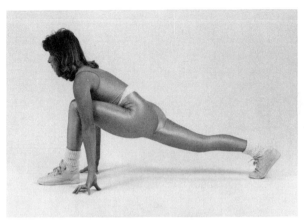

a. Hip flexor stretch

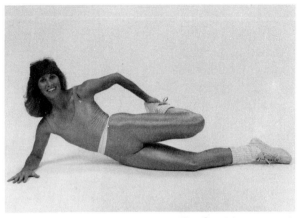

b. Quadriceps stretch

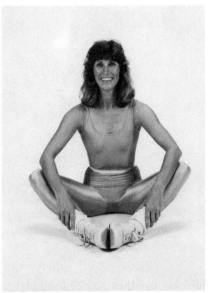

c. Hip adductor stretch

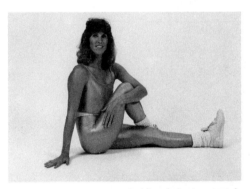

d. Hip abductor stretch

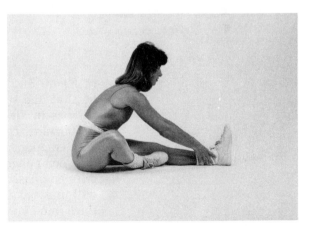

f. Hamstring stretch

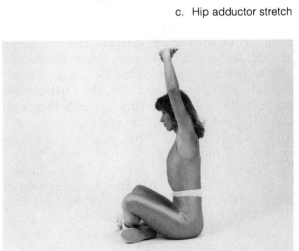

e. Shoulder extensor stretch

FIGURE 5–34 (continued)

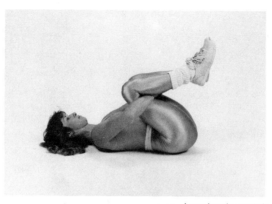

g. Low-back stretch

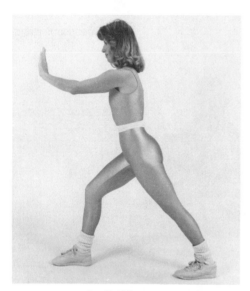

h. Calf (gastrocnemius) stretch

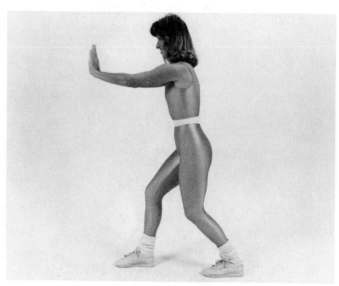

i. Calf (soleus) stretch

in Figure 5–31, should be substituted. The quadriceps femoris may be stretched standing, as illustrated in Figure 5–31, or lying on the side, as in Figure 5–34(b). In either position, the pelvis should not tip forward. This stretch may be used to emphasize either the single-joint components of the quadriceps, the vasti muscles, or the double-joint component, the rectus femoris, and other hip flexors. If the exerciser emphasizes bringing the heel to the buttocks, the vasti muscles will undergo greater stretch. If the exerciser emphasizes bringing the thigh into hyperextension, the rectus femoris and other hip flexors will be stretched more. In a stretch for the hip adductors (Fig. 5–34c), the exerciser sits with the soles of the feet touching and leans forward from the waist, gently pressing the knees toward the floor. The hip abductors may be stretched by sitting with one knee bent and crossed over the other leg (Fig. 5–34d). The exerciser pulls the bent knee across the body (hip adduction) while keeping the bottom of the pelvis (ischial tuberosity) in contact with the floor on that side. If the class includes rigorous shoulder-strengthening routines, additional shoulder flexibility exercises (Fig. 5–34e) may be needed.

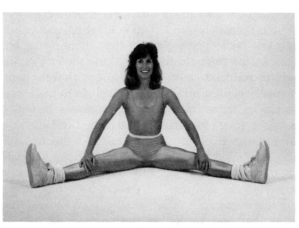

a. Straddle stretch (frequently difficult for beginners).

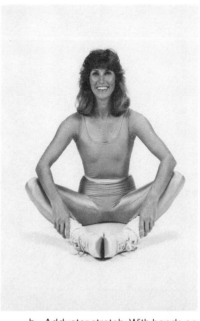

b. Adductor stretch: With hands on ankles, press knees to floor.

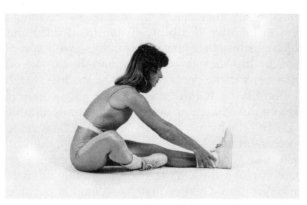

c. Single-leg hamstring stretch: Lean forward over extended knee.

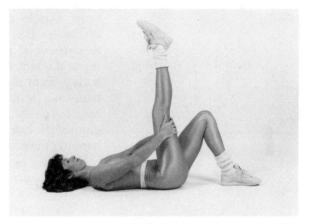

d. Supine hamstring stretch: With opposite leg bent, grasp leg below knee and pull toward chest, keeping leg straight.

FIGURE 5–35 Modifications of the straddle stretch

Modifying Stretches and Exercise Progress

Like strength, flexibility varies widely among people and among joints and muscles within the same person. An individual may be cardio-vascularly fit, muscularly strong, and yet inflexible in certain muscle groups. Some positions are particularly rigorous and can produce discomfort in less flexible people. If participants show discomfort, the instructor should modify exercises and substitute less stressful variations.

For less flexible participants, stretch positions are often safer and more effective if they isolate the stretch to a single muscle group, if they do not require flexibility at other joints, if they have a built-in mechanism to allow variation in intensity, and if they do not require tricky balance. In the supine hamstring stretch (Fig. 5–29b), for example, balance is easy because the back is supported on the floor. This position with the back flat and supported also limits involvement of the low back in the stretch and helps isolate stretching to the hamstring muscle group. Furthermore, the exerciser's ability to bend the knee, which slackens the hamstring, and to vary the angle of the leg as it is brought toward the chest allows the exerciser to control stretch intensity. In contrast, hamstring stretches that use forward trunk flexion (Fig. 5–29a) place the stretch on several muscle groups, including the calf and low back. The weight of the whole upper body produces the force elongating the hamstrings, making the stretch intensity high and difficult to control. In addition, people with tight hamstrings and low-back muscles cannot bring the trunk close to the legs, and so the force stretching the hamstrings actually increases in less flexible persons. Furthermore, they often cannot reach the floor and so cannot use hand support on the floor to reduce stress to the low back. Finally, this position is often awkward and requires tricky balance for less flexible exercisers, who often resort to undesirable compensations to achieve stability, such as shifting the weight back on the feet and hyperextending the knees.

As we can see, designing stretches for less flexible participants, especially beginners, makes it important to choose positions carefully. Two effective ways of modifying stretches are to change the relationship of the body with gravity or to simplify the movement, involving fewer muscle groups. For example, the straddle stretch illustrated in Figure 5–35a is frequently uncomfortable for beginners. Although this stretch is intended to increase flexibility in the hamstrings and hip adductors, the proper position to achieve this stretch—with upper-body weight in front of the hip sockets—requires more low-back and hamstring flexibility than many participants possess. The straddle stretch may be modified by simplifying it into stretches for single muscle groups, the hamstrings and hip adductors. Other modifications include bending the knees to slacken the hamstring (Fig. 5–35b) or flexing the hip to alter passive constraints at the hip joint (Figs. 5–35b and c). People who are too tight to sit with the trunk leaning forward can keep the stretching knee bent slightly, allowing the bottom of the pelvis to move back to the proper position. Or they may use a supine position with the stretching knee slightly bent (Fig 5–35d).

As flexibility increases, stretches can progress to include more muscle groups and more complex positions. However, it is still important to keep participants focused on technique and relaxing their muscles, not on keeping their balance. It is always important not to jeopardize the back or other joints. Many simple "beginning" stretches are effective enough to be carried over into advanced classes. Unlike strength exercises, in which positions must be altered to ensure adequate overload as participants' strength improves, stretches may progress simply by further approximating the appropriate body segments; for example, by leaning forward with the trunk in the straddle stretch (Fig. 5–35a) or by bringing the leg farther toward the chest in the supine hamstring stretch (Fig. 5–35d).

SUMMARY

Safe and effective class design requires a specific structuring of exercises so that the appropriate overload is provided to help achieve the desired gains. Instructors should balance each segment of the class—warm-up, aerobics, calisthenics, flexibility—in terms of muscles used and in terms of maximizing benefits while minimizing risks. Understanding basic kinesiology is necessary to anticipate problems, to know how to cue exercises, and to design movements. If instructors frequently explain and demonstrate modifications of exercises, participants can work at the appropriate intensity for their level of fitness. Instructors should move beyond emphasizing just quantity toward the fitness gains that come from emphasizing specificity and performance quality.

REFERENCES

American College of Sports Medicine. "The Recommended Quantity and Quality of Exercise for Developing and Maintaining Fitness in Healthy Adults." *Medicine and Science in Sports* 10 (1978): vii–x.

Anderson, T., and J. T. Kearney. "Effects of Three Resistance Training Programs on Muscular Strength and Absolute and Relative Endurance." *Research Quarterly in Exercise and Sport* 53 (1982): 1–7.

Astrand, P., and K. Rodahl. *Textbook of Work Physiology.* New York: McGraw-Hill, 1977.

Burkett, L. "Causative Factors in Hamstring Strains." *Medicine and Science in Sports* 2 (1970): 39–42.

Clippinger-Robertson, K. "Prevention of Low Back Injuries in Athletes: Putting Theory into Practice." In *Proceedings of the International Symposium of Biomechanics in Sports*, ed. J. Terauds. Del Mar, Calif.: Research Center for Sports, 1986.

Clippinger-Robertson, K., R. Hutton, D. Miller, and D. Nichols. "Mechanical and Anatomical Factors Relating to the Incidence and Etiology of Patellofemoral Pain in Dancers." In *The Dancer as Athlete*, ed. C. Shell. Champaign, Ill.: Human Kinetics Publishers, 1986.

Cooper, K. *The Aerobics Program for Total Well-Being.* New York: Evans, 1982.

DeVries, H. *Physiology of Exercise.* Dubuque, Iowa: Brown, 1966.

Fox, E. L. *Sports Physiology.* Philadelphia: W. B. Saunders, 1984.

Gerson, R. "Point-Counterpoint: Calisthenics Before Aerobics." *Dance Exercise Today* (May/June 1985): 26–28.

Jones, A. "Point-Counterpoint: Aerobics Before Calisthenics." *Dance Exercise Today* (May/June 1985): 27–28.

Kendall, H., F. Kendall, and P. Wadsworth. *Muscle Testing and Function.* Baltimore: Williams and Wilkins, 1971.

Liemohn, W. "Factors Related to Hamstring Strains." *American Journal of Sports Medicine* 18 (1978): 71–76.

Nieman, D. *The Sports Medicine Fitness Course.* Palo Alto, Calif.: Bull Publishing, 1986.

Philips, G., and K. Clippinger-Robertson. "Has the Bend Been Banned?" *Aerobics and Fitness* (January/February 1987): 20–26.

Pollock, M. L., L. Gettman, C. Mileses, M. Bah, J. Durstine, and R. Johnson. "Effects of Frequency and Duration of Training on Attrition and Incidence of Injury." *Medicine and Science in Sports* 9 (1977): 31–36.

Pollock, M. L., J. H. Wilmore, and S. M. Fox. *Exercise in Health and Disease.* Philadelphia: W. B. Saunders, 1984.

Shellock, F. "Physiological Benefits of Warm-Up." *Physician and Sportsmedicine* 11 (1983): 134–39.

Soderberg, G. *Kinesiology: Application to Pathological Motion.* Baltimore: Williams and Wilkins, 1986.

White, A., and M. Panjabi. *Clinical Biomechanics of the Spine.* Philadelphia: Lippincott, 1978.

SUGGESTED READING

Kendall, H., F. Kendall, and P. Wadsworth. *Muscle Testing and Function.* Baltimore: Williams and Wilkins, 1971.

Pollock, M., J. H. Wilmore, and S. M. Fox. *Exercise in Health and Disease.* Philadelphia: W. B. Saunders, 1984.

Testing and Modifying for Individual Needs

Larry S. Verity

Larry S. Verity, Ph.D., is assistant professor of physical education and director of the Adult Fitness Program at San Diego State University. He is certified by the American College of Sports Medicine and is the director of the ACSM Health Fitness Instructor and Exercise Specialist workshops held in San Diego.

6

IN THIS CHAPTER:

- Physical fitness assessments: Tests for evaluating cardiorespiratory endurance, body composition, and muscular strength, muscular endurance, and flexibility.

- Modifying an exercise program for individual needs: overexercising and underexercis-
ing, arthritis, obesity, chondromalacia patella, low-back pain, diabetes mellitus, cardiovascular disease, hypertension, colds and flu.

- Modifying an exercise program for the older adult.

While every aerobic dance-exercise program contains certain basic components, there is no such thing as a generic exercise program that is appropriate for all participants. An instructor must be prepared to modify a program based on the needs of individual participants. This chapter discusses fitness testing as an important way of determining individual strengths and weaknesses, and presents guidelines for modifying an exercise program for specific populations. Used in conjunction with health screening and class observation, these guidelines can help improve both the safety and effectiveness of a dance-exercise class.

FITNESS TESTING

Physical fitness is the ability of the heart, blood vessels, lungs, and muscles to function at an optimal level. A physically fit person can perform daily activities, enjoy an active lifestyle, and confront unforeseen emergencies without undue fatigue. A physical fitness assessment usually includes a battery of tests focusing on the areas of fitness addressed in a dance-exercise class: (a) cardiorespiratory endurance, (b) body composition (lean body mass and fat mass), and (c) musculoskeletal fitness (muscular strength, muscular endurance, and flexibility).

Although there are numerous tests for assessing each fitness area, many require elaborate equipment and specially trained professionals to administer and therefore are not appropriate for a typical dance-exercise setting. Other tests readily available to the instructor are simple to administer, but they lack norms by which the instructor can determine a participant's fitness level relative to others of the same age and sex. The tests discussed in this chapter are inexpensive, easy to administer, and provide the instructor with an objective and fairly reliable means of evaluating a participant's fitness against established norms.

Unlike health screening, which should be an essential part of every dance-exercise program, fitness testing is not absolutely necessary. However, assessing the fitness of participants before they begin an exercise program has several advantages:

1. A participant's fitness level in each of the three major areas of testing can be used to determine initial class placement, especially for beginners who often overestimate their abilities.

2. The tests provide a performance baseline against which to measure improvement, thus serving as a valuable motivational tool.

3. Along with individual fitness goals, test results help instructors tailor the exercise program for each participant. For example, an instructor might encourage one person to spend extra time on flexibility and another on upper body strength.

4. The testing process provides an additional opportunity for identifying medical problems or health risks and referring participants to other health professionals if necessary.

Fitness tests are usually administered after health screening and medical clearance (see Chapter 4) and before a participant begins to exercise. Follow-up tests are usually conducted every 3–6 months. Before the scheduled testing date, instructors should ask participants to prepare as follows:

1. Wear comfortable, loose-fitting clothes, such as jogging attire.

2. Do not eat for at least 2 hours and preferably 3 hours before the test.

3. Do not consume alcohol or coffee or use tobacco for about 3 hours before the test.

4. Avoid heavy exercise on the day of the test.

An instructor who chooses to use fitness tests must first become thoroughly familiar with the procedures for administering and interpreting each test. The following discussion describes the procedures for a variety of fitness tests.

Cardiorespiratory Endurance

Tests for cardiorespiratory endurance measure the amount of work the body can undertake, or the ability of the body to use oxygen to sustain aerobic activity. There are two basic approaches to testing for cardiorespiratory fitness. **Maximal exercise tests** measure a person's maximal aerobic capacity ($\dot{V}O_2$ max) and require a total effort to the point of voluntary exhaustion. A graded exercise test using a treadmill or bicycle ergometer is an example of maximal testing. The advantage of this

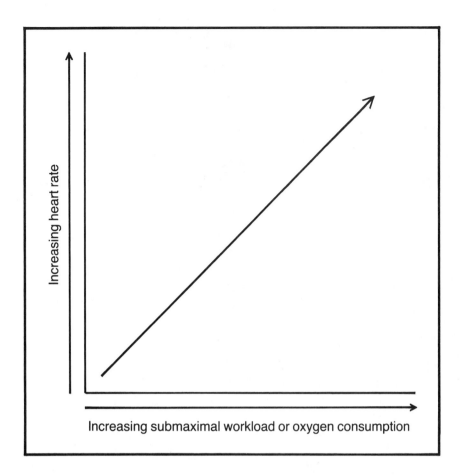

FIGURE 6–1 Relationship between heart rate, oxygen consumption, and workload during submaximal exercise

test is its accuracy. The disadvantages are that it requires a high level of participant motivation, must be performed under closely supervised, controlled conditions, and requires highly trained personnel and special equipment, such as 3-channel ECGs and oxygen/carbon dioxide analyzers. Obviously these tests are more appropriate for a laboratory or sports medicine center than for a dance-exercise class.

Although not as accurate as maximal tests, **submaximal tests** are both safer and easier to administer. A submaximal test requires the participant to perform at approximately 70%–80% of heart rate reserve for a given period of time, and the test is terminated before exhaustion. The heart rate is taken either during or immediately after testing to estimate $\dot{V}O_2$ max. This estimate is based on the assumption that a linear relationship exists between heart rate, oxygen consumption, and workload. As shown in Figure 6–1, an increase in exercise workload causes a proportional change in oxygen consumption requirements and is associated with a linear rise in submaximal heart rate. Therefore, submaximal tests such as the step test can be used to evaluate cardiorespiratory endurance.

SUBMAXIMAL STEP TEST. A 3-minute **step test** developed by Dr. Fred Kasch of San Diego is used by YMCAs for testing exercise participants (Golding, Meyers, and Sinning 1982). The following equipment is needed to administer this test:

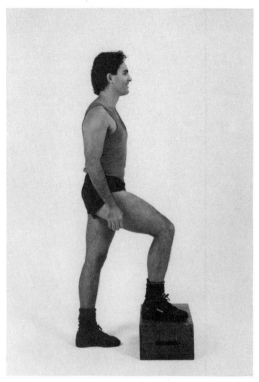

(a) Right foot up

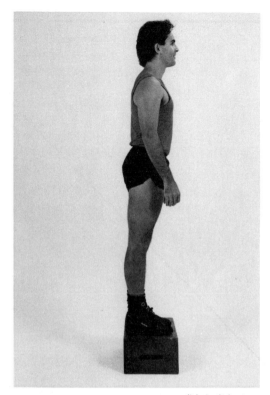

(b) Left foot up

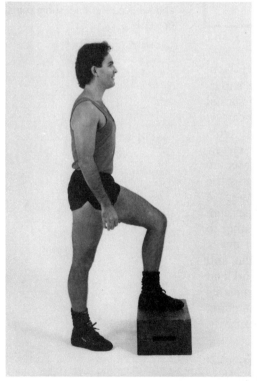

(c) Right foot down

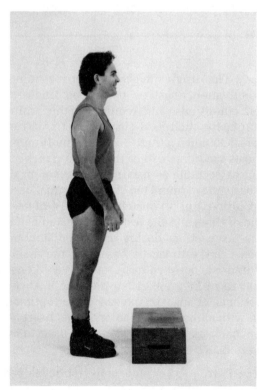

(d) Left foot down

FIGURE 6-2 Step test

Table 6-1

NORMS FOR THE 3-MINUTE STEP TEST
1-MINUTE RECOVERY HEART RATE

Beats Per Minute

	Men (age 20-46)	Women (age 20-46)
Excellent	81-90	79-84
Good	99-102	90-97
Above Average	103-112	106-109
Average	120-121	118-119
Below Average	123-125	122-124
Fair	127-130	129-134
Poor	136-138	137-145

Source: Adapted from YMCA, *Y's Way to Fitness* (Chicago: The YMCA of USA, 1982). Reprinted with permission from the YMCA of the USA.

- a 12-inch (30 centimeter) step bench
- a metronome for accurate pacing
- a timing clock
- a stethoscope for measuring heart rate (optional but highly recommended)

Before testing, the instructor should explain the purpose of the test and demonstrate how it is to be performed. The participant is to step up and down on the 12-inch bench at a rate of 24 steps per minute for 3 minutes. The metronome, used to maintain an appropriate stepping pace, should be set at 96 clicks per minute. One complete stepping cycle is equivalent to 4 clicks of the metronome, as follows (see Fig. 6-2):

- click #1—right foot up
- click #2—left foot up
- click #3—right foot down
- click #4—left foot down

Before testing begins, the participant should be allowed to practice stepping at the desired rate and should be warned to stop exercising if he or she experiences dizziness or light-headedness, nausea, severe shortness of breath, or just the need to stop. The instructor administering the test should watch for signs of discomfort, such as profuse sweating, a very red face, or the inability to speak in response to a question.

Immediately following the 3-minute period, the participant should be asked to sit down on the bench. Within 5 seconds, the instructor should begin to count the heart rate for 1 full minute, by using either a stethoscope (the preferred method) or by palpating the radial or carotid artery (see Chapter 9). This postexercise heart rate reflects the cardiovascular system's ability to recover from exercise. Then, using Table 6–1, the instructor can compare the participant's cardiovascular fitness against the norms established for men and women aged 20–46. For example, a 30-year-old woman with a recovery heart rate of 123 beats per minute would be considered "below average" in cardiovascular fitness.

The instructor should take special precautions before using the step test with participants who are obese or who have arthritis or chronic knee disorders. Unless the participant has clearance from a physician and can step up and down without difficulty or pain, he or she should not take the test because the stepping activity may exacerbate preexisting conditions. Anyone who experiences problems during the test should obtain medical clearance before continuing with testing or exercise. Suggesting another cardiovascular endurance test for people with orthopedic limitations would be illogical, however, because problems will probably occur with most weight-bearing tests.

There may be as much as a 10%–20% error in estimating $\dot{V}O_2$ max using the step test. The estimated maximum heart rate (220 − age) for any given age can vary by as much as 24 beats per minute. Also, at any workload, oxygen uptake can vary by as much as 15% between subjects. However, despite the possibility of error in estimating $\dot{V}O_2$ max, this test provides a reasonable measure of cardiorespiratory endurance and can be used to measure improvement as the exercise program progresses. Normally, those who engage in regular aerobic exercise recover faster from an exercise session than infrequent or nonexercisers. Therefore, follow-up testing will usually show a lower recovery heart rate, which indicates an improvement in the cardiovascular system's ability to recover from exercise.

FIELD TEST (1.5-MILE WALK/RUN). **Walk/run tests** of 1.5 miles, used routinely to assess aerobic fitness, are based on the notion that the faster a participant can walk/run a specified distance, the greater his or her aerobic capacity. This test is relatively easy to administer to a large group and requires only a measured distance of 1.5 miles over a smooth surface (a ¼-mile track is preferred) and a timing device. Because this test requires an all-out effort, only persons who are healthy and at least moderately active should participate.

Before administering the test, the instructor should provide an appropriate warm-up consisting of walking or light jogging and static stretching. After the warm-up, the instructor should gather all participants at the starting point and explain that they should exert a near-maximum effort during the test. For reasons of safety, however, it should be made clear that the participants should not run to complete exhaustion and that they should stop at any time if necessary. Everyone should start at the same time. As each person completes a lap, the elapsed time should be announced. After the test, completion time for each participant should be recorded and everyone should continue walking for several minutes to prevent dizziness or light-headedness.

Based on the completion time for the 1.5-mile run, a general fitness category can be identified using Table 6–2. Improving the cardiorespiratory function through aerobic dance-exercise will reduce the time needed to complete the test. This timed-distance test is a practical means of assessing cardiorespiratory fitness. However, because the results

Table 6–2

1.5-MILE WALK/RUN TEST TIME (MINUTES)

Age Groups

Fitness Category	13–19	20–29	30–39	40–49	50–59
I. Very Poor (men)	>15:31*	>16:01	>16:31	>17:31	>19:01
(women)	>18:31	>19:01	>19:31	>20:01	>20:31
II. Poor (men)	12:11–15:30	14:01–16:00	14:44–16:30	15:36–17:30	17:01–19:00
(women)	16:55–18:30	18:31–19:00	19:01–19:30	19:31–20:00	20:01–20:30
III. Fair (men)	10:49–12:10	12:01–14:00	12:31–14:45	13:01–15:35	14:31–17:00
(women)	14:31–16:54	15:55–18:30	16:31–19:00	17:31–19:30	19:01–20:00
IV. Good (men)	9:41–10:48	10:46–12:00	11:01–12:30	11:31–13:00	12:31–14:30
(women)	12:30–14:30	13:31–15:54	14:31–16:30	15:56–17:30	16:31–19:00
V. Excellent (men)	8:37– 9:40	9:45–10:45	10:00–11:00	10:30–11:30	11:00–12:30
(women)	11:50–12:29	12:30–13:30	13:00–14:30	13:45–15:55	14:30–16:30
VI. Superior (men)	<8:37*	<9:45	<10:00	<10:30	<11:00
(women)	<11:50	<12:30	<13:00	<13:45	<14:30

* > means "more than"; < means "less than".

Source: Cooper, K. H. *The Aerobics Program for Total Well-Being.* (New York: Bantam Books, 1982.) Reprinted with permission.

of the test depend on a participant's motivation, pacing ability, and degree of body fat, it is not always a true measure of $\dot{V}O_2$.

Body Composition

The assessment of body composition determines the relative percentage of lean body mass (muscle and bone) and fat mass (adipose tissue). Obesity is the excess storage of fat in the body. Obesity is associated with numerous health problems, including heart disease, diabetes, hypertension, and gallbladder disease; it is also associated with reduced endurance during exercise, increased risk for injury, and decreased exercise efficiency at submaximal workloads. Therefore, it is important to assess body composition as part of the overall fitness evaluation and to refer obese participants to appropriate weight-control specialists. This initial assessment of percent body fat also provides a baseline against which to measure changes in body composition as the exercise program progresses.

With aerobic exercise, body fat tends to decrease, while lean body mass either remains constant or increases. Therefore, it is not uncommon for a participant in an exercise program to lose fat but not body weight because the lean body mass increases. Standardized height-and-weight tables based on age and frame size assess the degree of excess weight but do not evaluate body composition. For example, according to these tables, a 5-foot, 2-inch male bodybuilder weighing 175 pounds would be overweight for his height, even if his percentage of body fat is very low, because muscle tissue is heavier, or denser, than fat tissue.

AEROBIC DANCE-EXERCISE INSTRUCTOR MANUAL

Hydrostatic weighing and skinfold measurements are the most widely used methods of assessing body composition. Although hydrostatic, or underwater, weighing is considered the most accurate, it requires expensive equipment, time, and trained personnel, and is impractical for a dance-exercise class. Fortunately, skinfold measurements, which require relatively inexpensive equipment and little time, can closely approximate hydrostatic weighing.

There is a relationship between the fat located in depots directly under the skin (subcutaneous fat) and body density. A high body density indicates greater muscle tissue, while a low body density indicates greater fat tissue. Thus, when skinfolds are taken, a higher value indicates a greater amount of fat stored beneath the skin and therefore a lower body density.

Skinfold calipers measure the thickness of the skinfolds in millimeters (mm). The procedure for measuring skinfolds is precise and should be followed carefully.

1. Identify the anatomical location of the skinfold.

2. Grasp the skinfold by the thumb and forefingers of the left hand.

3. Grasp the caliper in the right hand, hold it perpendicular to the skinfold, and place the pads about ¼-inch from the thumb and forefingers.

4. Release the caliper, allowing it to exert full tension on the skinfold.

5. After 1–2 seconds, read the dial.

6. Take 2 or more measurements, at least 15 seconds apart, at each skinfold site, until a consistent reading within 1 millimeter is obtained.

Improper site selection and inexperience are the most common causes of error in using skinfold measurement. Therefore, an instructor should become thoroughly familiar with this technique before using it in an actual testing situation.

There are more than 100 different equations for estimating body composition on the basis of skinfold measurements. Most are population-specific; that is, they are based on norms established for subjects of a certain age and sex. The best equations for the general population seen in dance-exercise classes have been developed by Jackson and Pollock (1985). These equations are based on the sum of skinfold measurements at three sites. For women, the skinfold sites are as follows (see Fig. 6–3 a,b):

1. Suprailium (Fig. 6–4): a diagonal skinfold taken above the crest of the ilium at the intersection of an imaginary anterior axillary line. Some experts recommend that this skinfold be taken more laterally.

2. Thigh (Fig. 6–5): a vertical skinfold taken midway between the hip and knee joints on the anterior, or top, of the thigh.

3. Triceps (Fig. 6–6): a vertical skinfold taken halfway between the acromial (shoulder) and olecranon (elbow) processes at the midline of the upper arm.

Testing and Modifying for Individual Needs

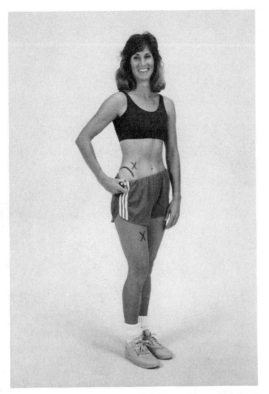

(a) Suprailium and thigh

(b) Triceps

FIGURE 6-3 Skinfold sites for women

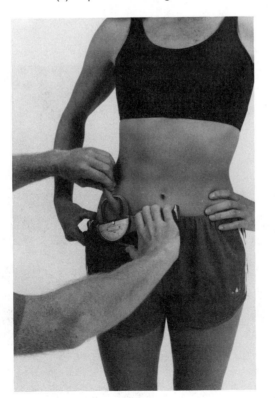

FIGURE 6-4 Suprailium skinfold for women: Grasp a diagonal skinfold just above the crest of the ilium, where an imaginary anterior axillary line intersects.

FIGURE 6–5 Thigh skinfold for women

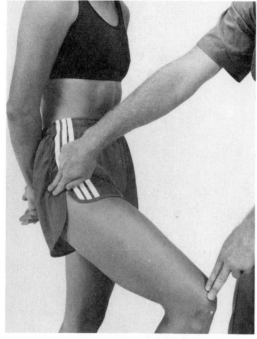

(a) Locate the hip and the knee joints and find the midpoint on the anterior (top) of the thigh.

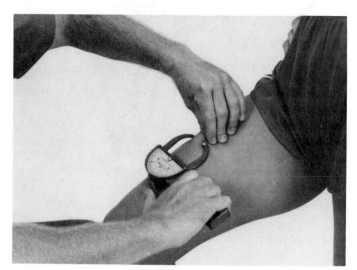

(b) Grasp a vertical skinfold with the thumb and forefinger and pull it away from body.

FIGURE 6–6 Triceps skinfold for women

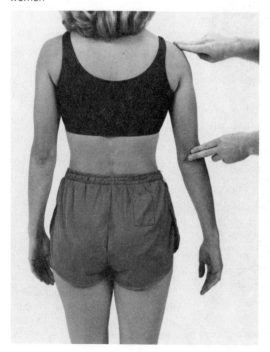

(a) Locate site midway between the acromial (shoulder) and olecranon (elbow) processes.

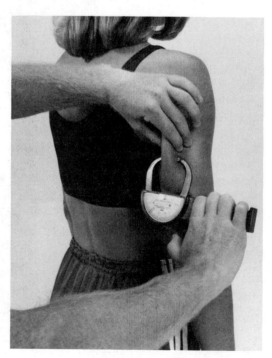

(b) Grasp a vertical fold on the posterior midline of the upper arm.

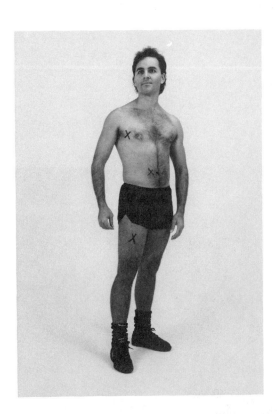

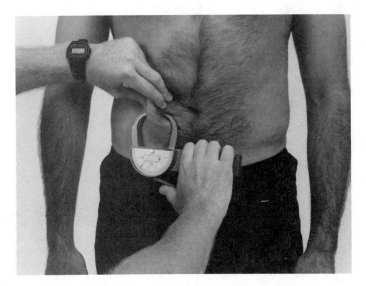

FIGURE 6–7 Skinfold sites for men: chest, abdomen, and thigh

FIGURE 6–8 Abdominal skinfold for men: Grasp vertical skinfold 2–2.5 centimeters lateral (left) of the umbilicus.

For men, the skinfold sites are as follows (see Fig. 6–7):

1. Abdomen (Fig. 6–8): a vertical skinfold taken about 2–2.5 centimeters lateral to the umbilicus.

2. Thigh (Fig. 6–9): a vertical skinfold taken midway between the hip and knee joints on the anterior, or top, of the thigh.

3. Chest (Fig. 6–10): a diagonal skinfold taken halfway between the anterior axillary line (crease of underarm) and nipple.

As a general rule, skinfolds are taken on the right side of the body. This test should never be administered when the skin is moist or immediately after exercise because the values will be larger.

After obtaining accurate skinfold measurements for each site, add the three figures, and refer to Table 6–3 for women or Table 6–4 for men to obtain an estimate of the participant's body fat percentage. For example, a 34-year-old woman with skinfold values of 20 millimeters for the suprailium, 24 millimeters for the thigh, and 12 millimeters for the triceps has a total of 56 millimeters for all three sites. According to the table, she has an estimated body fat of 23.4%. Table 6–5 interprets the body fat levels in terms of health and fitness. The woman with 23.4% body fat is classified as "plump."

With the percent body fat calculation obtained through skinfold measurements, participants can then use a formula to calculate desirable body weight. If they continue to exercise to maintain lean body mass and eat properly for gradual weight loss (see Chapter 3), this desirable body weight can represent a realistic fitness goal and a practical way of measuring progress. This method of calculating desirable

FIGURE 6-9 Thigh skinfold for men

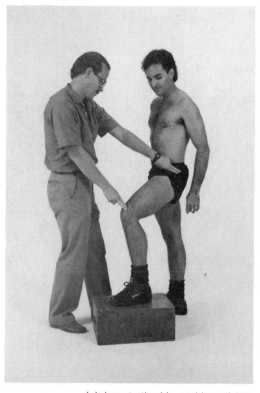

(a) Locate the hip and knee joints and find the midpoint on the anterior (top) of the thigh.

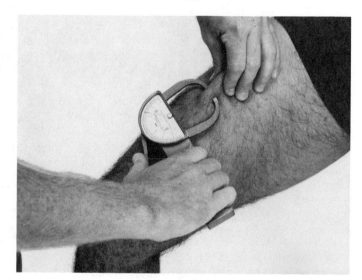

(b) Grasp a vertical skinfold with the thumb and forefinger and pull it away from body.

FIGURE 6-10 Chest skinfold for men

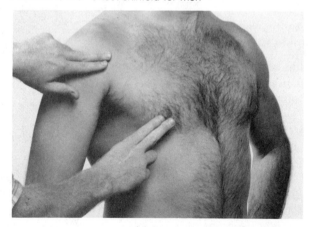

(a) Locate the site midway between the anterior axillary line and nipple.

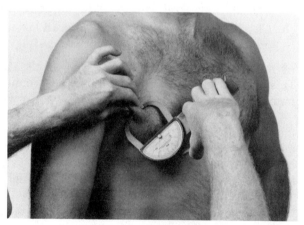

(b) Grasp a diagonal skinfold.

Table 6-3

**PERCENT FAT ESTIMATE FOR WOMEN:
SUM OF TRICEPS, SUPRAILIUM, AND THIGH SKINFOLDS**

Age Groups

Sum of Skinfolds (mm)	Under 22	23-27	28-32	33-37	38-42	43-47	48-52	53-57	Over 57
23-25	9.7	9.9	10.2	10.4	10.7	10.9	11.2	11.4	11.7
26-28	11.0	11.2	11.5	11.7	12.0	12.3	12.5	12.7	13.0
29-31	12.3	12.5	12.8	13.0	13.3	13.5	13.8	14.0	14.3
32-34	13.6	13.8	14.0	14.3	14.5	14.8	15.0	15.3	15.5
35-37	14.8	15.0	15.3	15.5	15.8	16.0	16.3	16.5	16.8
38-40	16.0	16.3	16.5	16.7	17.0	17.2	17.5	17.7	18.0
41-43	17.2	17.4	17.7	17.9	18.2	18.4	18.7	18.9	19.2
44-46	18.3	18.6	18.8	19.1	19.3	19.6	19.8	20.1	20.3
47-49	19.5	19.7	20.0	20.2	20.5	20.7	21.0	21.2	21.5
50-52	20.6	20.8	21.1	21.3	21.6	21.8	22.1	22.3	22.6
53-55	21.7	21.9	22.1	22.4	22.6	22.9	23.1	23.4	23.6
56-58	22.7	23.0	23.2	23.4	23.7	23.9	24.2	24.4	24.7
59-61	23.7	24.0	24.2	24.5	24.7	25.0	25.2	25.5	25.7
62-64	24.7	25.0	25.2	25.5	25.7	26.0	26.7	26.4	26.7
65-67	25.7	25.9	26.2	26.4	26.7	26.9	27.2	27.4	27.7
68-70	26.6	26.9	27.1	27.4	27.6	27.9	28.1	28.4	28.6
71-73	27.5	27.8	28.0	28.3	28.5	28.8	29.0	29.3	29.5
74-76	28.4	28.7	28.9	29.2	29.4	29.7	29.9	30.2	30.4
77-79	29.3	29.5	29.8	30.0	30.3	30.5	30.8	31.0	31.3
80-82	30.1	30.4	30.6	30.9	31.1	31.4	31.6	31.9	32.1
83-85	30.9	31.2	31.4	31.7	31.9	32.2	32.4	32.7	32.9
86-88	31.7	32.0	32.2	32.5	32.7	32.9	33.2	33.4	33.7
89-91	32.5	32.7	33.0	33.2	33.5	33.7	33.9	34.2	34.4
92-94	33.2	33.4	33.7	33.9	34.2	34.4	34.7	34.9	35.2
95-97	33.9	34.1	34.4	34.6	34.9	35.1	35.4	35.6	35.9
98-100	34.6	34.8	35.1	35.3	35.5	35.8	36.0	36.3	36.5
101-103	35.3	35.4	35.7	35.9	36.2	36.4	36.7	36.9	37.2
104-106	35.8	36.1	36.3	36.6	36.8	37.1	37.3	37.5	37.8
107-109	36.4	36.7	36.9	37.1	37.4	37.6	37.9	38.1	38.4
110-112	37.0	37.2	37.5	37.7	38.0	38.2	38.5	38.7	38.9
113-115	37.5	37.8	38.0	38.2	38.5	38.7	39.0	39.2	39.5
116-118	38.0	38.3	38.5	38.8	39.0	39.3	39.5	39.7	40.0
119-121	38.5	38.7	39.0	39.2	39.5	39.7	40.0	40.2	40.5
122-124	39.0	39.2	39.4	39.7	39.9	40.2	40.4	40.7	40.9
125-127	39.4	39.6	39.9	40.1	40.4	40.6	40.9	41.1	41.4
128-130	39.8	40.0	40.3	40.5	40.8	41.0	41.3	41.5	41.8

Source: Jackson, A. and M. Pollock. "Practical Assessment of Body Composition." *The Physician and Sportsmedicine* (May 1985): 86. Reprinted with permission from McGraw-Hill, Inc.

Aerobic Dance-Exercise Instructor Manual

Table 6-4

**PERCENT FAT ESTIMATE FOR MEN:
SUM OF CHEST, ABDOMEN, AND THIGH SKINFOLDS**

Age Groups

Sum of Skinfolds (mm)	Under 22	23-27	28-32	33-37	38-42	43-47	48-52	53-57	Over 57
8-10	1.3	1.8	2.3	2.9	3.4	3.9	4.5	5.0	5.5
11-13	2.2	2.8	3.3	3.9	4.4	4.9	5.5	6.0	6.5
14-16	3.2	3.8	4.3	4.8	5.4	5.9	6.4	7.0	7.5
17-19	4.2	4.7	5.3	5.8	6.3	6.9	7.4	8.0	8.5
20-22	5.1	5.7	6.2	6.8	7.3	7.9	8.4	8.9	9.5
23-25	6.1	6.6	7.2	7.7	8.3	8.8	9.4	9.9	10.5
26-28	7.0	7.6	8.1	8.7	9.2	9.8	10.3	10.9	11.4
29-31	8.0	8.5	9.1	9.6	10.2	10.7	11.3	11.8	12.4
32-34	8.9	9.4	10.0	10.5	11.1	11.6	12.2	12.8	13.3
35-37	9.8	10.4	10.9	11.5	12.0	12.6	13.1	13.7	14.3
38-40	10.7	11.3	11.8	12.4	12.9	13.5	14.1	14.6	15.2
41-43	11.6	12.2	12.7	13.3	13.8	14.4	15.0	15.5	16.1
44-46	12.5	13.1	13.6	14.2	14.7	15.3	15.9	16.4	17.0
47-49	13.4	13.9	14.5	15.1	15.6	16.2	16.8	17.3	17.9
50-52	14.3	14.8	15.4	15.9	16.5	17.1	17.6	18.2	18.8
53-55	15.1	15.7	16.2	16.8	17.4	17.9	18.5	19.1	19.7
56-58	16.0	16.5	17.1	17.7	18.2	18.8	19.4	20.0	20.5
59-61	16.9	17.4	17.9	18.5	19.1	19.7	20.2	20.8	21.4
62-64	17.6	18.2	18.8	19.4	19.9	20.5	21.1	21.7	22.2
65-67	18.5	19.0	19.6	20.2	20.8	21.3	21.9	22.5	23.1
68-70	19.3	19.9	20.4	21.0	21.6	22.2	22.7	23.3	23.9
71-73	20.1	20.7	21.2	21.8	22.4	23.0	23.6	24.1	24.7
74-76	20.9	21.5	22.0	22.6	23.2	23.8	24.4	25.0	25.5
77-79	21.7	22.2	22.8	23.4	24.0	24.6	25.2	25.8	26.3
80-82	22.4	23.0	23.6	24.2	24.8	25.4	25.9	26.5	27.1
83-85	23.2	23.8	24.4	25.0	25.5	26.1	26.7	27.3	27.9
86-88	24.0	24.5	25.1	25.7	26.3	26.9	27.5	28.1	28.7
89-91	24.7	25.3	25.9	26.5	27.1	27.6	28.2	28.8	29.4
92-94	25.4	26.0	26.6	27.2	27.8	28.4	29.0	29.6	30.2
92-97	26.1	26.7	27.3	27.9	28.5	29.1	29.7	30.3	30.9
98-100	26.9	27.4	28.0	28.6	29.2	29.8	30.4	31.0	31.6
101-103	27.5	28.1	28.7	29.3	29.9	30.5	31.1	31.7	32.3
104-106	28.2	28.8	29.4	30.0	30.6	31.2	31.8	32.4	33.0
107-109	28.9	29.5	30.1	30.7	31.3	31.9	32.5	33.1	33.7
110-112	29.6	30.2	30.8	31.4	32.0	32.6	33.2	33.8	34.4
113-115	30.2	30.8	31.4	32.0	32.6	33.2	33.8	34.5	35.1
116-118	30.9	31.5	32.1	32.7	33.3	33.9	34.5	35.1	35.7
119-121	31.5	32.1	32.7	33.3	33.9	34.5	35.1	35.7	36.4
122-124	32.1	32.7	33.3	33.9	34.5	35.1	35.8	36.4	37.0
125-127	32.7	33.3	33.9	34.5	35.1	35.8	36.4	37.0	37.6

Source: Jackson, A. and M. Pollock. "Practical Assessment of Body Composition." *The Physician and Sportsmedicine* (May 1985): 87. Reprinted with permission from McGraw-Hill, Inc.

Table 6−5

PERCENT BODY FAT—CLASSIFICATIONS

Classification	Male	Female
Unhealthy	<3%	<8%
Lean	4%–7%	9%–14%
Healthy	8%–15%	15%–22%
Plump	16%–19%	23%–27%
Fat	20%–24%	28%–33%
Obese (overfat)	>24%	>33%

Note:

Average college male = 15%   Average college female = 25%
Average middle-aged   Average middle-aged
American male = 23%   American female = 32%

Source: Nieman, D.C. *The Sports Medicine Fitness Course.* (Palo Alto, California: Bull Publishing Company, 1986.) Reprinted with permission.

body weight is preferable to standardized height-and-weight tables because the weight is calculated on the basis of body composition instead of poundage alone.

$$\text{desired body weight} = \text{lean body mass}/1.00 - \% \text{ fat desired}$$
$$\text{lean body mass} = (1.00 - \% \text{ fat}) \times \text{body weight}$$

For example, a 150-pound woman with 30% body fat wishes to reduce her body fat to 25%. Her desirable body weight can be computed as follows:

$$
\begin{aligned}
\text{lean body mass} &= (1.00 - .30) \times 150 \text{ lbs} \\
&= .70 \times 150 \text{ lbs} \\
&= 105 \text{ lbs} \\
\text{desired body weight} &= 105 \text{ lbs} / (1.00 - .25) \\
&= 105 \text{ lbs} / .75 \\
&= 140 \text{ lbs}
\end{aligned}
$$

Thus, if this woman continues to exercise as she loses 10 pounds, her body fat will decrease from an estimated 30% to an estimated 25%.

Musculoskeletal Fitness

The evaluation of musculoskeletal fitness involves three basic components: muscular strength, muscular endurance, and flexibility. The principal reason for assessing musculoskeletal fitness is to identify potential problems that participants may experience in a dance-exercise program. For example, a participant with poor flexibility may be unable to assume certain exercise positions, while a participant with poor upper body strength may be unable to perform even modified push-ups. An instructor who is aware of each participant's musculoskeletal fitness can provide appropriate modifications in the exercise program.

FIGURE 6–11 Using the hand-grip
dynamometer

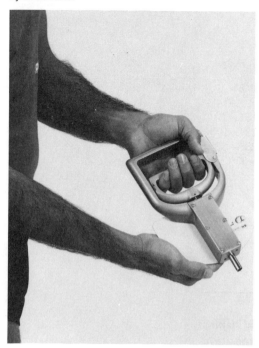

(a) Grip the dynamometer so the
second joint of the hand fits firmly
under the handle.

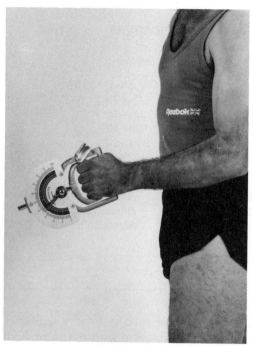

(b) Holding the hand in front of the
body with the arm bent, grip as
tightly as possible for 2–3 seconds.

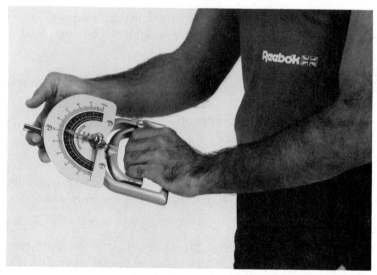

(c) Read the score from the dial.

Table 6-6

NORMS FOR GRIP STRENGTH (RIGHT + LEFT HANDS = KG)

Age Groups

Age	17–19	20–29	30–39	40–49	50–59	60–65
MALES						
Excellent	>119	>123	>125	>122	>113	>107
Good	101–118	105–122	106–124	103–121	96–112	90–106
Minimum	82–100	87–104	88–105	85–102	78–95	73–89
Below Minimum	63–81	68–86	69–87	66–84	61–77	57–72
Poor	<62	<67	<68	<65	<60	<56
FEMALES						
Excellent	>78	>71	>72	>73	>67	>60
Good	61–77	59–70	60–71	59–72	55–66	50–59
Minimum	45–60	47–58	48–59	45–58	44–54	39–49
Below Minimum	28–44	35–46	36–47	32–44	32–43	28–38
Poor	<27	<34	<35	<31	<31	<27

Excellent	95th percentile and above
Good	75th–95th percentile
Minimum	25th–75th percentile
Below Minimum	5th–25th percentile
Poor	Below 5th percentile

Source: Adapted from 1977 Canadian Public Health Association Project (3,464 subjects). Developed by and reproduced with the permission of Fitness and Amateur Sport, Canada.

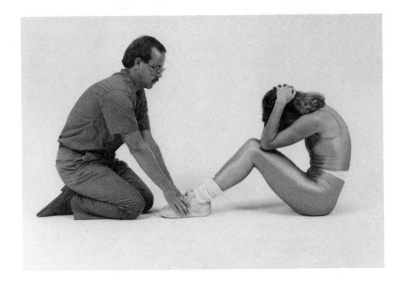

FIGURE 6-12 Timed bent-knee sit-up test

AEROBIC DANCE-EXERCISE INSTRUCTOR MANUAL

Table 6–7

NORMS FOR THE TIMED, BENT-KNEE SIT-UP TEST

Category	Men	Women
Super	79–91	64–72
Excellent	69–76	58–62
Good	62–67	52–56
Average	52–59	46–50
Fair	44–50	40–44
Poor	35–41	34–38
Very Poor	21–32	24–32

Source: Adapted from B. Getchell, *Physical Fitness: A Way of Life,* 3rd ed. (New York: John Wiley & Sons, 1983.) Reproduced with permission from Macmillan Publishing Co.

FIGURE 6–13 Push-up test

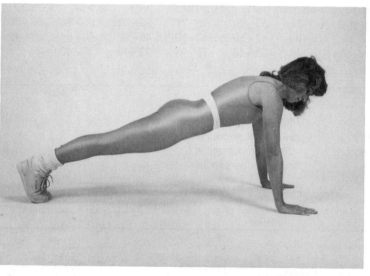

(a) Standard position

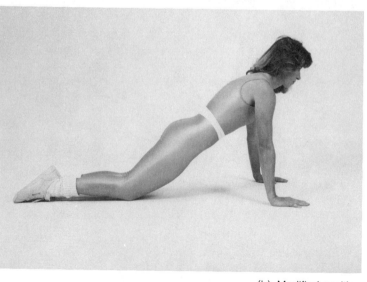

(b) Modified position

MUSCULAR STRENGTH.   Muscular strength is the maximum amount of force that a muscle can produce. Although barbells or multistation weight machines provide an easy means of measuring strength, they are not practical for most dance-exercise studios. Instead, dynamometers—instruments capable of measuring the force of a muscle contraction—are widely used to assess muscular strength.

The **hand-grip dynamometer** measures the static gripping strength of either hand. Because strength is specific to each muscle group, the hand-grip test measures only grip strength. However, grip strength provides an estimate of general strength, because the hands represent an important and frequently used muscle group. The grip-strength test may not be appropriate for people with high blood pressure or cardiac problems. Participants often hold their breath (the Valsalva maneuver) while performing this test, which increases blood pressure and makes the heart work harder.

The grip-strength test should be administered as follows:

1. Ask the participant to dry both hands.

2. Adjust the dynamometer so that the second joint of the hand fits firmly under the handle to allow for a proper grip (Fig. 6–11a.).

3. Make sure the hand to be tested is in front of the body with the arm bent.

4. Have the participant grip the dynamometer as tightly as possible for 2–3 seconds, keeping the arm motionless (Fig. 6–11b).

5. Read the score from the dial on the dynamometer (Fig. 6–11c) and record the score in kilograms.

6. Allow 2–4 practice and repeat trials.

7. Have the participant switch hands and repeat the procedure.

8. The score is the sum of the best right hand and left hand grip-strength scores.

Table 6–6 provides the norms for evaluating the score. For example, a 30-year-old woman with a grip-strength score of 35 for the right hand and 30 for the left hand has a total score of 65. According to the table her grip strength is "good," which places her in the 75th–95th percentile.

MUSCULAR ENDURANCE.   Muscular endurance refers to the ability of a group of muscles to exert a force either repeatedly or statically over time. Most tests of muscular endurance also measure strength to some degree. Tests that have proved reliable and easy to administer include the 2-minute, timed, bent-knee sit-up test and the push-up test.

The 2-minute, timed, bent-knee sit-up test (Fig. 6–12) evaluates abdominal endurance as well as strength. The procedure for administering this test is as follows:

1. Ask the participant to lie on his or her back with feet flat, knees flexed at 90 degrees or less, and heels about 12–18 inches from the buttocks.

2. Both hands should be clasped firmly behind the back of the head.

3. The feet can be held firmly on the ground by a partner.

4. During the sit-up phase, the participant's hands should remain clasped behind the head, the low back should be perpendicular to the floor, and the elbows should reach or pass the knees in the up position.

AEROBIC DANCE-EXERCISE INSTRUCTOR MANUAL

5. The midback should touch the floor in the down position.

6. The participant can be allowed to rest in the appropriate down position.

Count the number of correct sit-ups performed during the 2-minute period and compare the total to the norms presented in Table 6–7.

A push-up test assesses the endurance and strength of the upper body. The push-up technique used during the test usually differs for men and women. Most men will perform the push-ups in the standard position, while most women will use the modified or bent-knee position. However, the procedures for administering the test are the same.

1. Ask the participant to assume the appropriate up position (see Fig. 6–13). The body should be straight and the hands about shoulder width apart.

2. The body should remain rigid throughout the down phase, with the chest coming to within 3 inches of the floor. (A partner can place a fist on the floor beneath the participant's chest as a general guide.)

3. From the down phase, the participant must return to the up position with the arms straight.

4. The participant is only permitted to rest in the up position.

Count the total number of push-ups the participant performs until he or she becomes exhausted. Table 6–8 provides the norms for the push-up test.

FLEXIBILITY.   Flexibility, defined as the range of motion of a given joint, is influenced by the ligaments, muscles, and tendons around the joint. The **sit-and-reach test** is a simple and economical test for evaluating the flexibility of the low back. Low-back flexibility is particularly important in light of the growing problem of low-back pain in the United States. Participants with tight lower back muscles probably have tight hamstring muscles as well although the flexibility of these muscles isn't directly tested.

The sit-and-reach test uses a flexibility box (Fig. 6–14) about 12 inches high with a ruler along the top to measure the degree of flexibility. The ruler extends 25 centimeters beyond the box for participants who are not flexible enough to reach their feet. The sit-and-reach test should be administered as follows:

1. Before the test, provide an adequate warm-up (walking and static stretching).

2. Ask the participant to assume the starting position with feet flat against the box and legs straight.

3. One hand should be placed over the other, with the fingertips even and the arms extended forward along the ruler. Reach as far forward as possible. Hold the position for a few seconds.

4. If the hands reach unevenly, retake the trial. Allow approximately 4 trials and record the most distant point reached.

The norms established for both sex and age are identified in Table 6–9. It is important to remember that the results of the sit-and-reach test do not indicate total body flexibility—only the flexibility of the low back.

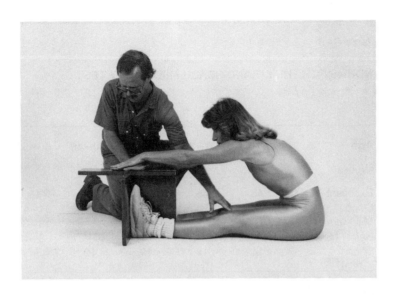

FIGURE 6–14 Sit-and-reach flexi-bility test

Table 6–8

NORMS FOR PUSH-UP

	Age Groups					
Age	**17–19**	**20–29**	**30–39**	**40–49**	**50–59**	**60–65**
Males: Standard position						
Excellent	>51	>43	>37	>31	>28	>27
Good	35–50	30–42	25–36	21–30	18–27	17–26
Minimum	19–34	17–29	13–24	11–20	9–17	6–16
Below Minimum	4–18	4–16	2–12	1–10	0–8	0–5
Poor	<3	<3	<1	0		
Females: Modified position						
Excellent	>32	>33	>34	>28	>23	>21
Good	21–31	23–32	22–33	18–27	15–22	13–20
Minimum	11–20	12–22	10–21	8–17	7–14	5–12
Below Minimum	0–10	1–11	0–9	0–7	0–6	0–4
Poor		0				

Source: 1977 Canadian Public Health Association Project. Developed by and reproduced with permission from Fitness and Amateur Sport, Canada.

Table 6-9

NORMS FOR THE SIT-AND-REACH FLEXIBILITY TEST*

	Age Groups					
Age	**17-19**	**20-29**	**30-39**	**40-49**	**50-59**	**60-65**
Males						
Excellent	>48	>45	>45	>43	>42	>41
Good	37-47	36-44	34-44	32-42	31-41	29-40
Minimum	26-36	25-35	24-33	22-31	19-30	18-28
Below Minimum	15-25	15-24	13-23	11-21	8-18	6-17
Poor	<14	<14	<12	<10	<7	<5
Females						
Excellent	>43	>41	>38	>35	>32	>28
Good	40-42	38-40	35-37	31-34	27-31	25-27
Minimum	37-39	34-37	31-34	28-30	23-26	21-24
Below Minimum	34-36	31-33	28-30	24-27	18-22	17-20
Poor	<33	<30	<27	<23	<17	<16

Source: 1977 Canadian Public Health Association Project. Developed by and reproduced with permission from Fitness and Amateur Sport, Canada.

*Note: Footline set at 25 centimeters.

PROGRAM MODIFICATIONS FOR SPECIAL POPULATIONS

To design an exercise program for each participant, the instructor uses information from a variety of sources. The results of a physical fitness assessment, as discussed above, identify areas that need improvement. The health-screening process (see Chapter 4) alerts the instructor to medical conditions that require modification in the exercise program. Equally important are the participant's individual goals, which can vary widely (see Chapter 10). Based on this information, the instructor can individualize an exercise program using the **FITT principle:**

- Frequency (F): the number of exercise sessions per week
- Intensity (I): how hard the participant exercises during each session as measured by heart-rate-monitoring techniques (see Chapter 9)
- Time (T): duration of an exercise activity at a specific intensity
- Type (T): usually classified as weight-bearing or non-weight-bearing activities (In aerobic dance-exercise, "type" can refer to low-impact versus traditional aerobics and class emphasis such as muscular strength, flexibility, or cardiovascular endurance.)

For example, an instructor would recommend that an unfit, sedentary person who scores low on all fitness assessments begin his or her exercise program by building up muscular strength, endurance, and flexibility before subjecting the body to the impact of aerobics. For a participant whose main goal is to lose body fat, an instructor may recommend low-intensity, long-duration cardiovascular exercise, provided the participant has adequate musculoskeletal strength and endurance. For a participant with a chronic knee problem, the instructor would recommend avoiding certain types of activities and modifying others to reduce stress on the knee. Some specific modifications an instructor may want to make within each segment of an aerobic dance-exercise class are discussed in Chapter 5.

Note that in cases involving physical limitations or medical disorders, the instructor's role is to modify exercises to help participants, who have medical clearances from their physicians, work safely toward their exercise goals. An instructor should never try to treat a disorder or prescribe an exercise program for rehabilitation purposes.

Overexercising and Underexercising

Some necessary modifications related to motivation and individual personalities cannot be predicted. Some participants may exercise beyond the limits of their physical ability, while others may fail to progress because they exercise below their target heart-rate range. Therefore the instructor needs to observe participants during each session and to monitor their progress closely. The following are observable signs of overexercising:

- profuse sweating
- very red face
- breathlessness, or difficulty responding verbally to a question
- inability to keep up with the exercise routine
- facial expression signifying distress

An instructor who observes these signs in an exercise participant should intervene to decrease the intensity of the activity. Intensity can be reduced by (a) slowing the tempo of the music, (b) minimizing arm movement, (c) reducing the frequency and height of kicks or knee lifts, and (d) shortening the duration (see Chapter 5). A participant who is overexercising may have been placed in a class beyond his or her ability level. Incorrect class placement is especially likely if no fitness assessment was performed and if class placement was based on the participant's own assessment of his or her ability. Transferring to a less advanced class may solve the problem.

Instructors may also prevent participants from overexercising by cautioning them against the "more is better" approach and explaining that moderate, regular exercise will realize greater long-term gains than bursts of intense activity, which may lead to injury or illness. Overexercisers who do not allow the body to recover properly between sessions may experience the following symptoms:

During exercise:

- dizziness
- significant breathlessness
- nausea
- excessive heart rate
- undue fatigue
- tightness in the chest

After exercise:

- sleeping difficulties
- joint soreness or pain
- loss of appetite
- elevated heart rate (over 120 beats per minute) 5 minutes after exercise

Participants experiencing these symptoms should reduce their exercise frequency to allow the body to recover. Because instructors themselves are at high risk for overexercising, those who teach aerobic dance-exercise should also be alert to these symptoms and monitor their exercise levels.

In contrast to the overexerciser who pushes too hard, the under-exerciser doesn't work hard enough. Signs of underexercising include

- not fully participating in the exercise routine, or halfhearted effort when participating
- failure to achieve the target heart rate
- little if any perspiration
- little change in facial color
- failure to progress

A participant who seems to participate fully in class with no visible signs of exertion may have been placed initially in the wrong class. In this case, changing to a more advanced class or modifying the routine to increase intensity will solve the problem. For those participants who are simply not working hard enough, the instructor should make sure they have realistic short-term fitness goals (see Chapter 10). A partic-ipant whose goals are too high may become discouraged. Someone whose goals are too low may not feel sufficiently challenged or ade-quately motivated to work harder.

Instructors can help most underexercisers by working with them to clarify their fitness goals and by showing them how to increase exercise intensity. Participants who are not underexercisers but who still fail to show improvement may not be attending class regularly. Instructors should then explain the important role exercise frequency plays in improving physical fitness.

Arthritis

There are two basic forms of arthritis: osteoarthritis and rheumatoid arthritis. **Osteoarthritis,** the most common form, is caused by a degen-eration of the cartilage of the bones that form the joints. This form of arthritis is usually associated with the aging process. The pain of arthritis often results in disuse of the affected joints, decreased range of motion, and muscular atrophy. **Rheumatoid arthritis** is an autoimmune disease that causes an inflammatory response in the tissues.

Although the conditions that precipitate the two forms of arthritis differ, the necessary exercise modifications are similar. In general, an exercise program for arthritics should include exercises to increase range of motion and develop strength, and an aerobics component that minimizes weight-bearing activities. Aqua-aerobics or swimming may be preferable to low-impact aerobics, which reduces impact stress but uses knee bends and upper body movements that may stress arthritic joints. Arthritics who are overweight or obese should also reduce their body fat levels because extra weight places added stress on the joints.

The following program modifications are suggested for a participant with arthritis:

1. Provide an extended warm-up to improve joint mobility.

2. Emphasize range-of-motion exercises.

3. Develop cardiorespiratory fitness through aqua-aerobics or swimming (the buoyant effect of the water minimizes stress on the joints), or a low-impact aerobics program modified to reduce stress on commonly-affected joints such as knees and shoulders.

4. Begin the exercise program slowly and build it gradually.

5. Decrease intensity and duration of exercise and increase frequency to impose less stress on the joints.

6. Stop any exercise that causes undue pain.

7. Do not use wrist or leg weights, which increase stress on the joints.

8. Ask the participant not to exercise during inflammatory episodes of rheumatoid arthritis.

If an arthritic participant consistently experiences pain during exercise, he or she should see a physician and obtain a medical clearance before returning to class.

Overweight/Obese

The body composition assessment will tell the instructor which participants are overweight or obese. As mentioned earlier, an overweight person may not be obese, and someone who is obese can still be within the normal range for weight according to standardized tables. Usually, however, an obese person will be carrying extra weight and will require a modified exercise program.

The average body fat for young men is approximately 15% of body weight; for young women the average is 25%. Using these percentages as a reference, an instructor would consider as overweight a participant whose percent body fat exceeds these values by 5%. Obesity is defined as above 25% body fat for men and above 33% for women.* Obesity is associated with a number of medical problems, including hypertension, diabetes, high total cholesterol, and high levels of LDL-cholesterol (see Chapter 3). Excessive weight also increases the possibility of musculoskeletal injuries and overexertion during exercise.

---

*Other sources define obesity as over 23% body fat for men and over 30% for women.

It is important for the instructor to realize that an obese person must work much harder to walk, climb stairs, or perform other daily activities than a person of normal weight. The cardiovascular demands of any activity are usually greater in obese persons, and because moving around is difficult, their muscles may have atrophied from limited activity. It is essential, therefore, to modify an exercise program for an obese participant.

The following modifications are recommended for an obese participant:

1. Use low-impact aerobics to develop cardiovascular fitness, if there are no contraindications such as joint pain with walking and/or standing or previous surgery. If low-impact activities are difficult, recommend non-weight-bearing exercise such as aqua-aerobics, stationary cycling, or swimming.

2. Be aware that an obese person may have poor coordination and balance. Begin with simple step patterns and movements.

3. Use low-intensity (60%–70% maximal heart rate reserve) and long-duration (30–50 minutes) exercise a minimum of 3 times per week to help burn body fat. Encourage the participant to engage in aerobic activity 4 or 5 times per week.

4. Encourage the participant to make dietary changes under the guidance of a qualified professional.

5. Prohibit the use of weight-loss gimmicks, such as rubber suits or plastic wraps (see Chapter 3).

6. Caution obese participants against exercising in excessive heat. They have more difficulty dissipating heat and are at high risk for heat exhaustion.

Chondromalacia Patella

Chondromalacia is a degenerative process in which the back surface of the patella gradually wears away, causing pain around the knee. Weight-bearing activities or exercises that require full flexion and extension of the knee, such as knee bends, precipitate the pain. Chondromalacia patella is most often seen in women. (See Chapter 11 for more information.)

The following program modifications are recommended for participants with chondromalacia patella:

1. Determine which motions cause pain—walking, jogging, range-of-motion exercises, crossover steps—and develop an exercise routine that avoids these movements.

2. If climbing stairs causes pain, do not use the step test as part of the fitness assessment. Stationary cycling is also contraindicated.

3. Use isometric exercises and single-leg raises to strengthen the muscles around the patella.

4. When symptoms appear, reduce frequency of activity.

If pain persists or becomes worse, refer the participant to an orthopedic physician or other health professional specializing in exercise-related injuries.

Low-Back Pain

An estimated 80% of the people in industrialized countries suffer from some form of back pain. Many injuries are a combination of poor posture and poor body mechanics, such as lifting heavy objects using the arms and back instead of the legs. In a dance-exercise class, many participants with low-back problems will also be overweight and sedentary. Therefore it is important for the instructor to identify participants who are experiencing low-back pain or who may be prone to low-back problems. A low score on the sit-and-reach test indicates poor low-back flexibility, which should be addressed in an exercise program.

The following modifications are recommended for participants with existing or potential low-back problems (see Chapter 11 for more information):

1. Include daily flexion exercises to stretch the low-back muscles and hamstrings.

2. Strengthen the abdominals, using abdominal curls and pelvic tilts (never double-leg raises or straight-leg sit-ups).

3. Use low-impact activities to prevent jarring.

4. Stress the importance of the warm-up period.

5. Remind the participant to keep the knees flexed at all times.

6. Avoid the use of hand and ankle weights.

7. Avoid movements, such as high knee-lifts, twisting the upper body, or hyperextension of the trunk, which may aggravate low-back problems.

8. Emphasize the importance of moderate, regular exercise to maintain strength and flexibility.

9. Stop any exercise that causes pain.

Diabetes Mellitus

There are two types of diabetes: type I, or insulin-dependent diabetes (formerly called juvenile diabetes) and type II, or non–insulin-dependent diabetes (formerly called adult onset diabetes) (see Table 6–10). Type I diabetics must take insulin injections to control their blood glucose level. Type II diabetics usually control their blood glucose levels through oral medication.

In normal persons, the hormone insulin is released from the pancreas in response to high glucose (blood sugar) levels, especially after ingesting a meal. Insulin promotes the entry of glucose into the body's cells and thereby lowers the blood glucose level to normal. However, in diabetes, insulin is unable to regulate glucose effectively, leading to high blood glucose levels, or hyperglycemia. More specifically, type I diabetics produce insufficient insulin to regulate blood glucose; type II diabetics are able to produce adequate amounts of insulin, but because cellular tissues are not sensitive to insulin, the glucose is unable to enter the cells.

The therapeutic triad used to control blood glucose levels consists of diet, medication (insulin injections or oral agents), and exercise. Physical exercise has an insulinlike effect on the body and promotes

AEROBIC DANCE-EXERCISE INSTRUCTOR MANUAL

Table 6-10

COMPARISON OF TYPE I AND TYPE II DIABETES

	Type I	Type II
synonym	insulin-dependent (juvenile onset)	non-insulin dependent (adult onset)
age at onset	under 20 years old	over 40 years old
obesity/overweight	very uncommon	common (80% are obese)

the entry of glucose into the cells. Thus a bout of exercise can actually lower the glucose level of a diabetic. However, a type I diabetic who has taken too much insulin or has not eaten properly is at risk for hypoglycemia, or low blood sugar (see Chapter 14 for symptoms and treatment). The likelihood of hypoglycemia is also increased if the type I diabetic injects insulin into an active limb just before exercise. The increased blood flow to the active muscles speeds the entry of the insulin into the body's cells.

The type II diabetic is usually obese and would benefit from an exercise program similar to that described earlier for obese persons. However, there are certain problems that can develop in type II diabetics that are not apparent in nondiabetic obese persons. The obese diabetic may experience loss of sensation in the distal extremities and poor circulation in the lower extremities as a consequence of the disease process. Both conditions can be exacerbated by weight-bearing activity.

Diabetes is not an excuse to avoid exercise. Instead, it should be an incentive for engaging in an exercise program. With proper medical clearance, instructor awareness, and program modifications, exercise can be part of a safe and effective approach to improving glucose control for the diabetic.

The following are general guidelines for dance-exercise instructors working with diabetics:

1. Although important, exercise should not be viewed as the single means of achieving glucose control for the diabetic. Diet and medication are also essential therapies for attaining glucose control.

2. With appropriate precautions (correct timing of meals and injections before exercise), type I diabetics are capable of participating in the same exercise program as nondiabetics.

3. Caution type I diabetics not to inject insulin into a muscle that soon will be used in exercise (i.e., do not inject insulin into the quadriceps and then ride a bicycle).

4. Easily digestible carbohydrates, such as candy or fruit juice, should be available at all times for diabetics who may experience hypoglycemia.

5. Obese type II diabetics should initially follow the exercise guidelines for nondiabetic obese participants.

6. Ask diabetic participants to discuss their exercise programs with their physicians and make any modifications recommended by the physician.

Cardiovascular Disease

Cardiovascular disease is the major health problem in the United States, contributing to over half of all deaths each year. There are many forms of cardiovascular disease, including coronary heart disease, stroke, and hypertension (see Chapters 4 and 14 for further information). Exercise can play an important role in preventing cardiovascular disease and in rehabilitating cardiac patients. By providing education, encouragement, and safe, effective exercise programs, the dance-exercise instructor can help participants improve their cardiovascular fitness and thus reduce further progression of the disease. However, participants recovering from heart attacks, surgery, stroke, or similar conditions should exercise only within the confines of special programs run by qualified medical professionals. Participants with cardiovascular disease should enter a traditional dance-exercise class only after they have sufficiently recovered from their disease and only if they obtain medical clearance to exercise from their physician.

Although exercise is not a panacea for cardiovascular disease, it does provide important preventive and rehabilitative functions, including increased work capacity, lower blood pressure, reduced anxiety, and improved sense of well-being. The following program modifications are recommended for a participant who has suffered from cardiovascular disease:

1. Obtain written medical clearance stating that the person may participate in a specific dance-exercise program (including intensity, duration, frequency, and type of activity) and documenting the physician's recommendations for exercise (see Chapter 4).

2. Begin with a thorough warm-up and increase intensity gradually.

3. Maintain a low to moderate level of intensity during aerobics for at least 20 minutes.

4. Provide a thorough cool-down to prevent possible hypotension.

5. Emphasize rhythmic activities using large muscle groups and refrain from those that bring about the Valsalva maneuver.

6. Carefully observe the participant's responses and be particularly alert for signs of dizziness, loss of facial color, shortness of breath or difficulty breathing, and unusual fatigue or loss of vigor.

7. Monitor heart rates frequently to ensure the participant is exercising at the appropriate intensity.

8. Identify any medications that the participant is taking and determine their effect on heart-rate response to exercise and any possible side effects.

9. Be certified in CPR (a requirement for IDEA Foundation certification).

Hypertension

Hypertension, or high blood pressure, is the most prevalent form of cardiovascular disease. The force of the blood as it is pumped from the heart exerts excessive pressure against the arterial walls, creating a blood pressure that is chronically elevated above a desirable level. A consistent reading above 140 mmHg systolic (force generated when the heart contracts) and above 90 mmHg diastolic (the amount of pressure when the heart relaxes) is considered hypertensive. A normal reading is 120/80 mmHg.

AEROBIC DANCE-EXERCISE INSTRUCTOR MANUAL

There are three important facts an instructor should know about hypertension: (a) in approximately 90% of all hypertensives, the cause of the disease is unknown; (b) hypertension is known as a "silent killer" because there are no identifiable symptoms; and (c) hypertension is a primary risk factor for coronary heart disease. Therapy for hypertension includes reducing the consumption of sodium, alcohol, and saturated fat; losing weight; exercising regularly; quitting smoking; and reducing stress. Many hypertensives also take medication to help control blood pressure.

It is extremely important that participants with hypertension receive medical clearance from their physicians before beginning an exercise program. In most people, physical exercise increases the systolic blood pressure but causes little change in the diastolic blood pressure. However, during exercise both systolic and diastolic blood pressure tend to increase in hypertensives. Such an increase places an excessive workload on the heart and can be dangerous.

The following program modifications are recommended for the hypertensive participant:

1. Obtain written medical clearance from the participant's physician.

2. Provide a thorough and gradual warm-up.

3. Maintain a low to moderate intensity level during aerobics.

4. Identify any medications the participant is taking, determine their effect on the heart-rate response to exercise, and adjust the target heart-rate accordingly (see Chapter 9).

5. Avoid static exercises, such as isometrics, which induce the Valsalva maneuver and are particularly dangerous for hypertensives.

6. Avoid sustained exercise involving upper body work above shoulder level. This activity will also raise the blood pressure, particularly when hand-held weights are used.

7. Avoid weight-lifting regimens that include high intensity and low repetitions.

8. Remind participants to breathe properly, especially during such exercises as sit-ups, when they should exhale on the way up.

9. Provide a thorough cool-down to prevent pooling of blood in the lower extremities, dizziness, and possible fainting (medication taken to lower blood pressure may combine with the effects of exercise, causing hypotension).

Colds and Flu

While everyone catches an occasional virus, frequent colds and flu can be a sign of overtraining. Excessive stress placed on the body over a prolonged period lowers resistance to disease. Therefore, instructors should remind participants to listen to their bodies. Sickness, like pain, is a sign to slow down.

A dance-exercise class is not a place for someone who is sick. Just as participants must rest an injury to the musculoskeletal system, they must rest the body while it recovers from a virus. To continue to exercise further stresses the system and may make the illness worse or delay recovery. Participants taking cold medications may place themselves in additional jeopardy because some medications increase the heart rate, both at rest and during exercise. Aerobic exercise also exacerbates intestinal problems and can increase the risk of dehydration. Therefore, the best advice an instructor can give to a participant with a cold or the flu is to do themselves and the class a favor and rest. When ready to begin exercising again, the participant should start at a reduced intensity and duration and increase their workload gradually.

THE OLDER ADULT

It is estimated that by the year 2000, one out of eight Americans will be over 65 years of age. Aging is part of a process that starts with conception. At about age 30, a person begins to experience a gradual, usually subtle, decline of the characteristics associated with fitness, including cardiovascular endurance, muscular strength and endurance, and flexibility. After 60, the signs of aging become more obvious, and there is substantial evidence that this natural decline can be magnified by a sedentary lifestyle. Fortunately, research has also shown that exercise can significantly slow down the natural aging process, as well as remove negative residuals caused by sedentary habits. With exercise, an older adult can have the physiological capacity of a much younger person.

Body Composition

Body composition tends to undergo a major change with age. It is common for people to gain weight steadily until their fifth or sixth decade, probably due to decreased activity and/or a decreased **basal metabolic rate** (BMR), or resting energy expenditure. Even a small decrease in caloric expenditure can lead to a steady weight gain over the years. Unfortunately, this weight gain usually represents an increase in body fat and a decrease in lean body mass. An aerobic dance-exercise program can improve body composition by maintaining lean body mass, increasing the basal metabolic rate, and decreasing body fat.

Skeletal Muscle and Strength

Muscle mass is directly related to strength. After age 30, a progressive decline in muscle mass and strength may be noticed in both men and women. There is a decrease in the number and size of muscle fibers, as well as a decrease in the contractile elements of skeletal muscle, primarily fast twitch fibers (see Chapter 1). Increased physical exercise can improve strength by increasing muscle mass.

Relative strength gains from weight training tend to be similar for young and old adult men: however young men increase strength predominantly by hypertrophy, or increasing the size of the muscle fiber, while older men increase strength through enhanced recruitment of muscle fibers (Montani and deVries 1981). Thus, the degree of muscular development following a strength-training program will be less in older men than in younger men.

All movements should be tailored to meet the needs of the individual. For example, participants with kyphosis or neck problems should avoid sit-ups or curl-ups. Pliés should be modified or omitted for exercisers with arthritis in the knees, and push-ups are inadvisable for exercisers who have problems with their wrists or shoulders. An exercise program for older participants who do not have cardiovascular problems, such as hypertension, or orthopedic problems, such as arthritis, can include 1-lb wrist weights. However, the pace of an exercise program to develop strength should be very gradual and should stress controlled movements and proper alignment.

Flexibility

With age, joint flexibility may decrease, sometimes as a result of the aging process itself and sometimes as a result of arthritis and related musculoskeletal conditions, which are among the most common disorders affecting people over 65 (Kart, Metress, and Metress 1978). The ability of some older adults to perform normal daily activities is limited by joint range of motion. Inactivity can compound the problem. Although some joints are limited in motion by bony structures, the primary limitation is associated with soft tissues, such as muscles, tendons, and ligaments. Many experts believe that exercise can keep the tissues strong. However, it is important to structure flexibility exercises so the vulnerable joints are not placed at risk.

An exercise program for older adults should be careful not to place unnecessary stress on arthritic joints. For example, the hands and knees position would be inadvisable for a person with pain in the wrists or knees. Some older adults in an exercise program may try to ignore pain, believing it to be a natural result of aging. Instructors should stress that pain is the body's signal to discontinue a movement and encourage participants to listen to their bodies. It is usually possible to find a safer, pain-free approach to accomplishing the same fitness goal.

For most older participants, the use of walking patterns, general stretches and static stretching during the warm-up and cool-down phases of a class can increase range of motion. However, older adults may need to spend much more time warming up—some as much as 20 minutes or more—than younger exercisers. Instructors should advise participants who need more than the 5–10 minutes usually allotted for the warm-up to arrive early and begin their warm-up before class. Participants with extremely limited mobility may require a physical therapy program or special classes. Therefore, the instructor should be aware of the physical limitations of older participants and refer them when necessary to other health professionals.

Bone Structure

Bone mass may decrease with age, particularly in women. Decreased bone mass accompanied by an increased susceptibility to fractures is called osteoporosis (see Chapter 3). Osteoporosis involves most bones of the body and often is not discovered until the person suffers a fracture. Although the loss of bone mass is not fully understood, it appears to be related to a number of factors, including physical inactivity, estrogen deficiency in menopausal women, smoking, inadequate calcium intake, and extreme thinness. Adequate calcium intake and exercise are the two best weapons against osteoporosis. Like muscles, bones must be exercised to stay strong. Studies have shown that immobility leads to bone loss, and that the stress of weight-bearing exercise builds up bone mineral mass.

A person with diagnosed osteoporosis should not be in a traditional dance-exercise class, for a fall or even a simple twisting movement can cause a fracture. Those at risk for osteoporosis, which affects an estimated 25%–35% of women past menopause, should begin exercise at a low level of intensity, build gradually, and minimize impact as much as possible. It is also important to wear shoes with proper support and to take special care to avoid movements that might cause a fall.

Maximal Oxygen Consumption

Aerobic capacity represents the integrative function of the heart rate, stroke volume, lung ventilation, and oxygen use by the tissues. The single best measure of aerobic capacity is maximal oxygen consumption. In the normal aging process, maximal oxygen consumption declines about 8%–10% per decade after age 30. This decline is believed to result from a corresponding decrease in maximal heart rate, which affects the amount of blood pumped from the heart per minute. Aerobic capacity decreases almost twice as fast in sedentary and overweight persons as in active persons.

There is growing evidence that regular exercise may delay the age-related decline in maximal oxygen capacity (Kasch, Wallace, and Van Camp 1985). Of primary importance is the fact that aerobic capacity can be improved in sedentary older adults through a mild to moderate exercise program consisting of 3–4 sessions per week on alternate days, for a minimum of 20 minutes, at an intensity of 50%–60% maximal oxygen consumption (Smith and Gilligan 1983), which is roughly equivalent to 60%–70% maximal heart rate reserve. It is important for instructors to remember, however, that some participants may need to begin at an intensity below 60% maximal heart rate reserve, or a duration of 10 minutes or less, and build gradually toward these goals. Others may have a good aerobic capacity but lack the muscular endurance to perform the routines.

When performing aerobic routines, older exercisers are more likely to suffer from extremes of heat and cold. They may be more likely to suffer from heat exhaustion as a result of changes in the body's capacity to perspire. Therefore, they should not exercise when it is too hot or too humid, and they should avoid warm, stuffy rooms. In cool environments, older adults may become chilled, partially as a result of diminished blood flow to the skin. The instructor should advise participants to layer their clothing so they can add or remove layers as necessary to remain comfortable.

Although older adults can demonstrate improvements in maximal oxygen consumption similar to that of their younger counterparts, it may take longer to achieve such enhanced function. Overall, an older adult participating in an aerobics program may enjoy some or all of the following improvements in cardiorespiratory fitness: a decrease in submaximal heart rate at a similar workload, a faster recovery heart rate, and a decreased systolic blood pressure at rest and during exercise. However, most older adults will progress more slowly and will not progress as far as younger exercisers.

In addition to these physiological benefits, an older adult can experience the psychological and social benefits of a regular aerobic exercise program. These benefits include decreased anxiety and tension, improved self-confidence and self-esteem, and the sense of well-being. Many older adults will not exercise alone but enjoy exercising in a group that also provides social contact. For this population exercise can play an important role in reducing the anxiety of growing older and the stress caused by lifestyle changes. Because inactivity ages the body as well as the brain, older adults who exercise may not only have more control over their bodies, they may also feel more alert.

Exercise Modifications for the Older Adult

The approach to developing an exercise program for older adults is similar to that for the rest of the population. The instructor needs to take a health history, conduct a fitness assessment and design a program using the FITT principle. However, because the different systems of the body age at different rates, and because older participants are more likely to have medical problems than younger participants, the exercise program should, in general, be more personalized. For example, a 65-year-old woman may have the cardiovascular system of a 40-year-old but be hampered during aerobics by an arthritic condition that limits her mobility. Similarly a 60-year-old man may have good muscular strength but also have a heart condition that requires him to work at a low intensity during aerobics.

When working with older adults, instructors may want to take a more in-depth health history. Class placement is very important, not only for regulating exercise intensity but to ensure adequate supervision. Above all, the instructor needs to use a conservative approach, especially at first, to developing an exercise program for the older adult. Before entering an exercise program, all men over 40 years of age and women over 45 should obtain a physician's approval (see Chapter 4). The following program modifications are recommended for older adults:

1. Conduct a thorough and progressive warm-up, from 5–20 minutes or more for some participants. (Some exercisers may have to come to class early to begin their warm-up.)

2. Begin at a low level of intensity and progress very gradually to a mild to moderate level.

3. For participants with arthritis or other orthopedic problems, obtain a medical clearance and only include those activities recommended by the physician or physical therapist.

4. Emphasize alignment and balance throughout the workout.

5. Never use weights with a participant who has arthritis or other orthopedic problems, unless the participant has a clearance to use weights from his or her physician.

6. Observe participants at all times for signs of distress or over-exercising.

7. Give cues for breathing throughout the exercise period. (While they are concentrating, many participants will forget to breathe, especially when they are learning something new.)

8. Encourage older adults to move at their own pace, and allow them extra time to learn new movements.

9. Remind participants to listen to their bodies and stop any movement that causes pain.

10. Because many older adults have poor posture, emphasize exercises that improve posture.

11. To avoid overuse of muscles and joints, carefully sequence the movement patterns of each routine and the class as a whole.

12. Limit the number of repetitions, especially those involving the knee and shoulder joints.

13. Emphasize the importance of hydration, and encourage water breaks.

14. For participants who have vision or hearing problems, stay in their line of sight and speak loudly, slowly and clearly (do not yell). If necessary, repeat instructions in another way.

15. Caution older adults against exercising in the heat, and advise them to layer their clothing when exercising in cool environments.

In summary, an instructor working with older adults should take special care to start at each participant's level of fitness and ability. To do so means that the instructor must know the participants—their physical and postural problems, their attitudes toward exercise, and their general levels of health—and build from there. It is important to pay more attention to keeping all movements in balance, neither over-stretching or overstrengthening the muscles. The older adult may require a more thorough introduction to all new exercises and more feedback as they progress. The time needed to build endurance and improve fitness is different for each person, and the instructor needs to be patient and offer frequent encouragement.

SUMMARY

No exercise program is appropriate for all participants. Therefore, an instructor must be prepared to modify a program in light of each participant's fitness goals, abilities, and medical history. As discussed in Chapter 4, medical clearance is necessary for participants with medical conditions that may make exercise dangerous. While not absolutely essential, physical fitness assessments provide valuable information on participants' strengths and weaknesses and provide a performance baseline against which to measure improvement. Fitness tests appropriate for a dance-exercise setting include (a) the step test and 1.5-mile walk/run for cardiovascular fitness, (b) skinfold measurements for body composition, (c) the grip-strength test for muscular strength, (d) the 2-minute, timed, sit-up test and the push-up test for muscular endurance, and (e) the sit-and-reach test for low-back flexibility.

Using the results of the fitness assessment and information from the health screening process, an instructor can individualize an exercise program using the FITT principle (frequency, intensity, time or duration, and type of activity). For example, participants with hypertension should avoid isometric exercises and should maintain a low to moderate level of intensity during aerobics. Instructors should make a special point of reminding hypertensives to breathe properly and to undergo a thorough and gradual warm-up and cool-down. For participants with arthritis, instructors should emphasize range-of-motion exercises, while decreasing the intensity and duration, and increasing the frequency of low-impact aerobics to impose less stress on the joints. Such program modifications, combined with close observation of participants to detect signs of overexercising or underexercising, will ensure a safe and effective workout for the vast majority of people.

REFERENCES

Golding, L. A., C. R. Meyers, and W. E. Sinning. *The Y's Way to Physical Fitness.* Chicago: National Board of YMCA, 1982.

Jackson, A. S., and M. L. Pollock. "Practical Assessment of Body Composition." *The Physician and Sportsmedicine* (May 1985): 76–90.

Kart, C. S., E. S. Metress, and J. F. Metress. *Aging and Health: Biological and Social Perspectives.* Menlo Park, California: Addison-Wesley, 1978.

Kasch, F., J. P. Wallace, and S. Van Camp. "Effects of 18 Years of Endurance Exercise on the Physical Work Capacity of Older Men." *Journal of Cardiopulmonary Rehabilitation* (July 1985): 308–12.

Montani, T. and H. deVries. "Neural Factors versus Hypertrophy in the Time Course of Muscle Strength Gain in Young and Old Men." *Journal of Gerontology* 36 (1981): 294–97.

Smith, E. L. and L. Gilligan. "Physical Activity Prescription for the Older Adult." *The Physician and Sportsmedicine* (August 1983): 91–101.

SUGGESTED READING

American College of Sports Medicine (ACSM). *Guidelines for Exercise Testing and Prescription.* Philadelphia: Lea and Febiger, 1986.

Cooper, K. H. *The Aerobics Program for Total Well-Being.* New York: Bantam Books, 1982.

deVries, H. A. *Physiology of Exercise: For Physical Education and Athletics.* 4th ed. Dubuque, Iowa: William C. Brown, 1986.

Getchell, B. *Physical Fitness: A Way of Life.* 3rd ed. New York: John Wiley & Sons, 1983.

McArdle, W. D., F. I. Katch, and V. L. Katch. *Exercise Physiology: Energy, Nutrition and Human Performance.* 2nd ed. Philadelphia: Lea and Febiger, 1986.

Nieman, D. C. *The Sports Medicine Fitness Course.* Palo Alto, Calif.: Bull Publishing Company, 1986.

Pollock, M. L., J. H. Wilmore, and S. M. Fox. *Exercise in Health and Disease: Evaluation and Prescription for Prevention and Rehabilitation.* Philadelphia: W. B. Saunders, 1984.

Exercise and Pregnancy: Physiological Considerations

Janet P. Wallace

Janet P. Wallace, Ph.D., is associate professor of clinical exercise physiology and program director of the Adult Fitness Program at Indiana University. She serves on the certification committee for the American College of Sports Medicine and conducts research on the role of exercise in health, disease and aging.

7

IN THIS CHAPTER:

- The physiology of pregnancy: the metabolic system, the circulatory system, the respiratory system, and the musculoskeletal system.

- Principles of exercise during pregnancy and postpartum: contraindications, frequency, intensity, duration, progression, and precautions.

A pregnant woman is not fragile; neither is she incapacitated. Most women are able to exercise during pregnancy and many choose to do so. A pregnant woman, however, is different physiologically from a woman who is not pregnant. In addition to the obvious changes in shape and weight, she experiences more subtle changes in hormones and cardiac output. It is necessary therefore to tailor the mode, intensity, and duration of any exercise program to the specific needs of the pregnant woman.

The purpose of this chapter is to provide a basic understanding of pregnancy and the postpartum period so that a dance-exercise instructor can respond to the needs of pregnant and postpartum exercisers and can recognize warning signs that indicate a woman should see her doctor. It is extremely important to understand that the information here does not qualify an exercise leader to conduct specialized prenatal or postnatal exercise classes. It is also important to realize that scientific and medical knowledge regarding exercise during pregnancy and postpartum is in its infancy. Because this knowledge is still developing, what is written here today may be modified tomorrow.

THE PHYSIOLOGY OF PREGNANCY

The growth and development of a new life requires the interaction of many of the body's systems. Exercise requires these complex interactions as well. In fact, pregnancy and exercise "share" certain body systems, including the metabolic system, the circulatory system, the respiratory system, and the musculoskeletal system. Because exercise and pregnancy depend on common systems, they can affect each other. For example, pregnancy changes the muscular and skeletal systems which are the basic systems of balance and movement. On the other hand, exercise produces heat which may also disturb the developing fetus. This section describes how these common systems interact when a pregnant woman exercises.

The Metabolic System

Metabolism is energy expenditure. Energy is required to grow a baby *and* to exercise. Fuel is needed to produce that energy or to do work. Glucose or sugar is the major fuel for pregnancy. Exercising muscles also use glucose, especially at the start of a workout and when the exercise is hard. After 20 minutes, easy to moderate exercise will rely more on fats than on glucose. Because both pregnancy and exercise demand glucose, low blood sugar (hypoglycemia) may occur in pregnant women who exercise strenuously or for long periods.

Exercise produces waste products like lactic acid and carbon dioxide, and changes the body to a more acidic state. The amount of the waste products produced depends on how hard a person exercises; the harder the work, the more waste produced. All of these waste products can be delivered to the **fetus** through the **placenta.** The fetus does take protective action; however, the mother can keep the waste to a minimum by controlling how hard she exercises.

The Circulatory System

The purpose of the circulatory system is to deliver nutrients, gases like oxygen and carbon dioxide, waste products of metabolism, and heat. The developing fetus needs nutrients and oxygen to grow, and the exercising muscles also need nutrients and oxygen for work. Similarly, the fetus produces waste products during its growth and development, and the muscles produce waste products and heat during exercise. Both the waste products and heat must be disposed of by the circulatory system.

The arteries and veins are the rivers of the circulatory "delivery" system. Plasma (the fluid part of blood) is the medium of transport, carrying the nutrients, waste, and heat. The gases ride on red blood cells that travel like boats through the plasma. Together the plasma and red blood cells form the blood or the total blood volume.

The blood is of no use if it sits stagnant like a swamp; it must move to deliver its goods. The current for blood flow is generated by the pumping action of the heart. The cardiac output is the total amount of blood the heart pumps each minute. This current is determined by how much blood the heart pumps with each beat (the stroke volume) and how many times the heart pumps per minute (the heart rate).

Because of the increased metabolic demands of pregnancy, more blood vessels are formed and total blood volume increases 40%. Plasma accounts for most of the increase. The red blood cells also increase, but not in proportion to the plasma. Therefore, in the circulatory system of a pregnant woman, there are fewer red blood cells or transportation vehicles at any one spot than in a nonpregnant woman. When there are fewer red blood cells in a single area, the blood cannot carry as much oxygen. The ability of the blood to carry oxygen is called the oxygen carrying capacity. When the oxygen carrying capacity becomes too low, a condition called anemia exists. Anemia during pregnancy is not a problem for most women, especially if they increase their iron intake. However, for some women, anemia reduces the oxygen carrying capacity to a level where the fetus may not get enough oxygen. In this case, exercise may be contraindicated.

Because of the larger blood volume and the growing baby, cardiac output increases during pregnancy. This increase in stroke volume and heart rate, similar to that found during very easy exercise, reflects the fact that fetal growth takes work. Thus, the pregnant woman can never achieve a state of rest, as she could achieve before pregnancy or will achieve again after pregnancy.

When a system needs blood, the body directs, or shunts, the blood to that area. For example, when muscles need the blood, the stomach, liver, and kidneys give up some of theirs. During pregnancy, more blood is directed to the uterine artery for the fetus to receive nourishment and grow. Yet, if the mother exercises, the exercising muscles also need the blood flow. Scientists do not know if the fetus gives up its share of the blood flow to the exercising muscles; some animal studies show a decrease in uterine blood flow during exercise and others do not. In any case, scientists propose that, in a normal healthy pregnancy, the fetus can give up a little less than half of its blood supply for the duration of a typical exercise class without any problems.

The circulatory system also plays an important role in temperature regulation. If the body were perfect, all the energy it produces would end up as work. But the body is not perfect—it produces heat when it exercises. Heat production during exercise is like waste production. The harder the exercise, the higher the body temperature. In addition, temperature regulation becomes more difficult as pregnancy progresses. One recent study (Jones 1985) observed women exercise throughout pregnancy: Skin temperatures were higher in the third trimester than in the first, even though the total amount of work performed during exercise decreased significantly as pregnancy progressed. In a normal environment, temperature regulation appears to be adequate. However, in a hot, humid environment a pregnant exerciser may have more difficulty regulating body temperature than a nonpregnant exerciser.

The fetus usually stays one degree hotter than the mother. Because it has no way of getting rid of heat, the fetus must depend entirely on the mother's ability to cool off. Animal studies have indicated that chronic exposure to heat in early pregnancy may cause defects of the neural tube, the part of the embryo that develops into the brain and spinal cord. Although neural tube defects are rare (2 per 1,000 births in the United States) and have a variety of causes, including rubella and exposure to radiation, pregnant women should be aware of the problem and avoid chronic exposure to heat.

Exercising in the heat places greater demands on a pregnant woman's circulatory system in still another way. To cool off, the body must sweat. One of the functions of the circulatory system is to deliver hot blood to the skin so that when the sweat evaporates, the heat goes away from the body. When a pregnant woman exercises, more blood is shunted to the skin, increasing the possibility that the fetus will not receive enough blood.

AEROBIC DANCE-EXERCISE INSTRUCTOR MANUAL

Excess sweating can deplete the body of water, a state called dehydration. Dehydration may precipitate premature labor later in pregnancy and can lead to difficulties with breast-feeding. Therefore it is important for pregnant women to be conscious of the environment and to take precautions against the heat.

The Respiratory System

The circulatory system is a good oxygen-delivery network, but it needs help loading oxygen and unloading carbon dioxide. The lungs bring oxygen into the body and load it onto the red blood cells. Then they unload carbon dioxide and remove it from the body. The kidneys help unload other waste, and the sweat glands help unload heat.

As the fetus grows, the uterus rises in the abdominal cavity. Near the end of pregnancy, the uterus pushes the diaphragm upward, creating a feeling of dyspnea, or shortness of breath, in some women. At the same time, physiological changes occur that improve the oxygen–carbon dioxide exchange between mother and fetus. The rib cage also expands, and the movement of the diaphragm increases. Therefore, although the respiratory rate remains the same during pregnancy, **tidal volume** (the amount of air that passes in and out of the lungs in an ordinary breath) actually increases.

A pregnant woman is able to meet the increased ventilatory needs of mild exercise. However, the maternal respiratory system is not able to compensate effectively for high-intensity, or anaerobic, exercise (Artal et al. 1986).

The Musculoskeletal System

Changes in the breasts and the abdomen of a pregnant woman alter the balance point of the body (the center of gravity), making the body more unstable. When the center of gravity changes, the body often has to "relearn" how to stand or to move.

The change in the center of gravity puts extra work on the muscles to keep the body "in balance" at rest or for any kind of movement. In addition, the enlarged abdomen creates a lower back curvature called lordosis, which results in low-back pain for many women. The low-back pain will increase as body weight increases in the last trimester. A good fitness program will provide exercises to relax the lower back and help ease low-back pain.

The skeletal system must also change during pregnancy: the ribs must be elevated to make room for the fetus, and the pelvic region must widen for birth. Because the bones cannot stretch, **relaxin,** a pregnancy hormone, loosens the joints. As a result, the pelvis and all the joints of the body become looser. This increased joint laxity may increase the potential for injury during physical activity and must be considered when leading exercises for pregnant participants.

PRINCIPLES OF PRENATAL AND POSTPARTUM EXERCISE

The purpose of an exercise program during pregnancy is to maintain physical fitness and to prepare for labor and delivery, not to improve athletic performance nor to participate in competitive activities. A dance-exercise instructor working with a pregnant exerciser should consider

Table 7–1

ACOG GUIDELINES FOR EXERCISE DURING PREGNANCY AND POSTPARTUM

The following guidelines are based on the unique physical and physiological conditions that exist during pregnancy and the postpartum period. They outline general criteria for safety to provide direction to patients in the development of home exercise programs.

Pregnancy and Postpartum

1. Regular exercise (at least 3 times per week) is preferable to intermittent activity. Competitive activities should be discouraged.

2. Vigorous exercise should not be performed in hot, humid weather or during a period of febrile illness.

3. Ballistic movements (jerky, bouncy motions) should be avoided. Exercise should be done on a wooden floor or a tightly carpeted surface to reduce shock and provide a sure footing.

4. Deep flexion or extension of joints should be avoided because of connective tissue laxity. Activities that require jumping, jarring motions or rapid changes in direction should be avoided because of joint instability.

5. Vigorous exercise should be preceded by a 5-minute period of muscle warm-up. This can be accomplished by slow walking or stationary cycling with low resistance.

6. Vigorous exercise should be followed by a period of gradually declining activity that includes gentle stationary stretching. Because connective tissue laxity increases the risk of joint injury, stretches should not be taken to the point of maximum resistance.

7. Heart rate should be measured at times of peak activity. Target heart rates and limits established in consultation with the physician should not be exceeded.

8. Care should be taken to gradually rise from the floor to avoid orthostatic hypotension. Some form of activity involving the legs should be continued for a brief period.

9. Liquids should be taken liberally before and after exercise to prevent dehydration. If necessary, activity should be interrupted to replenish fluids.

10. Women who have led sedentary lifestyles should begin with physical activity of very low intensity and advance activity levels very gradually.

11. Activity should be stopped and the physician consulted if any unusual symptoms appear.

Pregnancy Only

1. Maternal heart rate should not exceed 140 beats per minutes.

2. Strenuous activities should not exceed 15 minutes in duration.

3. No exercise should be performed in the supine position after the fourth month of gestation is completed.

4. Exercises that employ the Valsalva maneuver should be avoided.

5. Caloric intake should be adequate to meet not only the extra energy needs of pregnancy, but also of the exercise performed.

6. Maternal core temperature should not exceed 38°C.

Source: American College of Obstetricians and Gynecologists. *Exercise during Pregnancy and the Postnatal Period (ACOG Home Exercise Programs).* Washington, D.C.: ACOG, 1985. Reprinted with permission.

the mode, frequency, duration, intensity, and progression of an exercise program. The American College of Obstetricians and Gynecologists (1985) has set forth guidelines for exercising safely during pregnancy and the postpartum period (see Table 7–1). Although an exercise program should be tailored to the needs of the individual, these guidelines provide good general information.

Table 7–2

CONTRAINDICATIONS FOR EXERCISE DURING PREGNANCY

ABSOLUTE CONTRAINDICATIONS	RELATIVE CONTRAINDICATIONS
Heart disease	High blood pressure
Ruptured membranes	Anemia or other blood disorders
Premature labor	Thyroid diseases
Multiple gestation	Diabetes
Bleeding	Palpitations or irregular heart rhythms
Placenta previa	Breech presentation in the last trimester
Incompetent cervix	Excessive obesity
History of 3 or more spontaneous abortions or miscarriages	Extreme underweight
	History of precipitous labor
	History of intrauterine growth retardation
	History of bleeding during present pregnancy
	Extremely sedentary lifestyle

Contraindications for Exercise during Pregnancy

Before beginning or continuing an exercise program, a pregnant woman must be evaluated for contraindications or signs that she should not exercise. A physician is the only person qualified to evaluate these contraindications. Table 7–2 lists the absolute and relative contraindications for exercise during pregnancy. Whether a woman chooses to begin an exercise program during her pregnancy or wishes to continue an existing program, she must obtain a written medical clearance from her physician.

Women with absolute contraindications should not exercise. Women with relative contraindications may exercise if their physicians approve; however, they should be in supervised exercise programs with specially trained instructors, not in classes for the general public. A pregnant woman who does not have an obstetrician or is not under the care of a physician or health professional should not be allowed in an exercise class and should not be given an exercise program.

Exercise Frequency, Intensity, and Duration

There is no scientific literature investigating the minimal amount of exercise (frequency, intensity and duration) necessary to maintain cardiovascular fitness during pregnancy. For the majority of the nonpregnant population, 2–3 aerobics sessions per week for 20–30 minutes is adequate to maintain, if not improve, fitness. The American College of Obstetricians and Gynecologists (1985) suggests a 15-minute period as the maximum duration for maintaining cardiovascular fitness during pregnancy. Three to four sessions per week is appropriate for relaxation and strengthening exercises. Exercises for the lower back can be done whenever relief is required, which means that they may be more frequent near the end of the pregnancy.

Exercise intensity should be low, well below the anaerobic threshold. An intensity of 50%–60% maximal functional capacity (maximal oxygen consumption) will prevent excessive buildup of exercise by-products and heat which could be delivered to the growing fetus. Intensity can be guided by target heart rates, perceived exertion, and the talk test (see Chapter 9 for more information on these methods).

Measures of exercise intensity may need modification, especially if nonpregnant target heart rates are used. During pregnancy the heart rate is never at rest and the maximal heart rate decreases. No formula can be devised at this time to estimate changes in maximal heart rates during pregnancy. If nonpregnant heart rates are used to predict exercise heart rates, the target could be 10–20 beats too high, and the pregnant exerciser would be working too hard.

The American College of Obstetricians and Gynecologists has chosen a maximum target heart rate of 140 beats per minute for pregnant women because exercising above that level may increase the body temperature above the critical temperature (Pers. com., Art Ulene November 1984). However, there is no scientific basis for choosing a single target heart rate that would be applicable to all pregnant women under all environmental conditions. Target heart rates are most valid when the true resting and the true maximal heart rates have been measured. Because pregnancy changes both resting and maximal heart rates, and because most pregnant women will not have their maximal heart rate measured or predicted accurately, other means of guiding exercise intensity are preferable.

Ratings of perceived exertion (RPE) may be a better monitor of exercise intensity. Although the use of perceived exertion during pregnancy has not been adequately investigated, it may be a safer method. The instructor must teach each participant how to use perceived exertion as a measure of intensity during exercise. RPE measures how hard the participant works. The rating of 6 represents the participant's exertion "at rest," while 20 is the "hardest" the participant has ever, or will ever, work. The recommended 50%–60% of maximum functional capacity correlates with 13–14 on the RPE scale.

Another useful guide of exercise intensity is the talk test. If a pregnant exerciser cannot carry on a conversation during exercise, she is exercising too hard. The talk test keeps her under the anaerobic threshold. Exercising above the anaerobic threshold causes shortness of breath and, thus, difficulty in talking.

Exercise Progression

The progression of physical activity is an important aspect of any exercise program. During pregnancy, however, progression may be better described as "regression." The instructor should know when to slow down the exercise program. During the first trimester, physical fitness will decrease. Some women will perceive that the same amount of work will require more effort than before pregnancy and they will adjust their efforts accordingly. Other women, who try to continue prepregnancy activity levels, will need instruction on decreasing their efforts.

In the second trimester, physical fitness will increase, although never to prepregnancy levels. A pregnant exerciser may be able to exert more effort during this trimester, however. If the exercise is comfortable for the pregnant participant and within the recommended guidelines, she should be allowed to continue. Remind her that she must not try to do the same amount of work she did before she was pregnant.

As body weight increases in the third trimester, physical fitness will again decrease and the amount of work a pregnant exerciser does should be decreased as well. During this time, weight-bearing activities may become uncomfortable, and a gradual transition to non-weight-bearing activities such as swimming and stationary cycling may become a reasonable alternative. A progressive exercise program for pregnancy may move from traditional aerobics to low-impact aerobics (see Chapter 13), then alternate low-impact aerobics with a walking program, and finally shift to a total walking program. Most changes in exercise mode depend on the participant's comfort. Some women have been able to participate in regular dance-exercise classes and even lead classes until childbirth. Most women, however, need guidance for change.

Precautions for Exercise during Pregnancy

Physiological changes during pregnancy require modifications in the exercise program. The problems discussed below may occur in an unmodified program. An exercise program for pregnant women should always err on the side of caution, and dance-exercise instructors who have pregnant students should be particularly alert to the following physiological conditions.

EXERCISING IN THE SUPINE POSITION. When a pregnant woman lies on her back, the weight of the fetus may obstruct the flow of blood back to her heart and head. For this reason, exercise in the supine position has been contraindicated after the fourth month (American College of Obstetricians and Gynecologists, 1985). Symptoms of obstructed blood flow include light-headedness or dizziness. If a participant becomes light-headed in the supine position, roll her on to her side until she feels better. Then help her slowly sit up.

Some women continue to exercise in the supine position because they do not "feel" the symptoms of low blood flow to the head. It is important to note that only one study has investigated blood flow to the fetus during exercise in the supine position (Morris 1956). This study found that the blood flow to the fetus decreased. Therefore, the fetus may experience negative effects even though the mother does not. As stated earlier, scientists theorize that in a normal healthy pregnancy, the fetus can give up a little less than half of its blood supply for a short time without any problems. However, the instructor should still caution a pregnant woman against supine exercise and suggest safer alternatives.

THERMOREGULATION. Everything that happens in the human body can be broken down into a chemical reaction. If the body temperature deviates even 6–7 degrees from normal, these chemical reactions cannot take place. Because of the hormone changes and the growing fetus, the body temperature of a pregnant woman usually starts 1–2 degrees higher than that of a nonpregnant woman. It is extremely important that pregnant exercisers take every precaution against overheating during exercise in a warm environment.

As stated earlier, frequently elevating the body temperature to over 102°F in the first trimester may increase the likelihood of neural tube defects in the fetus. Studies associating an increase in body temperature with neural tube defects have dealt primarily with chronic heat exposure, not the heat generated by exercise. However, it is still wise for a pregnant exerciser to be conservative, because the heat generated during exercise can exacerbate chronic heat exposure.

Later in pregnancy, dehydration from chronic heat exposure may precipitate premature labor. Temperature regulation also remains important in postpartum, especially if the mother is breast-feeding her infant. If a nursing mother becomes dehydrated from working in the heat, milk production will be difficult. Drinking plenty of fluids before, during, and after exercise is one of the best precautions.

The best measure to prevent heat-related problems during pregnancy is education. The instructor should make certain that pregnant participants are aware of potential problems, and that they follow established guidelines for exercising in the heat (see Chapter 1). The instructor should also alert pregnant exercisers to the signs and symptoms of heat intolerance, which include (a) chills, (b) throbbing pressure in the head, (c) unsteadiness, (d) nausea, (e) dry skin, and (f) clammy skin.

If a heat-related problem does occur, the instructor should follow this procedure:

1. Have the pregnant exerciser stop exercising and find a cool place for her to cool down.

2. Give her cool fluids.

3. Refer her to her obstetrician.

4. If her response is extreme (dry or clammy skin and chills), call an ambulance.

JOINT LAXITY. During pregnancy most women will be more flexible than at any other time in their lives. If a pregnant exerciser applies the same effort in range-of-motion exercises as before pregnancy, increased joint laxity may lead to injury. The pregnant woman should not overstretch and should perform all exercises in a controlled manner. The focus of a flexibility program during pregnancy should be to stretch the muscles worked during strength and endurance activities, to counteract muscle cramping or muscle soreness, and to relax the lower back. Improving joint range of motion should not be the primary focus during pregnancy.

LOW BLOOD SUGAR. Low blood sugar (hypoglycemia) should not occur during exercise if a pregnant woman eats regular and nutritious meals. Low blood sugar usually occurs in insulin-dependent diabetics who exercise. Diabetes is a relative contraindication for exercise during pregnancy. Although most diabetic women will be screened out of regular dance-exercise programs, one type of diabetes does exist only during pregnancy. The signs and symptoms of low blood sugar (see Table 7-3) are the same for both pregnancy and diabetes. If these symptoms occur, the instructor should follow this procedure:

1. Have the participant stop exercising.

2. Give simple carbohydrates, preferably in liquid form, such as orange juice.

3. Let the participant rest.

4. Refer her to her obstetrician.

5. If the response is extreme—loss of consciousness or convulsions—transport her to the hospital.

Table 7–3

SIGNS AND SYMPTOMS OF LOW BLOOD SUGAR

Drowsiness	Faintness	Hand tremors
Sweating	Dizziness	Excessive hunger
Fatigue	Irritability	Unsteady gait
Apathy	Blurred vision	Confusion
Loss of consciousness	Double vision	Convulsions
Headache	Nervousness	Inability to concentrate
Slurred speech	Poor coordination	

Exercise Programming for the Postpartum Period

The physiological changes of pregnancy remain until 6–8 weeks after birth. Hormones will not return to normal levels in nursing mothers until they stop breast-feeding. Many of the guidelines for exercise during pregnancy still apply to the postpartum period.

MODE.   All exercise modes for physical fitness, including aerobic activities, can be resumed after pregnancy. Few women are able to resume activity within a week after delivery; more women begin to exercise again around the sixth week. Each woman should consult with her obstetrician to determine the best time to resume exercise.

Most women resume their exercise program by walking for 6 to 8 weeks and gradually switch to the mode of exercise they prefer. Those women who resume dance exercise early in the postpartum period report the sensation of their uterus falling. The uterus is not actually falling, however, and the sensation should disappear once the muscles regain their former tone. During this time, the Kegel exercises described in Chapter 8 become most important and most effective.

Abdominal exercises are still important to firm up the muscle tone of the stomach. Continuing the lower back exercises will help control low-back pain, and additional instruction in lifting and carrying should help prevent low-back problems and fatigue. Abdominal and lower back exercises used in nonpregnant classes can be safely incorporated into the postpartum exercise program.

FREQUENCY, DURATION, AND INTENSITY.   Exercise frequency, duration, and intensity will depend on the fitness and goals of the new mother. To maintain fitness, a postpartum exerciser will probably have to exercise 2–3 times per week for 20–30 minutes. To improve fitness, she may have to increase the frequency to 3–4 times per week and the duration to 30 minutes. If she also wants to lose excess fat gained during pregnancy, her exercise program should emphasize long-duration, low-intensity exercise 4–5 times per week.

Exercise intensity during pregnancy was low. Any increase in intensity should be made gradually and as comfort dictates. One study suggests that nursing mothers should exercise at an intensity below the anaerobic threshold. Wallace and Rabin (1986) found lactic acid, a byproduct of anaerobic exercise, in mother's milk. A few mothers have reported difficulties with breast-feeding after vigorous exercise. However, aerobic exercise (exercise below the anaerobic threshold) should not cause difficulty for the nursing infant.

SUMMARY

Exercise can be beneficial during pregnancy. Because safety for the mother and the fetus is very important, the early guidelines for exercise during pregnancy are often conservative. As our knowledge and experience expands, these guidelines may change. The guidelines presented here provide basic criteria for an instructor who wants to incorporate a pregnant participant in a regular dance-exercise class. Instructors will require further training and experience to be qualified to conduct specialized prenatal classes.

REFERENCES

American College of Obstetricians and Gynecologists. *Exercise During Pregnancy and Postnatal Period (ACOG Home Exercise Programs)*. Washington, D.C.: ACOG, 1985.

American College of Sports Medicine. "Position Statement: Prevention of Heat Injuries during Distance Running." *Medicine and Science in Sport 7*, no. 1 (1975): vii–viii.

American College of Sports Medicine. *Guidelines for Exercise Testing and Prescription*. Philadelphia: Lea & Febiger, 1986.

Artal, R., and R. A. Wiswell. *Exercise in Pregnancy*, Baltimore: Williams & Wilkins, 1986.

Artal, R., R. A. Wiswell, Y. Romem, and F. Dorey. "Pulmonary Responses to Exercise in Pregnancy," *American Journal of Obstetrics and Gynecology* 154 (1986): 378–83.

Gorski, J. "Exercise during Pregnancy: Maternal and Fetal Responses. A Brief Review." *Medicine and Science in Sport and Exercise* 17 (1985): 407–16.

Jones, R. L., J. J. Botti, W. M. Anderson, and N. L. Bennett. "Thermoregulation during Aerobic Exercise in Pregnancy." *Obstetrics and Gynecology* 65 (1985): 340–45.

Morris, N., S. Osborn, H. Wright, and A. Hart. "Effective Uterine Blood Flow during Exercise in Normal and Pre-eclamptic Pregnancies." *Lancet* 2 (1956): 481–84.

Wallace, J. P., and J. Rabin. "Lactic Acid Accumulation in Mother's Milk during Maximal Exercise." *Medicine and Science in Sport and Exercise*, 18 (1986): 547.

Exercise and Pregnancy: The Dance-Exercise Class

Cameron Kelly

8

Cameron Kelly, B.S., a prenatal exercise expert and childbirth educator, is founder of Dynamic Pregnancy Program, the largest prenatal and postpartum fitness program on the East Coast. She has served as Northeast Regional Representative for the IDEA and as a judge for the Crystal Light National Aerobic Competition.

IN THIS CHAPTER:

- Attainable fitness goals during pregnancy.
- Instructor guidelines for accepting pregnant exercisers.

- Integrating pregnant women into conventional classes: advice for pregnant participants, preparing class members, modifying class components.

All women should discuss their prenatal fitness plans with their obstetricians. However, dance-exercise instructors can provide much useful, basic information about exercise during pregnancy in response to the questions frequently asked by participants. Instructors who choose to work with pregnant exercisers in conventional dance-exercise classes must be aware of the normal discomforts experienced during pregnancy and ways to modify a conventional class to achieve maximum safety, comfort, and effectiveness. Instructors should also realize that exercise during pregnancy remains controversial and that research on the subject is inconclusive. Therefore, participants need to use their own common sense when exercising. Instructors should respect individual differences among their pregnant participants and should give them the additional support and guidance they require.

As described in Chapter 7, many body systems are affected by both pregnancy and exercise. The primary goal for a pregnant exerciser who remains in a conventional dance-exercise class should be to maintain the fitness of these systems. If the movements, specific exercises, or intensity of the dance-exercise class are producing a negative impact, such as backache, sciatica, heartburn, or edema, the participant should be advised to discontinue the class despite the other benefits she may be receiving. Even a fit, healthy woman experiences many common discomforts when she is pregnant. Dance exercise should make a pregnant woman feel better about herself and her body, not create further discomfort.

ATTAINABLE FITNESS GOALS

To experience success in a dance-exercise class, a pregnant participant must begin with informed and realistic fitness goals. By working out conscientiously and safely, improving her nutrition, increasing rest and relaxation, eliminating bad health habits, and receiving regular pre-natal care, a woman may become healthier during pregnancy than ever before. Many pregnant women develop a greater interest in health and fitness due to their concern for the baby growing inside them and their desire to provide the best possible environment for fetal growth. Health and fitness habits developed during pregnancy often remain into new motherhood and beyond.

CARDIOVASCULAR FITNESS.   Cardiovascular fitness can be maintained or even improved during pregnancy while working out at a necessarily lower target heart rate of 140 beats per minute or less. If a pregnant woman incorporates aerobic exercise into her fitness plan, she will enjoy a greater work capacity without undue fatigue and will have more energy to get through the day.

IMPROVED MUSCULAR STRENGTH.   Research has shown that women can improve their muscular strength during pregnancy. Since muscles are the stabilizers that support the joints loosened by pregnancy hor-mones, a pregnant woman may reduce her risk of injury with increased muscular strength. Muscular development will lead to muscular effi-ciency, slowing the onset of fatigue and lessening its degree. The devel-opment of upper body strength during pregnancy is also of great prac-tical benefit to a woman who will soon be carrying a baby weighing 6–9 pounds in her arms.

IMPROVED POSTURE.   A pregnant woman may improve her posture significantly by developing her musculoskeletal system. Pregnancy lor-dosis strains the muscles and ligaments of the vertebral column. Strengthening the abdominal muscles counteracts this lordosis. Devel-opment of muscular strength in the upper body can prevent round shoulders, increasing the pregnant woman's capacity for a full breath. Improvement in the postural muscles will also increase a pregnant exerciser's stability.

INCREASED FLEXIBILITY.   Increasing flexibility by enhancing the bal-ance of opposing muscle groups is a desirable and attainable fitness goal during pregnancy. Even though circulating pregnancy hormones loosen the joints, range of motion also depends on the balanced devel-opment of muscles that work in pairs. If a woman is engaged in an aerobics or strength development program that focuses on specific muscles, she must also do flexibility exercises to prevent these short-ened muscles from pulling unevenly on the joints. Increased flexibility can also lessen reduced joint mobility of the extremities due to water retention.

GREATER BALANCE AND EASE OF MOVEMENT.   Although a pregnant exerciser should not expect to improve her agility during her preg-nancy, she may find that her changing shape, weight gain, and loosened joints have less impact on her grace and agility if she participates in a regular, comprehensive exercise program. The repetitious move-ments of dance exercise can help improve her kinesthetic sense, result-ing in greater balance and ease of movement.

ENHANCED SELF-CONCEPT.   Enhanced body image and self-concept are easily met psychological goals for the pregnant student who exercises regularly in a supportive environment. By avoiding excess weight gain and learning to deal comfortably with her healthy increase in weight, she will not feel alienated from her body. Moving gracefully through dance patterns, recognizing small but continual gains in muscular strength and flexibility, and benefiting from improved circulation will give her a psychological lift and help her cope with the limitations she may encounter as her body changes. By reducing anxiety, exercise can also diminish stress.

PREPARATION FOR THE BIRTH PROCESS.   There is no scientific evidence to support the view that exercise will make labor easier or shorter, or that it will reduce the incidence of maternal or fetal complications. However, a fitness program during pregnancy can contribute to a woman's preparation for labor and the birth of her baby. Exercise will result in improved endurance or stamina, which is an asset during labor. She will be better able to use correct muscles with the right amount of force and relax muscles that are not directly involved in the different stages of labor. The pregnant exerciser can expect to tone major muscle groups throughout the body, which will give her a greater number of positions to choose from to enhance comfort during labor. Exercise will also increase her awareness of correct breathing and its impact on muscular efficiency. The ability to breathe with control is a great benefit to a woman's management of her own labor.

GUIDELINES FOR ACCEPTING PREGNANT EXERCISERS INTO A CONVENTIONAL CLASS

Most obstetricians recommend that a healthy pregnant woman continue the physical activities she pursued before pregnancy for as long as she feels comfortable doing so. Pregnancy is not the time to take up a new sport or to train for competition. Most women who have exercised previously can expect to participate safely in a class with their nonpregnant peers. However, most regular dance-exercise classes are not appropriate for a previous nonexerciser. The best option for these women is to join a specialized pregnancy exercise class.

Instructor Considerations

Before accepting pregnant women into their classes, instructors should consider the impact on nonpregnant participants. Answering the following questions can help instructors decide whether their classes can accommodate a pregnant exerciser.

1. *Is the class small enough to allow the instructor to give a pregnant exerciser the supervision and encouragement she needs?* Individual attention may be difficult in a class with more than 20 participants.

2. *What is the nature of the present clientele?* Will they support or resent a pregnant exerciser? Will nonpregnant participants object to the instructor devoting class time and attention to supervising one person? Will nonpregnant participants object to any necessary restructuring of the class to accommodate the needs of the pregnant exerciser?

3. *Does the instructor's or the studio's insurance policy cover teaching pregnant participants?* Can additional coverage be purchased if necessary?

4. Does the studio or spa have any objections to including pregnant women in a conventional dance-exercise class?

5. Is a bathroom readily accessible? Pregnant women need to void frequently, particularly when exercising.

Instructors who feel their classes cannot provide a safe, supportive environment for a pregnant exerciser should refer her to another program.

Screening Potential Participants

An instructor who decides to include pregnant women in a dance-exercise class must carefully screen each potential participant.

1. *Set up an interview to discuss her pregnancy fitness goals and her reasons for wanting to remain in a conventional dance-exercise class.* Review the impact of pregnancy on her body systems and outline realistic fitness goals. Keep in mind that weight loss is not an acceptable pregnancy fitness goal. Instructors should carefully consider whether they are willing to take responsibility for a pregnant woman who may be trying to prove something to herself and others by making it through her entire pregnancy in a conventional class. A woman who alludes to this goal may not be willing to listen to her body and make the necessary modifications in her workout. Some women want to exercise strenuously during pregnancy to keep from "showing" for as long as possible. Intensive abdominal exercises will not achieve this result and may cause discomfort or back pain. If a pregnant participant exercises her abdominals in the supine position for extended periods, she faces additional potential risks (see Chapter 7).

2. *Discuss the absolute and relative contraindications for pregnancy exercise according to the guidelines of the American College of Obstetricians and Gynecologists and clear her for the contraindications.* Require a note from her doctor agreeing with her decision to participate in the specific dance-exercise class (not exercise in general). Instructors may want to give the participant a card or brochure in case her obstetrician wants to call for more information about the content of the class.

3. *Record and have available the following information for a pregnant participant:* An emergency phone number (friend, spouse or other relative) where someone can be reached during class time, and the obstetrician's name, address, and phone number.

Orienting the Pregnant Participant

Before a pregnant woman begins or continues an exercise program, she should be familiar with the physiological changes of pregnancy and how these changes will affect her exercise program. The instructor should cover the following points with a pregnant participant.

1. *Discuss the impact of pregnancy on the cardiovascular system.* Explain that her resting heart rate will be 10–15 beats per minute higher than before pregnancy, and that her heart rate will elevate with less physical effort. Point out that her physical work capacity will decrease during the first trimester, increase during the second trimester (although not to prepregnancy levels), and decrease again during the third trimester. Discuss the impact of pregnancy on her musculoskeletal system, resulting in increased joint laxity and lordosis (see Chapter 7).

Table 8-1

WARNING SIGNS TO STOP EXERCISING

Fainting	Temperature extremes of very hot or cold and clammy
Vaginal bleeding	Gush of fluid from the vagina
Sharp pains in the chest or abdomen	Blurred vision
Extreme nausea	Marked swelling or fluid retention
Feeling of disorientation	Severe or continuous headaches

Table 8-2

COMMON DISCOMFORTS OF PREGNANCY

Heartburn	Stretch marks
Insomnia	Headaches
Leg cramps	Backaches
Urinary incontinence	Feeling unsexy
Self-consciousness about size	Nausea
Sciatica	Excess vaginal discharge
Bunions	Larger, heavier breasts
Constipation	Groin pains or spasms
Itching skin	Edema
Spider veins	Dry or oily skin
Excessive perspiration	Constant overheating
Fatigue	Fallen arches
Breast tenderness	Spreading buttocks
Varicose veins	Varicose veins of the vulva
Aching, swollen feet	
Propensity for vaginal yeast infections	

2. *Ask the participant to pay attention to how she feels during the first trimester when her body is adapting to its pregnant state.* Fatigue and nausea are common, even among physically fit pregnant women. Encourage her to rest often during the day when possible and to take breaks from her workout if she feels so inclined. Assure her that she will feel more like her old self during the second trimester and can resume her activities then.

3. *Emphasize the additional energy expenditure of pregnancy.* Advise the pregnant participant to discuss her diet with her doctor to ensure that her caloric intake is adequate to compensate for the additional calories burned during exercise. An active pregnant woman must have adequate iron in her diet to prevent anemia and she should discuss this subject with her doctor.

4. *Review the immediate pregnancy danger signs listed in Table 8–1. Inform the student that if she experiences any of these symptoms, exercise is definitely contraindicated until she is cleared by her obstetrician.*

5. *Discuss feelings and discomforts commonly experienced during pregnancy (see Table 8–2).* Every pregnant woman does not experience every discomfort listed, but few women avoid them all. While it is essential for a pregnant exerciser to be aware of the danger signs that require immediate medical guidance, it is also important to reduce anxiety about minor discomforts.

Recommending Specialized Prenatal Exercise Classes

Although some conventional dance-exercise classes can provide a suitable environment for a pregnant woman to continue her fitness routine, a woman who has not exercised regularly before pregnancy should be referred to a specialized prenatal exercise class. A woman who has exercised before pregnancy may also want to join a prenatal exercise class because of the specialized information and fitness routines offered.

Prenatal exercise classes address the comprehensive fitness needs of a pregnant woman, including corrective exercises for the musculoskeletal imbalances caused by pregnancy and special exercises to relieve pregnancy discomforts. These classes, which are designed to help a woman prepare physically for labor and delivery, can be choreographed more effectively and paced more appropriately when all participants share similar fitness goals. A discussion of the variety of exercises that can help alleviate the discomforts of pregnancy is outside the scope of this chapter, and leading these exercises requires extensive additional training.

In addition to the increased focus on childbearing muscles and fitness needs, a specialized class provides important emotional and social support. Consider the following benefits:

1. The pregnant exerciser will feel more comfortable with her changing shape if she is not comparing herself to nonpregnant classmates.
2. There will be less temptation to compete with nonpregnant peers who may be exercising at a higher intensity than recommended during pregnancy.
3. Exposure to women in later stages of pregnancy will provide an opportunity for the participant to prepare emotionally for forthcoming changes.
4. There will be opportunities to ask questions and share information about corollary pregnancy fitness issues such as nutrition.
5. The pregnant exerciser will gain confidence in her body and its ability to work hard during labor.
6. For postpartum women, a specialized class can counteract the stresses of poor body image, isolation, and feelings of inadequacy in early motherhood.

In some communities pregnant women have been directed to exercise classes that include the elderly, the infirm, and the handicapped. For the psychological reasons mentioned above, this solution is not appropriate because it reinforces the view that pregnancy is an illness, not a normal, healthy state of being.

INTEGRATING PREGNANT WOMEN INTO CONVENTIONAL CLASSES

In addition to modifying the exercises, there are many other necessary steps to consider when integrating a pregnant woman into a traditional dance-exercise class. These steps include providing practical advice for the pregnant participant and preparing the others in the class.

Advising the Pregnant Participant

Before the pregnant woman joins the class, the instructor should suggest the following ways of increasing her comfort during exercise and preventing possible problems.

1. *Eat a light snack before coming to class.* An easily digestible, high-carbohydrate snack will provide needed energy to complete the workout and will prevent the blood sugar level from plummeting.

2. *Drink fluids, preferably water, before, during, and after class to prevent dehydration.* Be especially careful during hot, humid weather.

3. *Wear a jogging bra or extrasupport bra specifically designed for an active woman.* During pregnancy the breasts enlarge due to the circulating hormones estrogen and progesterone. During exercise, larger, unsupported breasts will bounce against the chest. While there is no evidence that this bouncing will contribute to permanent sagging, it can be uncomfortable because the breasts are more tender during pregnancy. Select an all-cotton bra that will effectively absorb perspiration and that has wide shoulder straps and a back that does not ride up during movement. All plastic and metal fasteners and any elastic should be covered with fabric to prevent chafing.

4. *Wear good-quality aerobics shoes that support lateral motion.* Purchase new shoes to minimize impact to the joints during dance exercise. The shoes may need to be a half-size larger than usual because pregnancy often causes the feet to spread. Dancing barefoot is especially inappropriate during pregnancy because of increased weight and the propensity for ankle injury. Wear cotton athletic socks over stockings or tights to insure adequate cushioning and to absorb moisture and prevent blisters.

5. *Wear layers of clothing that can be removed during class.* A pregnant woman's metabolism will make her feel warm even before the warm-up is over. During exercise 75%–80% of the energy expended is transformed into heat which leaves the body by sweating. Dress to aid this process.

6. *Wear properly fitting support hose.* The extra support during exercise can help reduce edema of the feet and ankles and prevent pooling of blood in the varicose veins of the legs.

7. *Wear minipads if occasional "leaking" occurs with vigorous movement.* Urinary incontinence is common due to the increased pressure of the enlarged uterus on the bladder and weakened pelvic floor muscles. Kegel exercises performed regularly can help alleviate this problem.

8. *Bring a good quality exercise mat to class for additional cushioning during floor work.* A towel or carpet square is not adequate during pregnancy.

9. *Wear cotton panties, cotton tights, or tights with cotton inserts to help prevent itching caused by superficial fungus or monilia.* Hormonal changes during pregnancy are responsible for a significant increase in monilian infections, which are aggravated by tight noncotton garments. This problem is an even greater concern when the weather is warm and humid.

Preparing Other Participants

A supportive atmosphere is extremely important for a pregnant exerciser in a conventional class. To prevent well-meaning but perhaps upsetting or misleading comments from other participants, the instructor should take a few minutes to introduce the new participant (or announce her pregnancy if she is already a member of the class) and discuss some of the physiological implications of exercise during pregnancy. This is a good time to dispel some old wives' tales. For example, some participants may believe that extending the arms over the head can cause the umbilical cord to strangle the baby or that aerobic exercise will "shake the baby loose." The instructor should explain that the baby lies within a fluid-filled sac protected by the thick muscles of the uterus and covered by the tough skin, muscles, and connective tissue of the abdominal wall, and that both the baby and the cord are unaffected by movements of the mother's extremities.

By asking the pregnant student to report occasionally on the changes she is experiencing, the instructor can involve the whole class in the process of the pregnancy. Other participants are often excited about the course of events. The instructor can also enlist the class's help in providing the psychological support necessary to encourage the pregnant student to listen to her body and not compete with her former pregnant self. Let the class know that the participant will be working at her own pace and modifying exercises for her own health and comfort.

Modifying Class Components

Pregnancy is a dynamic state of being. Physiological changes taking place in the first trimester may disappear by the third trimester, and discomforts come and go as the pregnancy progresses. These changes necessitate continual modifications throughout the 9 months that a pregnant woman is in class. Modifying the workout only during the first trimester is not enough. Some pregnant exercisers continue their fitness routines until delivery. Significant changes must be made in the mode, frequency, intensity, and duration of the workout if the pregnant exerciser is to remain comfortable.

It is easier to integrate a pregnant woman into a class with a regular clientele. In a drop-in class with an ever-changing population, the instructor must take extra time to educate the pregnant exerciser so that she is well acquainted with her goals and limitations and can make her own modifications during each workout. Under these conditions, the instructor will not be able to supervise her constantly and other participants might not realize she is pregnant, so the exerciser will have to assume responsibility for adhering to program modifications and heeding warning signs.

WARM-UP. Because of joint laxity, a pregnant woman is more vulnerable to injury and must build up slowly to a peak cardiovascular workout. For this reason, the warm-up is even more important than usual. A pregnant participant should be encouraged to arrive on time and make the following modifications in her warm-up.

1. *Eliminate all ballistic stretching.* Substitute easy range-of-motion exercises or static stretching.

2. *Eliminate cross-body movements, such as touching the opposite elbow to the knee, because the abdomen interferes.* Substitute movement well within the pregnant woman's comfort limit.

3. *Eliminate forward bending movements, such as hamstring stretches and side lunges (spider legs).* These exercises may result in dizziness or heartburn. Substitute hamstring or gastrocnemius stretching in a standing position while leaning against the wall.

4. *Eliminate deep squats and hyperflexion of hips, knees, and ankles to avoid injury due to joint laxity.* Substitute hip circles and figure eights.

AEROBICS. During the aerobics segment, substitute low-impact choreography for traditional high-impact movements. In low-impact aerobics one or both feet must maintain contact with the floor at all times. Make sure the heels touch down after each movement instead of dancing on the balls of the feet. The pregnant exerciser can intensify the cardiovascular workout by increasing the involvement of the arms and upper body in large vigorous movements (see Chapter 13 for further discussion of low-impact aerobics).

The aerobics routine should also eliminate fast twists and turns. A pregnant woman may feel less agile and be prone to tripping during abrupt changes in direction. Suggest that she stand toward the back of the class, or over to the side, to prevent another participant from running into her during routines that require changes in direction. To prevent leg cramps, eliminate movements performed on the balls of the feet for long periods.

As stated in Chapter 7, heart rate may not be an accurate indication of a pregnant woman's exercise intensity. Therefore, instead of taking her pulse, a pregnant exerciser should use the talk test or the rating of perceived exertion scale (RPE) to monitor exercise intensity. A pregnant student should never exercise to the point of exhaustion, nor should she be gasping for air. Limit a pregnant student to 15 minutes of strenuous activity as recommended by the American College of Obstetricians and Gynecologists (1985). Also, suggest that she work slower than the rest of the class if necessary, possibly performing half the number of repetitions of each movement.

Light (no more than 1 lb), hand-held weights may be used during the aerobics portion of the class to increase the conditioning effect on the cardiovascular system and to promote upper body strength and muscular endurance. If a pregnant participant does use hand weights, make sure she keeps in mind the following safety and comfort tips:

1. Use controlled movements, instead of flinging the weights, to protect the joints.

2. Be careful not to hyperextend the joints.

3. Reduce the frequency of each set of repetitions, doing 5 instead of 10 and concentrating more on form and control.

AEROBIC DANCE-EXERCISE INSTRUCTOR MANUAL

4. Breathe out with each effort to prevent the Valsalva maneuver (forced exhalation against a closed glottis), which could significantly reduce the blood flow to the heart and brain, causing dizziness and fainting.

Never allow pregnant women to wear ankle weights during the aerobics segment. The increased weight of the pregnancy already places additional stress on the joints of the lower body. Added stress from ankle weights can cause serious injury and create great discomfort.

Before moving on to floor work, the instructor should make sure the pregnant participant undergoes a cardiovascular cool-down consisting of gentle, rhythmic movements.

CALISTHENICS.   The muscular conditioning or calisthenics component of a conventional dance-exercise class usually involves floor work. A pregnant woman is uncomfortable lying on her stomach after the first trimester and should not lie on her back after the fourth month. The hands-and-knees position may also cause discomfort to the wrists and knees because of the added weight of pregnancy. The best positions for maximum comfort and safety are side lying, sitting, or semirecumbent. Exercises can be modified for these positions. A pregnant woman should always stand up slowly after floor work to prevent hypotension.

After the fourth month, substitute reverse curls (Fig. 8–1) and pelvic tilts (Fig. 8–2) for abdominal exercise performed in the supine position. Pelvic tilts may be done in the standing, kneeling, sitting, and side-lying positions to gently tone the abdominals and to stretch the back muscles. Diaphragmatic breathing is also a mild abdominal toner. Have the woman bend forward slightly, flex her knees, and visualize her abdomen as a large balloon that expands as it fills with air and contracts as it deflates.

Push-ups tone the abdominal muscles by holding the pelvis in alignment against the force of gravity and preventing hyperextension of the lumbar spine. Even the modified push-up (Fig. 8–3) is a challenge for a pregnant woman, because the increased weight of the abdomen increases the resistance. If the modified push-up is too difficult, the pregnant exerciser can lower herself to the ground, roll to her side, and then push herself up.

Pregnant participants should eliminate deep squats or exercises performed in the cross-legged or tailor position for long periods. These positions hyperflex the knee and hip joints which can cause discomfort and injury due to joint laxity. These positions also can aggravate varicosities in the lower leg by impeding the return of blood.

During the floor-work portion of every class, the pregnant participant should **Kegel**, or contract the pelvic floor muscles—called the pubococcygeus or PC muscles—which are used to shut off the flow of urine. The buttocks and abdominal muscles are not used when performing Kegel exercises. To Kegel, contract the PC muscles for 3–5 seconds and then relax. Repeat up to 10 times. These exercises increase the circulation and the elasticity of the pelvic floor, which may help a pregnant woman avoid an episiotomy during delivery. Kegel exercises will certainly speed recovery after birth and are a great help to nonpregnant women who suffer urinary incontinence (leaking) when bouncing up and down during exercise.

Exercise and Pregnancy: The Exercise-Dance Class

FIGURE 8-1 Reverse curls

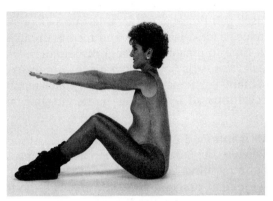

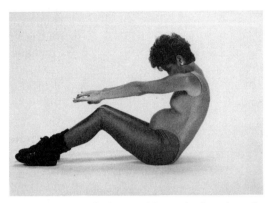

a. Sit straight, knees bent and arms straight out in front.

b. Lower chin to chest and gently roll back until hands are directly in front of knees. Place hands on knees for support before returning to upright position.

FIGURE 8-2 Pelvic tilt, hands-and-knees position.

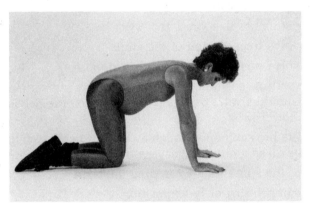

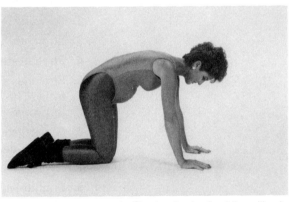

a. Begin with back flat to avoid hyperextension of lower back.

b. Slowly raise back while pulling in abdominals and tucking buttocks under. Return to beginning position and repeat.

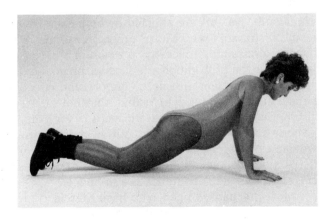

FIGURE 8-3 Modified push-up. Begin with hands directly beneath shoulders and back straight. Tilt pelvis to prevent hyperextension of lower back. Lower body down as far as is comfortable and push back up to starting position.

Finally, an instructor should caution a pregnant participant against isometric exercises and "going for the burn." If the breath is held, isometric exercises can create considerable internal pressure. "Going for the burn" creates excess lactic acid and results in muscle soreness. Pregnancy is no time to create additional discomforts.

In all phases of the calisthenics component, the instructor should observe the pregnant participant to make sure she maintains proper alignment and performs all movements in a controlled manner.

STRETCHES.   As mentioned earlier, the purpose of stretching during pregnancy is to ensure the balanced development of muscles that work in pairs. Without stretching, muscles developed through an aerobics or strength development program may pull unevenly on the joints. As with all other components of a dance-exercise class, stretching exercises must be modified to accommodate the physiological changes of pregnancy. A stretching program for a pregnant participant should avoid the following:

1. Ballistic stretches that may overstretch a joint and lead to injury. The pregnant woman may stretch to the point of maximum stretch when discomfort just begins to be felt. She should not stretch past that point, to the point of pain.

2. Forward bending stretches that stress the lower back.

3. Stretches that involve hyperflexion of the joints.

4. Stretches that involve nonsupported lateral flexion.

5. Stretches from a sitting position with both legs straight out in front. The knees should always be slightly bent to keep the pelvis in proper alignment.

6. Hyperflexion of the hips and knees, such as the hurdler's stretch, for extended periods. These positions may contribute to varicosities.

7. Hyperextension of the spine such as arching the back.

8. Double leg raises in a sitting or lying position.

9. Toe pointing, which may cause lower leg cramps.

10. Inverted postures, such as bicycling positions or shoulder stands.

SUMMARY

Many body systems are affected by both exercise and pregnancy. As a result, instructors who accept pregnant exercisers into a conventional dance-exercise class need to be aware of the common discomforts of pregnancy, the physiological effects of pregnancy, and how to modify an exercise program for safety, comfort, and effectiveness during pregnancy. Instructors need to realize that not all traditional classes are appropriate for a pregnant exerciser. It is very important that the class provide a supportive, noncompetitive atmosphere where the pregnant woman can exercise at her own pace. Before accepting a pregnant participant, instructors should also consider the impact on other exercisers, class size, and insurance requirements.

Most pregnant women who have exercised previously can participate safely in a conventional dance-exercise class if they modify their exercises properly and heed warning signs to stop exercising. Women who start exercising for the first time during pregnancy can best be accommodated in a specialized pregnancy exercise class.

Before a pregnant woman begins to exercise, the instructor should help her to set informed, realistic, and attainable fitness goals. Pregnant exercisers can improve cardiovascular fitness, posture, muscle strength, balance, ease of movement and even self-concept with regular participation in a comprehensive dance-exercise program. Under the instructor's guidance, the pregnant exerciser should modify each segment of her exercise routine and continue to make changes as pregnancy progresses. The modifications suggested in this chapter pertain to the most commonly used dance-exercise movements. An instructor who wishes to design or teach a specialized pregnancy exercise class will need extensive additional training.

REFERENCES

American College of Obstetricians and Gynecologists. *Exercise During Pregnancy and the Postnatal Period (ACOG Home Exercise Programs)*. Washington, D.C.: ACOG, 1985.

SUGGESTED READING

Artal, R., and R. A. Wisell *Exercise in Pregnancy*. Baltimore: Williams and Wilkins, 1986.

Gauthier, M. M. "Guidelines for Exercise During Pregnancy: Too Little or Too Much." *The Physician and Sportsmedicine* (April 1986): 162–69.

Monitoring Exercise Intensity

Donna Todd

9

Donna Todd, M.A., is an exercise physiologist who has taught dance exercise and trained dance-exercise instructors for 7 years. She is now the exercise physiologist at the La Costa Hotel and Spa.

IN THIS CHAPTER:

- The MET system of measuring intensity.
- Calculating and adjusting target heart rate: Karvonen formula, maximal heart-rate formula, pulse-taking techniques, adjusting target heart rate, recovery heart rate.

- Supplemental methods of measuring intensity: rating of perceived exertion (RPE), dyspnea scale, talk test.

When designing or modifying an exercise program, an instructor must consider four factors: exercise frequency, exercise intensity, time (duration) of exercise, and type (mode) of exercise. Intensity may be the most important of these factors. This chapter discusses the methods for determining, monitoring, and, when necessary, adjusting exercise intensity for each participant in an aerobic dance-exercise class.

Monitoring and adjusting exercise intensity is essential to both the safety and the effectiveness of an aerobic dance-exercise program. A participant who exercises at an intensity that is too low may show little or no improvement in cardiorespiratory fitness. Conversely, a participant who exercises at an intensity that is too high may become injured or overly fatigued or even find that exercise is too unpleasant to continue. Exercising within the appropriate intensity range improves cardiovascular fitness and reduces the likelihood of injury. Monitoring exercise intensity also provides motivation. A participant who monitors his or her exercise intensity regularly can document increasing cardiovascular fitness, which in turn serves as an incentive to continue with the exercise program.

Exercise intensity can be determined using one or more of the following techniques:

231

AEROBIC DANCE-EXERCISE INSTRUCTOR MANUAL

MET system

Karvonen formula

Maximal heart-rate formula

Rating of perceived exertion (RPE)

Dyspnea index

Talk test

As will be discussed below, some techniques are better suited than others to the dance-exercise setting. Which technique an instructor selects will most often depend on a participant's fitness level, health status, and past experience with monitoring exercise intensity.

THE MET SYSTEM

The **MET system** of monitoring exercise intensity is not commonly used in the dance-exercise community. However, the instructor should be aware of the system because professional literature often refers to this method of measuring intensity. In addition, some dance-exercise participants may have a specific MET level of activity prescribed by their physicians, and the instructor will need to work with these exercisers to ensure they remain within the appropriate intensity range.

Maximal oxygen consumption ($\dot{V}O_2$ max), or maximal functional capacity, is considered the best indicator of cardiorespiratory endurance capacity. $\dot{V}O_2$ max refers to the highest volume (V) of oxygen (O_2) that can be consumed per minute (the · above the V). $\dot{V}O_2$ max is measured during a graded exercise test, which is usually conducted in a laboratory or sports medicine center equipped with a treadmill or bicycle ergometer. As the workload on the treadmill or bicycle is increased gradually from light to maximal, or exhaustive, highly trained personnel using special equipment measure oxygen consumption, heart rate, and blood pressure response to exercise.

$\dot{V}O_2$ max can be expressed in **METs, or metabolic equivalents.** One MET is defined as the amount of oxygen required per minute under quiet, resting conditions (resting $\dot{V}O_2$), or 3.5 milliliters (ml) of oxygen per kilogram (kg) of body weight per minute (min^{-1}). An activity that requires 10 METs means that the oxygen cost of the exercise is equal to 10 times the energy expenditure at rest, or 35 ml/kg · min^{-1} (10 × 3.5). For example, a person weighing 50 kg and performing exercise requiring 10 METs would have a $\dot{V}O_2$ of 1.75 liters per minute (50 × 35 = 1,750 ml, or 1.75 liters). Table 9–1 shows MET values for various activities.

In a dance-exercise class, the level of exercise intensity should range from 50% to 85% of each participant's $\dot{V}O_2$ max, or maximal functional capacity (max METs). Therefore, a participant with a $\dot{V}O_2$ max of 35 ml/kg · min^{-1} would calculate max METs as follows:

$$\frac{35\,ml/kg/min\,(\dot{V}O_2\,max)}{3.5\,ml/kg/min\,(resting\,\dot{V}O_2)} = 10\,max\,METs.$$

With a maximum aerobic capacity of 10 METS, an average intensity range of 65%–80% can be calculated as follows:

$$
\begin{array}{r}
10 \ \textit{(max METs)} \\
\times \ \ .65 \ \textit{(lower intensity range)} \\
\hline
6.5 \ \text{METs,}
\end{array}
$$

$$
\begin{array}{r}
10 \ \textit{(max METs)} \\
\times \ \ .80 \ \textit{(higher intensity range)} \\
\hline
8.0 \ \text{METs}
\end{array}
$$

Therefore, using the MET system, this person would exercise at an intensity range of 6.5–8 METs, a moderate level of intensity for aerobic dance-exercise, which has a range of 6–9 METs. Because there are variations in metabolic efficiency within any given population, the MET values of activities should be treated as approximations and not as absolute values.

The MET system for establishing exercise intensity is especially useful for participants who need a clear guideline for selecting safe activities. This system is used predominantly with cardiac patients, pulmonary patients, or others who must avoid participation in activities that require excessive energy expenditure. For example, a person whose activity level should not exceed 5 METs would not choose racquetball as an exercise activity because racquetball requires 8–12 METs.

CALCULATING AND ADJUSTING TARGET HEART-RATE RANGE

Because heart rate increases proportionately with an increase in workload (Taylor et al. 1969), heart rate can indicate the stress placed on the cardiovascular system. Heart rate can be monitored easily by periodically taking the pulse during an exercise session and then adjusting the exercise intensity to bring the heart rate to a recommended level. This recommended heart-rate level is called the **target heart rate.** In dance-exercise classes, the two most common methods of determining target heart rate are the Karvonen formula and the maximal heart-rate formula.

Karvonen Formula

The **Karvonen formula** (Karvonen et al. 1957) is a relatively accurate and very popular method of determining target heart rate. The formula calculates a percentage of the **heart-rate reserve,** which is the difference between the resting heart rate and the maximal heart rate:

HR* reserve = maximal HR − resting HR.

Target heart rate is then determined as a percentage of the target heart-rate reserve, plus the resting heart rate:

target HR = % intensity (maximal HR − resting HR) + resting HR.

Before calculating an actual target heart rate using this formula, it is important to understand how to determine maximal heart rate, resting heart rate, and target heart-rate ranges.

---

*HR stands for "heart rate" in all equations in this chapter.

AEROBIC DANCE-EXERCISE INSTRUCTOR MANUAL

Table 9-1

LEISURE ACTIVITIES IN METs: SPORTS, EXERCISE CLASSES, GAMES, DANCING

	Mean	Range
Archery	3.9	3-4
Back Packing	–	5-11
Badminton	5.8	4-9+
Basketball		
Gameball	8.3	7-12+
Non-game	–	3-9
Billiards	2.5	–
Bowling	–	2-4
Boxing		
In-ring	13.3	–
Sparring	8.3	–
Canoeing, Rowing and Kayaking	–	3-8
Conditioning Exercise		3-8+
Climbing Hills	7.2	5-10+
Cricket	5.2	4.6-7.4
Croquet	3.5	–
Cycling		
Pleasure or to work	–	3-8+
10 mph	7.0	–
Dancing (Social, Square, Tap)	–	3.7-8.4
Dancing (Aerobic)	–	6-9
Fencing	–	6-10+
Field Hockey	8.0	–
Fishing		
From bank	3.7	2-4
Wading in stream	–	5-6
Football (Touch)	7.9	6-10
Golf		
Power Cart	–	2-3
Walking (carrying bag or pulling cart)	5.1	4-7
Handball	–	8-12+
Hiking (Cross-country)	–	3-7
Horseback Riding		
Galloping	8.2	–
Trotting	6.6	–
Walking	2.4	–
Horseshoe Pitching	–	2-3
Hunting (Bow or Gun)		
Small game (walking, carrying light load)	–	3-7
Big game (dragging carcass, walking)	–	3-14
Judo	13.5	–
Mountain Climbing	–	5-10+
Paddleball, Racquetball	9	8-12
Rope Jumping	11	
60-80 skips/min	9	–
120-140 skips/min	–	11-12

LEISURE ACTIVITIES IN METs: SPORTS, EXERCISE CLASSES, GAMES, DANCING (continued)

	Mean	Range
Running		
12 min per mile	8.7	–
11 min per mile	9.4	–
10 min per mile	10.2	–
9 min per mile	11.2	–
8 min per mile	12.5	–
7 min per mile	14.1	–
6 min per mile	16.3	–
Sailing	–	2–5
Scubadiving	–	5–10
Shuffleboard	–	2–3
Skating, Ice and Roller	–	5–8
Skiing, Snow		
Downhill	–	5–8
Crosscountry	–	6–12+
Skiing, Water	–	5–7
Sledding, Tobogganing	–	4–8
Snowshoeing	9.9	7–14
Squash	–	8–12+
Soccer	–	5–12+
Stairclimbing	–	4–8
Swimming	–	4–8+
Table Tennis	4.1	3–5
Tennis	6.5	4–9+
Volleyball	–	3–6

Source: American College of Sports Medicine. *Guidelines for Exercise Testing and Prescription*, 3rd ed. Philadelphia: Lea & Febiger, 1986. Reprinted with permission.

DETERMINING MAXIMAL HEART RATE.   Maximal heart rate is the highest heart rate a person can attain during heavy exercise. The most accurate way of determining maximal heart rate is to undergo a graded exercise test using an electrocardiogram. As mentioned earlier, graded exercise testing requires special equipment, a controlled setting, and trained personnel, and, therefore, is not practical for a dance-exercise setting. As a result, an **age-predicted heart-rate** formula is used in most classes:

$$\text{maximal HR} = 220 - \text{age}.$$

For example, a 40-year-old person would have an estimated maximal heart rate of 180 beats per minute (220 − 40). This formula is based on the assumption that 220 is the approximate maximal heart rate of a baby, and each year this rate decreases by one beat. Although this formula is practical for a class setting, it is not always accurate because maximal heart rates can vary at any given age by ± 10 beats per minute (Astrand and Rodahl 1977).

DETERMINING RESTING HEART RATE. **Resting heart rates** are determined most accurately just before getting out of bed in the morning (Taylor et al. 1963). The pulse should be taken for a full 60 seconds, or for 30 seconds and multiplied by 2. To ensure accuracy, the dance-exercise participant should measure the resting heart rate for 3 mornings and then take an average of the 3 readings.

In addition to its application in the Karvonen formula, periodic reevaluation of resting heart rate is useful for observing improvements in fitness. For many participants, resting heart rate will decrease as fitness increases because the heart will work more efficiently and pump more blood with each contraction. In fact, it has been shown that with regular exercise, the resting heart rate can decrease approximately 1 beat per minute every 1 or 2 weeks during the first 10–12 weeks of an exercise program (Pollock, Wilmore, and Fox 1984). Endurance athletes, such as cross-country skiers and marathon runners, often have resting heart rates of 40 beats per minute or lower, compared to sedentary persons who may have average resting heart rates of 80 beats per minute or higher (Fox and Matthews 1971).

Instructors should realize, however, that a low heart rate does not always reflect a high fitness level. Participants with heart disease (Hurst 1982), and participants who take a beta-adrenergic blocking agent (beta-blocker) for hypertension or migraine headaches, will experience lower heart rates both at rest and during exercise. Some extremely athletic people also have high resting heart rates. Because of this variability within the population, instructors should never use resting heart rate alone to evaluate fitness level.

DETERMINING TARGET HEART-RATE RANGES. As described earlier, training intensity should range from 50% to 85% of maximal oxygen consumption ($\dot{V}O_2$ max). Since a linear relationship exists between heart rate, oxygen consumption, and workload, **target heart-rate ranges** (also called training zones) are used to determine exercise intensity in most dance-exercise classes. Generally accepted ranges are 60%–80% of maximal heart-rate reserve (used in the Karvonen formula), or 70%–85% of maximal attainable heart rate (used in the maximal heart-rate formula). It is important to remember to use the correct intensity range for each formula.

The lower percentages represent the minimal threshold for improving cardiorespiratory fitness, while the higher percentages represent the upper limit of recommended exercise intensity. The instructor should match the appropriate intensity level with the health, fitness status, and exercise experience of each participant. For example, a participant who has attended a 1-hour aerobic dance-exercise class 3 days a week for several months may be able to tolerate an intensity of 70%–80% of maximal heart-rate reserve, while a beginning exerciser may feel more comfortable at an intensity of 60%–70%.

The instructor must remember, however, that target heart-rate ranges represent general guidelines only. Recommended ranges vary from source to source in the professional literature. Some are meant to encompass sedentary persons as well as the extremely fit, while others are geared toward the average healthy adult. Target heart-rate ranges also vary because none of the formulas is exact. Therefore, the instructor should not treat these ranges as if they were inscribed in stone. Some participants may have to begin exercising below the recommended ranges, and others may be fit enough to exceed their estimated training zones.

CALCULATING THE KARVONEN FORMULA.   Understanding these basics, the instructor can calculate target heart rate using the Karvonen formula:

target HR = % intensity $\times$ HR reserve + resting HR.

For example, a 50-year-old woman has a resting heart rate of 80, an age-predicted maximal heart rate of 170 (220 − 50), and a recommended intensity level of 65%–75% of maximum heart-rate reserve. Her target heart-rate range can be calculated as follows:

At 65% intensity:

$$
\begin{array}{rl}
170 & \textit{(predicted maximal HR)} \\
-\quad 80 & \textit{(resting HR)} \\
\hline
90 & \textit{(HR reserve)} \\
\times\quad .65 & \textit{(intensity)} \\
\hline
58.5 & \\
+\quad 80.0 & \textit{(resting HR)} \\
\hline
138.5 & \textit{(target HR).}
\end{array}
$$

At 75% intensity:

$$
\begin{array}{rl}
170 & \textit{(predicted maximal HR)} \\
-\quad 80 & \textit{(resting HR)} \\
\hline
90 & \textit{(HR reserve)} \\
\times\quad .75 & \textit{(intensity)} \\
\hline
67.5 & \\
+\quad 80.0 & \textit{(resting HR)} \\
\hline
147.5 & \textit{(target HR).}
\end{array}
$$

It is important for an instructor to calculate an upper and a lower limit of intensity (target heart-rate range) for each participant in the dance-exercise class so that the target heart rate can be adjusted as fitness increases. For example, the 50-year-old woman in the example would be given a range of 138.5–147.5 beats per minute, or 23−25 beats during a 10-second period. (Note that the numbers are rounded off during this last step of the calculation: 138.5 ÷ 6 = 23.083, or 23.) After exercising regularly for several months, she may want to adjust her heart rate to meet the upper limit so that she continues to gain substantial cardiorespiratory benefits.

The Karvonen formula is an accurate way of determining target heart rate, with an error of ± 5−10 beats per minute (Lamb 1984), and is recommended by the American College of Sports Medicine.

Maximal Heart-Rate Formula

The **maximal heart-rate formula** differs from the Karvonen formula in that the resting heart rate is not used in calculating the target heart rate:

target HR = maximal HR $\times$ % intensity.

Remember, if a participant does not know his or her maximal heart rate from a graded exercise test, it can be attained using the age-predicted formula.

For example, a 30-year-old man who wants to exercise at 70%–80% of his maximal heart rate would calculate his target heart-rate range as follows:

AEROBIC DANCE-EXERCISE INSTRUCTOR MANUAL

At 70% intensity:

$$\begin{array}{rl} 190 & \textit{(maximal HR: 220 − 30)} \\ \times \quad .70 & \textit{(intensity)} \\ \hline 133 & \textit{(target HR).} \end{array}$$

At 80% intensity:

$$\begin{array}{rl} 190 & \textit{(maximal HR: 220 − 30)} \\ \times \quad .80 & \textit{(intensity)} \\ \hline 152 & \textit{(target HR)} \end{array}$$

For a 10-second count, divide the target heart rate by 6 and round off to the closest whole number:

$$\frac{133}{6} = 22.17 = 22,$$

$$\frac{152}{6} = 25.33 = 25.$$

The target heart-rate range for this participant is 22–25 beats in a 10-second count.

Both the maximal heart rate and Karvonen methods have been used widely in the exercise community. The most common errors that occur in employing these methods include miscounting, taking too long to begin counting, and miscalculating the target heart rate. Therefore, an instructor should become thoroughly familiar with each method before introducing it in class. In addition, he or she should spend enough time with class participants to explain fully, and make sure they understand, the purpose and the techniques for establishing and monitoring exercise intensity.

1. Wrist.   The **radial pulse** can be felt on the radial artery of the wrist, in line with the thumb. Place the tips of the index and middle fingers (not the thumb, which has a pulse of its own) over the artery and press down lightly (Fig. 9–1).

2. Temple.   During exercise, a **temporal pulse** can be felt easily on either temple in front of the upper part of the ear. Press down lightly with the index and middle fingers (Fig. 9–2).

3. Neck.   The **carotid pulse** can be felt on the carotid artery, which is located on the neck just to the side of the throat (Fig. 9–3). Place the first two fingers gently on the side of the neck. Too much pressure placed on the carotid artery may stimulate a reflex mechanism that causes the heart to slow down. Participants should be extremely cautious when using this pulse point.

4. Chest.   The **apical pulse,** taken at the apex of the heart, can be felt most clearly after heavy exercise. Place the heel of the hand over the left side of the chest (Fig. 9–4).

The pulse can be taken for 6 seconds (and multiplied by 10), for 10 seconds (and multiplied by 6), or for 15 seconds (and multiplied by 4). The 10-second count is most accurate and therefore preferred (Pollock, Wilmore, and Fox 1984). The 6-second count is less accurate

Pulse-Taking Techniques

Instructors should teach participants how to monitor their heart rate by taking their pulse at one of four sites:

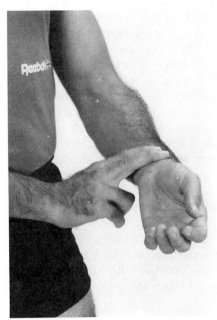

FIGURE 9–1 The radial pulse site

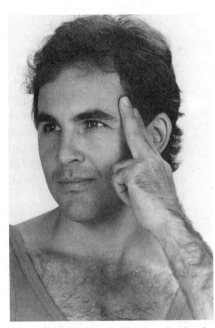

FIGURE 9–2 The temporal pulse site

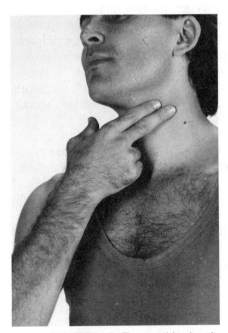

FIGURE 9–3 The carotid pulse site

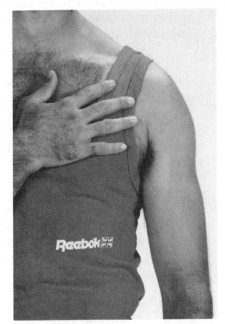

FIGURE 9–4 The apical pulse site

because there is a large margin of error if the pulse is miscounted, and the longest count, 15 seconds, should not be used on a well-conditioned exerciser whose heart rate may drop significantly within that time.

The first pulse usually is counted as 0 because the pulse beat represents one cardiac cycle, which begins on the first beat and ends on the second. Many instructors, however, begin counting at 1 instead. Although not preferred, this method is acceptable because it safely overestimates the actual heart rate. Whether an instructor chooses to begin at 0 or at 1, the most important thing is consistency.

Because heart rate begins to decrease soon after exercise stops, instructors should begin the count as soon as possible, preferably within 5 seconds (Pollock, Wilmore, and Fox 1984). Instructors should announce in advance that heart rates will be taken and should direct participants to continue moving while taking their pulse. Stopping suddenly may cause blood to pool in the extremities and result in light-headedness or fainting.

Instructors should encourage beginning exercisers to take their pulse rates every 5–10 minutes during a 20–30-minute workout. This practice will familiarize them with the relationship between heart rate and workload and help them to monitor their exercise intensity more effectively. Once a participant becomes more familiar with his or her body's response to exercise, heart rates can be taken less often, for example, every 10–15 minutes.

Adjusting Target Heart Rate

When participants exhibit signs of overexertion during exercise or fail to recover properly following the workout, the instructor may need to adjust their target heart rates, even after they have been appropriately calculated. Heart rates may also have to be adjusted for participants who have not attended class regularly, because training effects are lost with irregular exercise. Participants resuming exercise after an illness may need to reevaluate their target heart rate and change it according to how they feel. Similarly, as participants become more fit, they should adjust their target heart rates upward.

Instructors should be especially alert to unusual heart-rate responses in participants on medication (see Chapter 4). Beta-blockers, for example, tend to lower the heart rate both at rest and during exercise. However, the relationship between exercise intensity and percentage of maximal heart rate is roughly preserved when a person is taking a beta-blocker. Therefore the target heart-rate range can still be calculated, provided the person undergoes a graded exercise test while on beta blockers to determine maximal heart rate. For example, a man taking a beta-blocker has a desired target heart-rate range of 70%–80% of maximal heart-rate reserve. His resting heart rate is 55 and his maximal heart rate is 135, as determined by a graded exercise test. His target heart-rate range is calculated as follows:

$$
\begin{array}{r}
135 \ \textit{(maximal HR)} \\
- \ \ 55 \ \textit{(resting HR)} \\
\hline
80 \ \textit{(HR reserve)}
\end{array}
$$

$$.70 \times 80 = 56 \qquad 56 + 55 \ \textit{(resting HR)} = 111,$$
$$.80 \times 80 = 64 \qquad 64 + 55 \ \textit{(resting HR)} = 119.$$

Thus, 70%–80% of his maximal heart-rate reserve would be 111–19 (target heart-rate range), or 19–20 beats for a 10-second count.

Using the maximal heart-rate formula, the target heart-rate range for a desired intensity of 75%–85% is calculated as follows:

$$.75 \times 135 \; (max \; HR) = 101.25,$$
$$.85 \times 135 \; (max \; HR) = 114.75.$$

For a 10-second count, the target heart-rate range is 17–19 beats per minute.

The target heart-rate ranges are thus lower for anyone on beta-blockers, but the low ranges are appropriate because they represent the correct percentage of maximal capacity for the exerciser. Instructors may want to check the heart rate for these participants themselves, to ensure the readings are accurate.

Recovery Heart Rate

The **recovery heart rate** reflects how quickly the cardiorespiratory system is able to return to its preexercise condition. It has been used as an indicator of cardiovascular fitness, because a more fit person will recover faster from exercise than a less fit person (Wilmore 1977). However, recovery heart rates vary among participants and should not be used to compare one person with another.

After extended cardiovascular exercise, the heart rate decreases in two stages. There is a sharp drop within the first minute, then a leveling out, and then a slow, gradual return to normal. Most participants' heart rates will have recovered well within 2 minutes, maybe even to resting levels (McArdle, Hatch, and Hatch 1981). However, it may be best for instructors to take the recovery heart rate after 5 minutes to include those who have not sufficiently recovered within the shorter period. Whether the recovery heart rate is taken 2 minutes or 5 minutes after exercise, it is important to be consistent.

At the end of the cool-down period of an exercise session, the recovery heart rate should be below 120 beats per minute. Higher rates may indicate insufficient cool-down or a low fitness level; instructors should encourage participants to continue cooling down until heart rates drop sufficiently. As mentioned earlier, with improvements in fitness, the heart rate will return more quickly to its resting state after exercise.

A participant who fails to recover appropriately within 5 minutes after exercise may be exercising too vigorously. Irregular attendance or illness may also impede recovery. In these cases, intensity should be decreased and the target heart-rate range adjusted accordingly.

SUPPLEMENTAL METHODS OF MEASURING INTENSITY

Other methods of measuring exercise intensity can be used as adjuncts to heart-rate monitoring techniques. These methods include the rating of perceived exertion, the dyspnea scale, and the talk test.

Rating of Perceived Exertion

The **rating of perceived exertion (RPE)** scale is becoming increasingly more popular as an adjunct to heart-rate monitoring for determining exercise intensity (Noble 1982). The original RPE scale, developed by psychologist Gunnar Borg, allows participants to rate their effort on a scale from 6 to 20 (see Table 9–2). A rating of 7 is equivalent to an

AEROBIC DANCE-EXERCISE INSTRUCTOR MANUAL

Rating	Description
6	
7	Very, very light
8	
9	Very light
10	
11	Fairly light
12	
13	Somewhat hard
14	
15	Hard
16	
17	Very hard
18	
19	Very, very hard

TABLE 9–2 The rating of perceived exertion scale developed by Borg

Source: Borg, G.A.V., "Psychophysical Bases of Physical Exertion." *Medicine and Science in Sport and Exercise 14* (1982): 377–87. Reprinted with permission.

exertion level that is "very, very light"; a rating of 19 means the exerciser is working "very, very hard." In a typical dance-exercise class, ratings of 6–11 on the RPE scale are equivalent to the intensity levels in the warm-up and cool-down segments. Ratings of 12 and 13 are equal to approximately 60% of maximal heart-rate reserve, while 16 is equal to approximately 90% (Pollock, Wilmore, and Fox 1984). Therefore, an exercise intensity of 60%–80% of maximal heart-rate reserve corresponds to a range of 12 or 13 ("somewhat hard") to 15 ("hard") on the scale. In 1986, the American College of Sports Medicine released a revised RPE scale from 0 ("nothing at all") to 10 ("very, very strong"). This scale provides more verbal descriptions for rating the degree of exertion (see Table 9-3)

The RPE scale correlates highly with heart rate, ventilation, oxygen consumption ($\dot{V}O_2$), and blood lactate concentration (Borg 1982). For the beginning exerciser, the scale should be used in conjunction with heart-rate monitoring techniques for measuring exercise intensity. After the participant becomes familiar with the relationship between heart rate and the rating of perceived exertion, RPE can occasionally be used in place of heart rate to indicate exercise intensity. In addition, special population groups who do not have a normal heart-rate response to exercise, such as pregnant women, cardiac patients, diabetics, or hypertensives on beta-blockers, may find the RPE scale a useful guide to exercise intensity.

Instructors using the rating of perceived exertion should post the scale in full public view. A handout explaining how to use the scale may also be helpful. It is important to stress that using the RPE scale effectively requires practice. One way to cue participants is to announce that it is time to monitor heart rates, but before they begin their first pulse count, they should quickly select the number on the scale that reflects how they are feeling. Instruct the class to evaluate their overall feeling of effort, not focus on only one sensation, such as tired calf muscles. Over time, experienced exercisers will learn how to recognize

Rating	Description
0	Nothing
0.5	Very, very light (just noticeable)
1.0	Very light
2	Light (weak)
3	Moderate
4	Somewhat hard
5	Heavy (strong)
6	
7	Very heavy
8	
9	
10	Very, very heavy (almost max)

Source: Borg, G. A. V., "Psychophysical Bases of Perceived Exertion." *Medicine and Science in Sport and Exercise 14* (1982): 377–87. Reprinted with permission.

TABLE 9–3 Revised rating of perceived exertion scale

their feelings at each level of intensity as measured by heart rate, and how to transfer that knowledge to judge exercise intensity without actually counting heartbeats.

Although the RPE scale has been shown to be valid and reliable (Skinner 1973), studies have found that about 10% of the population either overrate or underrate their level of exertion (Morgan 1981). Thus, even though heart rate does reflect the subjective experience of physical exertion in many situations, RPE should not be the sole method used to judge intensity.

Dyspnea Scale

Dyspnea refers to shortness of breath, or labored breathing. The **dyspnea scale** monitors exercise intensity according to respiration effort.

1. Mild—noticeable to exerciser, but not to observer.

2. Some difficulty—noticeable to observer.

3. Moderate difficulty—exerciser can still continue.

4. Severe difficulty—exerciser cannot continue.

This scale is most often used for participants with asthma or impaired pulmonary function and those who feel limited because of breathlessness. The instructor should observe participants using the dyspnea scale and caution those who feel they are experiencing "severe difficulty" to reduce their exercise intensity. Again, this method should be used along with heart-rate or RPE methods for monitoring intensity.

Talk Test

The **talk test** is a simple but effective adjunct to heart-rate or RPE monitoring to determine exercise intensity. Exercisers should be able to breathe comfortably, deeply, and rhythmically during all class segments; in other words, they should be able to carry on a conversation while exercising. If exercisers are gasping or short of breath—if they cannot talk—they should reduce their exercise intensity. Because its accuracy varies within any given population, the talk test is best used in conjunction with heart-rate methods or the rating of perceived exertion for monitoring exercise intensity.

SUMMARY

Monitoring exercise intensity is essential to a safe and effective exercise program. Each participant in a dance-exercise class should work at an intensity level that is appropriate for his or her health status, fitness level, and exercise goals. The most commonly used method of measuring intensity is to monitor heart rate. The Karvonen formula is the most accurate and therefore the preferred method of calculating the target heart-rate zone. The maximal heart-rate method is less accurate but easier to calculate and very practical. Pulse beats should be counted at least twice during the aerobics segment of a class to ensure that participants are working within the appropriate heart-rate range.

Other measures of intensity can be used as adjuncts to heart-rate monitoring. The rating of perceived exertion (RPE) scale and the talk test are useful methods. The MET system, which calculates exercise intensity based on maximal oxygen consumption, is extremely accurate but inappropriate for most dance-exercise settings because special equipment and highly trained personnel are required.

Instructors should be alert to situations that require participants to adjust their intensity level or stop exercising. Participants who are overexercising, taking medications, or recovering from an illness may need to lower their target heart-rate range. Others will raise their intensity level as they become more fit. These necessary adjustments can be made only through accurate and consistent procedures for monitoring exercise intensity.

REFERENCES

American College of Sports Medicine. *Guidelines for Exercise Testing and Prescription.* 3rd ed. Philadelphia: Lea and Febiger, 1986.

Astrand, P. O., and K. Rodahl. *Textbook of Work Physiology.* 2nd ed. New York: McGraw-Hill, 1977.

Borg, G. A. V. "Psychophysical Bases of Perceived Exertion." *Medicine and Science in Sport and Exercise* 14 (1982): 377–87.

Fox, E. L., and D. K. Matthews. *The Physiological Basis of Physical Education.* 3rd ed. Philadelphia: W. B. Saunders, 1971.

Hurst, W. *The Heart.* New York: McGraw-Hill, 1982.

Karvonen, M., E. Kentala, and O. Mustalof. "The Effects of Training on Heart Rate: A Longitudinal Study." *Annales of Medicinae Experimentalis et Biologiae Fenniae* 35 (1957): 307–15.

Lamb, D. R. *Physiology of Exercise: Responses and Adaptions.* New York: Macmillan, 1984.

McArdle, W., F. Hatch, and V. Hatch. *Exercise Physiology, Energy, Nutrition and Human Performance.* Philadelphia: Lea and Febiger, 1981.

Morgan, W. P. "Psychophysiology of Self Awareness During Vigorous Physical Activity." *Research Quarterly in Exercise and Sport* 52 (1981): 385–427.

Noble, B. J. "Clinical Applications of Perceived Exertion." *Medicine and Science in Sport and Exercise* 14 (1982): 406–11.

Pollock, M. L., J. H. Wilmore, and S. M. Fox. *Exercise in Health and Disease.* Philadelphia: W. B. Saunders, 1984.

Skinner, J. S., R. Hursler, V. Bergsteinova, and E. R. Buskirk. "The Validity and Reliability of a Rating Scale of Perceived Exertion." *Medicine and Science in Sport and Exercise* 5 (1973): 94–96.

Taylor, H. L., W. Haskell, S. M. Fox, and H. Blackburn. "Exercise Tests: A Summary of Procedures and Concepts of Stress Testing for Cardiovascular Diagnosis and Function Evaluation." In *Measurements in Exercise Electrocardiography*, edited by H. Blackburn, 259–305. Springfield, Illinois: Charles C. Thomas, 1969.

Taylor, H. L., Y. Wang, L. Rowell, and G. L. Blomquist. "The Standardization and Interpretation of Submaximal and Maximal Tests of Work Capacity." *Pediatrics* 32 (1963): 703–22.

Wilmore, J. H. *Athletic Training and Physical Fitness.* Boston: Allyn and Bacon, 1977.

Teaching Dance Exercise

Lorna Francis

Lorna Francis, Ph.D., teaches physical education at San Diego State University and is the coauthor of the "Injury Prevention" column in *Dance Exercise Today*. Dr. Francis has lectured on and written numerous articles about the prevention of aerobic-dance injuries, and is involved in several nationwide research projects examining injuries among dance-exercise participants. An aerobic-dance instructor for 10 years, Dr. Francis is an injury prevention consultant for several organizations, including Feeling Fine Productions, Inc. and the Reebok Educational Division, and a member of the IDEA Foundation Committee on Standards and Certification in Dance Exercise.

10

IN THIS CHAPTER:

- The learning process: the nature of learning, learning strategies.
- Designing instruction: setting goals, planning lessons.
- Teaching class: teaching styles, teaching movement patterns, cueing.
- Motivating participants.
- Evaluating performance.

A safe and successful dance-exercise program depends on the instructor's ability to apply sound instructional principles and practices. In fact, effective teaching may well be the most important aspect of the dance-exercise instructor's role. Inadequate leadership is often cited by participants as a reason for dropping out of formal exercise programs (Nieman 1986, Franklin 1986). Unfortunately, many people believe that teaching is intuitive and spontaneous. Without proper training, however, an intuitive and spontaneous approach to teaching often results in ineffective leadership.

Over the years, researchers have provided invaluable information to help instructors effectively plan and implement their programs. Scientific investigation of teaching techniques has led to an understanding of the phenomenon of teaching and its impact on learning behavior. A theoretical approach to teaching has provided a way to identify role expectations for teachers and students. More important, a scientific approach has helped determine whether a teacher's actions result in the intended outcome. The purpose of this chapter is to provide exercise leaders with a sound teaching foundation by exploring the elements of effective teaching and how they apply to a dance-exercise setting.

THE LEARNING PROCESS

Many instructors do not appreciate the complexity of the process required to learn a new exercise or movement pattern. In a matter of seconds, the student must perceive and react to the proper cues, must remember similar situations and instructions on what to do, must determine the proper strategy and make the correct response, and finally, through feedback, must determine whether he or she performed the exercise correctly. This section examines the learning process and describes learning strategies that will facilitate the teaching of motor skills.

The Nature of Learning

Magill (1980) defines **learning** as an "internal change in the individual that is inferred from a relatively permanent improvement in performance of the individual as a result of practice" (p. 14). Instructors can therefore infer that learning has taken place when a person's performance shows less variability over time.

DOMAINS OF HUMAN BEHAVIOR.   Learning takes place in three domains of human behavior: cognitive, affective, and motor (Magill 1980). All three domains are important within the dance-exercise field.

The **cognitive domain** describes intellectual activities and involves the learning of knowledge. Studies have shown that education within an exercise program positively affects motivation and exercise compliance (Franklin 1986). Therefore, competent instructors should remain up-to-date on the latest research in exercise and related fields in an effort to inform their students and to respond intelligently to their questions or concerns. The **affective domain** describes emotional behaviors. Motivation to exercise depends on a person's feelings toward exercise (Nieman 1986). Instructors are therefore instrumental in helping participants develop positive attitudes about exercise. Finally, the **motor domain** refers to those activities requiring movement. Learning motor skills is the foundation of exercise classes.

Within the dance-exercise profession, the motor domain has been heavily emphasized, and limited attention has been given to the affective and cognitive domains. However, research has shown that teaching within all three domains is critical to exercise compliance.

STAGES OF LEARNING.   To teach effectively, an instructor must be aware of the various stages of learning. One of the most commonly cited learning models was developed by Fitts and Posner (1967), who theorized that there are three stages of learning for a motor skill: cognitive, associative, and autonomous. Within the first or **cognitive stage** of learning, the learners make many errors and have highly variable performances. They know they are doing something wrong, but they do not know how to improve their performance. At this stage, dance exercisers seem terribly uncoordinated and consistently perform exercises incorrectly. Learners in the second or **associative stage** have learned the basic fundamentals or mechanics of the skill. Their errors tend to be less gross in nature and they can now concentrate on refining their skills. During this stage, exercise participants are able to detect some errors and the instructor needs to make only occasional corrections. During the third or **autonomous stage,** the skill becomes automatic or habitual. Learners can now perform without thinking and can detect their own errors. Highly skilled dancers, for example, do not think about individual steps in a routine, but instead concentrate on the more difficult aspects of the choreography.

Learning Strategies

The kind and amount of information that dance-exercise participants can understand depends on what stage of the learning process they are in. For example, beginning dance exercisers see a choreographed routine as composed of many steps, each step demanding their full attention. Every step is critical. However, advanced dance exercisers see only a few steps as crucial, perhaps where the tempo changes or at the beginning of a difficult part of the dance. Because beginners are less skilled at determining what information they must attend to, the exercise instructor must provide them with specific information about what is important. For example, since maintaining the appropriate posture is necessary to properly execute many exercises and dance steps, instructors must constantly remind beginners to maintain correct exercise postures. Therefore, to employ appropriate teaching strategies, instructors need to be aware of each participant's stage of learning.

When teaching an exercise or movement pattern, instructors should determine which teaching approach will be most effective. They can use either a **part approach** where the skill is broken down into its components and participants practice each part, or a **whole approach** where participants practice the entire skill. The most efficient teaching method depends on the task complexity and the task organization of a skill (Magill 1980). **Task complexity** refers to the number of parts or components within a task and the level of information processing required to complete the task. A highly complex task has many components and requires much attention. Choreographed aerobics routines, for example, can be highly complex. Low-complexity tasks have few components and relatively limited attention demands. Many floor exercises are low in complexity. **Task organization** refers to the number of parts of the task that are interrelated. A task high in organization is composed of closely related components, such as the parts of a specific floor exercise. A task low in organization is composed of independent parts, such as the individual dance steps making up a routine.

Tasks or skills that are high in complexity and low in organization should be taught by practicing the parts. The part approach to teaching is therefore appropriate for aerobic dance-exercise routines. Instructors should teach each step in its simplest form. Once participants have mastered the steps, they should be placed in the proper sequence. Tasks or skills that are low in complexity but high in organization should be practiced in their entirety. The whole approach to teaching is therefore appropriate for most floor exercises. When teaching a floor exercise, instructors should explain the entire exercise in terms of the correct execution and then ask their students to perform the activity.

Feedback and Knowledge of Results

A very important part of learning is feedback and knowledge of results. **Feedback** is an internal response within a learner. During information processing, the correctness or incorrectness of a response is stored in memory to be used for future reference (Magill 1980). The instructor has little influence on this type of feedback. **Knowledge of results** or

KR is feedback from external sources such as the instructor. By providing appropriate feedback, exercise leaders can greatly influence a participant's performance. KR serves three important functions in learning: (a) it provides information about performance, (b) it serves as a motivator for further performances, and (c) it reinforces or strengthens correct responses. An instructor must determine the critical elements of a skill in order to know which aspects of the skill to evaluate. For example, if the primary objective of the class is to achieve target heart rate, the instructor should give KR that is specific to the intensity of movement.

Three types of statements can be used when giving KR: corrective statements, value statements, and neutral statements (Mosston 1981). **Corrective statements** are used when a learner's response is incorrect. The statement identifies the error and tells the learner how to correct it. For example, "You are raising your back too far off the floor during your curl-up—keep the lower back on the floor at all times." Corrective statements are the most effective type of KR for ensuring immediate improvement in performance. A **value statement** projects a feeling about a performance, using such words as "good," "well done," or "poor job." This type of statement can motivate or encourage a participant whose performance is still not altogether correct but is improving. For example, "Good, Mary, you are getting better." Finally, a **neutral statement** acknowledges the performance but does not judge or correct it. "I see you did 30 curl-ups" is an example of a neutral statement. All three statements have a place in the teaching environment, however, beginning instructors who have not yet developed effective skill analysis techniques often find themselves relying on value statements.

To determine the correctness of a performance, an instructor relies on kinesiological principles, past experience, and aesthetic standards (Mosston 1981). Kinesiological principles are used to determine which postures and movements are mechanically correct. For example, curl-ups are performed with the knees bent to reduce stress on the lower back and to isolate the abdominal musculature. Past experience is often used to correct a movement based on subtleties accumulated from observing many exercisers perform the same movement. Experienced instructors can often find just the right word or phrase to correct consistently inappropriate performances. Aesthetic standards are used to correct movements and postures determined to be culturally attractive. Dance movements are often corrected on the basis of aesthetic standards.

An important consideration when giving KR is the performer's stage of learning. In the early stages, performers cannot determine what they are doing wrong and therefore require a great deal of KR. On the other hand, proficient performers rely more on internal feedback and require little KR. Since beginners depend more heavily on visual cues than do experienced dance exercisers, instructors teaching multilevel classes should spend most of their time demonstrating beginning exercises and movement patterns, while occasionally demonstrating exercises for more advanced participants.

A person can attend to only a few cues at any given moment. Therefore, when giving KR instructors should limit the number of corrections offered at any one time. Positive reinforcement is very important in the early stages of learning. Instructors should use positive value statements when participants make a good attempt even if the performance is not yet correct. KR should always be given in a friendly manner and can be offered either publicly or privately to the individual. If several participants are performing a move incorrectly, the instructor should probably give feedback to the entire class. However, if one person consistently performs an exercise or movement incorrectly, the instructor should talk to that person privately, either when class participants are working individually or after class.

DESIGNING INSTRUCTION

Effectively designing a dance-exercise program involves setting goals and planning daily lessons. Lesson planning includes writing class objectives and selecting activities, selecting patterns of class organization, and considering facilities and equipment. Each element of designing instruction is addressed in this section. In addition, the process of selecting the appropriate music and movement patterns is examined.

Goal Setting

The effective use of goal setting facilitates both learning and performance of motor skills. The competent exercise instructor establishes program goals and aids participants in developing their personal goals. Program goals should reflect what the instructor expects students to gain from the program. Examples of program goals might include the following:

1. The participant will increase or maintain adequate aerobic fitness to acquire cardiorespiratory-related health benefits.

2. The participant will increase or maintain adequate and specific joint range of motion to prevent muscle imbalances and to provide appropriate range of motion for aerobic and floor-exercise movements.

3. The participant will increase or maintain adequate and specific muscular strength to prevent muscle imbalances and to provide adequate strength for aerobic movements.

Once the program goals have been established, instructors must set class objectives and plan daily activities that will result in the achievement and maintenance of program goals. These subjects are discussed in the next section.

Self-motivation depends on the degree to which participants perceive they control their own behavior (Nieman 1986). Therefore it is important that participants establish personal exercise goals. Instructors should help dance exercisers set goals that are realistic and make sure they understand what an exercise program can and cannot accomplish. Many participants expect instant results, particularly when their primary goal is weight loss. To ensure some immediate success, participants should establish short-term goals. For example, losing 1 lb per week is a short-term goal; losing 50 lbs is a long-term goal. Instructors also need to help participants maintain a good attitude and self-image as they work toward their goals. Once goals have been established, it is essential to monitor student progress. Periodic testing is discussed in the section on evaluating performance.

AEROBIC DANCE-EXERCISE INSTRUCTOR MANUAL

Lesson Planning

Planning and class preparation result in the efficient use of time, smooth progression of activities, and greater program variety. All too often, instructors who do not plan their lessons present the same music, exercises, and movement patterns day in and day out. Participants and instructors alike become bored with this daily routine.

It is particularly important that inexperienced instructors write out their daily class activities. While experienced instructors may no longer need to write a daily lesson plan, they should at least spend time before each class mentally preparing class activities. A daily lesson plan should consist of class objectives, planned activities and the time allotted for each activity, necessary equipment, and patterns of class organization. Figure 10–1 contains a sample lesson plan that can be modified to meet the needs of individual instructors and the objectives of specific classes.

CLASS OBJECTIVES. Just as exercise instructors need to establish program goals, they also need to develop more specific objectives for each class meeting. Class objectives state what instructors expect their participants to accomplish within each exercise session. The following are examples of class objectives:

1. The participant will maintain or increase cardiorespiratory fitness by exercising aerobically for 15 to 30 minutes at an intensity of 65%–75% maximal heart rate reserve.

2. The participant will increase or maintain adequate and specific flexibility by performing the following stretching exercises to their fullest range of motion: hamstrings, quadriceps, (and so on).

3. The participant will increase or maintain adequate and specific strength by performing the following exercises for 3 sets of 12 repetitions: leg lifts, curl-ups, (and so on).

Objectives help instructors focus on the purpose of each selected exercise and activity. In fact, novice instructors should list the purpose of each strength and flexibility exercise used in their classes. Knowing the benefits of each exercise will help instructors select appropriate class activities.

CLASS ACTIVITIES AND TIME ALLOCATION. The activities within a dance-exercise class can include the following:

- educational discussions (minilectures or daily fitness tips)
- warm-up and cool-down
- preaerobic and postaerobic stretching
- floor exercises
- cardiovascular activity (aerobic dance, aerobic calisthenics, or circuit training)

An important but often overlooked activity is a regularly planned educational discussion session that focuses on pertinent physiological, kinesiological, and nutritional information. These discussions, which should be concise and brief (5–10 minutes), can include such topics as exercise myths and misconceptions, the latest findings on fat utilization during exercise, and methods of reducing lower back pain. The

CLASS: Aerobic dance   **DATE: December 21, 1986   TIME: 9–10:15**

CLASS OBJECTIVES:

1. Participants will improve or maintain cardiorespiratory fitness by dancing aerobically for 15 to 25 minutes at 65%–75% heart-rate reserve.

2. Participants will improve or maintain flexibility by performing specific stretching exercises, holding for 15 seconds at maximum range of motion.

3. Participants will improve or maintain strength by performing specific strength exercises for 3 sets of 12 repetitions.

ACTIVITIES	TIME (minutes)	PATTERNS OF CLASS ORGANIZATION	EQUIP-MENT	MUSIC	COMMENTS
Discussion Spot-reducing	10				
Warm-up	3			Will vary according to season, age group, and participant interest.	Nice and easy
Preaerobic Stretch Hamstrings, Erector spinae, Quads, Gastrocnemius	4		Walls		Stretch to point of tightness not pain
Aerobic Dance-Exercise	25				Take EHR Check EHRs with a show of hands
Cool Down	3	(same as above)			Take RecHR
Floor Exercise Curl-ups, Shins, Leg lifts, Tricep extension	15		Mats, rubber bands		Slow and controlled
Postaerobic Stretch (Repeat preaerobic stretch)	10	(same as above)	Towels		Get exercisers to relax
Record Progress	4		Card file		Give praise/encouragement

FIGURE 10–1 Sample lesson plan

instructor can offer additional educational information during the workout by discussing the purpose of a particular segment or exercise while it is being performed. Educational handouts are also extremely valuable to participants and can serve as a motivator for continued attendance.

Strength and flexibility activities should be carefully planned. Specific stretching and floor exercises are discussed in Chapter 5. The selection of music and the selection of movement patterns for the warm-up, aerobics, and cool-down segments of the class are perhaps the instructor's most difficult tasks. These two very important activities are addressed in greater detail later in this chapter.

The time allotted for each activity varies according to the total class time available and according to the specific nature of the activity. Some activities will naturally require more time than others. Minimum and maximum time requirements for the warm-up, aerobics, and cool-down segments are discussed in Chapter 5. The time allotted for stretching and strengthening depends on the number of exercises to be performed.

Beginning and ending class on time is also important. Instructors who methodically plan their lessons will know the precise length of time for each activity. However, since unforeseen events such as a tape deck malfunction do occur, the competent instructor needs to be flexible and able to improvise at the last minute if necessary.

PATTERNS OF CLASS ORGANIZATION. Dance-exercise classes should be arranged to ensure the safety of participants and to enable everyone to hear the instructions and see the demonstrations. Patterns of class organization refer to the formations used by instructors to provide their students with maximum opportunities for learning and performing. In a typical dance-exercise class formation, the instructor stands at the front of the room and participants face him or her. While this formation can be effective, there is one major disadvantage. Usually the enthusiastic, experienced participants stand in the front of the room while the less experienced stay in the back. The result is a potentially unsafe situation, because it is difficult for an instructor to observe those in the back of the room. To resolve this problem, instructors can periodically move from the front to the sides and to the back of the class, asking participants to turn and face them in each new position. Another effective formation is for instructors to stand in the center of the room and have participants form a single or double circle around them. Exercise leaders using this formation should change their point of focus by rotating a quarter turn from time to time.

FACILITY AND EQUIPMENT CONSIDERATIONS. Not all instructors can choose the facility in which they teach. Ideally the dance-exercise facility should have the following items:

1. Good ventilation with a temperature range of 60°F–70°F.
2. A floor that will effectively absorb shock and will control undesirable medial-lateral motions of the foot.
3. Sufficient space for each student to move comfortably (with arms outspread, each participant should be able to take two large steps in any direction without touching another student).
4. Mirrors for participants to observe their own exercise positions and postures.
5. A raised platform for the instructor.

Equipment needs can include tapes, tape deck, microphone, mats, and props such as weights, rubber bands, and balls. Instructors should always arrive early to check that all equipment is in working order before class begins. Class time should never be spent cueing tapes or searching for props.

Selecting Music

Music not only provides the timing for exercise movements, it also makes a class more fun and helps to motivate participants. Because music is the basis of dance-exercise programs, instructors should be familiar with its fundamental elements, such as rhythm, beat, measure, meter, and tempo.

1. **Rhythm** is "the regular pattern of movement and/or sound" that can be felt, seen, or heard (Harris, Pittman, and Waller 1978, p. 39). Rhythm often dictates the style of a dance or exercise routine.

2. **Beats** are regular pulsations that have an even rhythm and occur in a continuous pattern of strong and weak pulsations (Fallon and Kuchenmeister, 1977).

3. A **measure** is "one group of beats made by the regular occurrence of the heavy accent" (Harris, Pittman, and Waller 1978, p. 39).

4. A **meter** organizes beats into musical patterns or measures such as 4 beats per measure (4/4). Most dance-exercise routines use music with a meter of 4/4 time (Fallon and Kuchenmeister, 1977).

5. **Tempo** is the "rate of speed at which music is played" (Harris, Pittman, and Waller 1978, p. 40). Dance-exercise instructors often determine the tempo of the music by counting the number of beats per minute.

The tempo of the music determines the progression of exercise and, because it dictates the speed of movement, the intensity of exercise. Using experience and common sense, instructors have adopted general guidelines for selecting the appropriate music tempo for the various components of a dance-exercise program. Slow tempos under 100 beats per minute are generally used for stretching, while tempos of 100–120 beats per minute are frequently used for warm-ups and cool-downs. Floor exercises are often performed to tempos of 110–130 beats per minute. However, the tempo for floor exercises should be slow enough for participants to control their movements. Aerobic dance activities are generally performed at a tempo of 130–160 beats per minute. Instructors must be cautious when choosing tempos over 140 beats per minute because participants need to move quickly at higher tempos. Encouraging students to perform smaller movements will help them preserve the control necessary for safety at high tempos. Beginners should never be expected to move at high tempos because they are not yet proficient enough to perform quick movements under control. Another consideration with fast-paced music is that participants with long arms and legs need more time to cover the same spatial area as participants with shorter limbs. For example, people with short arms can bring their arms above their heads more quickly than can people with long arms. Consequently, participants with long arms often appear to be uncoordinated unless they bend their elbows to keep in time with the instructor and the music.

Rhythm can dictate the style of movement. Instructors should select music that has a steady rhythm and a strong beat (with the exception of a slow stretch where bouncing to the beat must be avoided). The type of music selected will depend on the demographics of the exercise group and the creativity of the instructor. Staying open-minded is important. Instructors must not rely exclusively on their personal music preferences. The music style selected should reflect in part the interests of the age group. For example, young people may enjoy the top 40s, while an older group may prefer swing or big band music. Age should not be the only criterion for selecting music, however. In some parts of the country, gospel, folk, and country music are more appealing than rock and roll. Instructors may also want to consider the time of the year. At Christmas, for example, participants can be thoroughly delighted to exercise to "Rudolph The Red-Nosed Reindeer." For further variety, instructors can select music for special "theme days"— square dance, clogging, and polka music for a country music day or cha-cha, rumba, and samba music for a Latin music day. The greater the variety of music, the more enjoyment most participants will receive from a dance-exercise program.

To keep participants interested, instructors should change music frequently and avoid long pieces of music. For instructors who have trouble staying current with music selections, there are national music organizations designed to keep exercise leaders up-to-date. In addition, instructors can ask regular participants for suggestions.

Selecting Movement Patterns

Once the music has been selected, instructors must choose appropriate dance-exercise movements. The first consideration is whether the movement is safe, and even if an individual step is safe, the transition between that step and another may be hazardous. Therefore, instructors must also consider the safe sequencing of steps. Other chapters in this manual address contraindicated exercises, but for review purposes, instructors should keep in mind the following general guidelines when selecting dance-exercise steps.

1. Avoid movements that result in hyperextension of any joint.

2. Do not repeat a movement more than 4 consecutive times on one leg; in other words, alternate every 4 counts.

3. Avoid flinging the limbs at any time.

4. Make sure lateral foot moves are well controlled to avoid tripping or falling (especially on carpet).

5. Be cautious of lateral moves that use crossover steps (such as a grapevine), which can be particularly stressful to excessive pronaters during the weight-bearing phase of the crossover.

6. Avoid movements with forward trunk flexion, especially those movements that combine forward trunk flexion and rotation.

7. Never stretch muscles ballistically while performing movement patterns.

8. Avoid changing directions rapidly. Transitions between complex steps may require a movement sequence in place before changing directions.

9. Avoid continuous movement that requires participants to remain on the balls of their feet for extended periods.

Instructors teaching dance exercise should be familiar with the basic foundations of movement. Four **basic locomotor steps** use the feet as the base of support: walking (or stepping), running (or leaping), hopping, and jumping (Griffith 1982). All other steps are either variations or combinations of these basic steps. Common variations or combination steps include a two-step, polka, schottische, skip, slide, gallop, pony, cha-cha, and Charleston. A description of each of these steps follows.

Two-Step Step R (right) fwd (forward), close L (left), step R fwd. Begin next step on L foot. Rhythm: 1 and, 2

Polka Step R fwd, close L, step R fwd, hop R. Begin next step on L foot. Rhythm: 1 and, 2 and

Schottische Step R fwd, step L fwd, step R fwd, hop R. Begin next step on L foot. Rhythm: 1, 2, 3, 4

Skip Step R fwd, hop R. Begin next step on L foot. Rhythm: 1 and

Slide Step R sdw (sideways), close L. Begin next step on R foot. Rhythm: 1 and

Gallop Step R fwd, close left. Begin next step on R foot. Rhythm: 1 and

Pony Step R fwd or sdw, push off ball of L toe, step R pl (in place). Begin next step on L foot. Rhythm: 1 and, 2

Cha-cha Step R fwd, step L bwd (backward), step R pl, step L pl, step R pl. Begin next step on L foot. Rhythm: 1, 2, 3 and 4

Charleston Step R fwd, touch L fwd, step L bwd, touch R bwd. Begin next step on R foot. Rhythm: 1, 2, 3, 4

In addition to these steps, instructors can use low kicks, knee lifts, step touches, turns, jumping jacks, and hopscotches, to name a few. Instructors can increase their movement repertoire by borrowing steps from other dance forms, such as jazz, folk, modern, or ballet, or by using movements from various sports and games. All locomotor and stationary movements can be complemented with a variety of arm movements including swinging up and down or side to side, in circles, in opposition, in flexion, or with the hands punching, clapping, or snapping. To aid with verbal cueing, instructors should name all steps.

Two basic methods, known as freestyle and structured, are used to combine movement patterns and music. The **freestyle** method uses movements chosen randomly by the instructor during the aerobics segment of the class. Participants follow along by listening to verbal cueing and modeling the instructor. This method uses combinations of simple steps that are repeated throughout a piece of music. The **structured** method uses choreographed movements that are formally arranged step patterns, repeated in a predetermined order.

The freestyle method is spontaneous and requires less advanced preparation by the instructor. Movement patterns tend to be simpler and are repeated more often than in structured routines. While participants must still learn the movement patterns, they do not need to learn specific movement sequences. The disadvantages are that freestyle exercise can become monotonous, and participants may be unable to maintain appropriate exercise intensity as they anticipate the next unknown movement. It is particularly difficult for participants in the back of the class to anticipate the next move because they may have trouble seeing the instructor's feet.

Structured routines can be more challenging. Once participants have learned the routine, they become more confident and can concentrate on maintaining appropriate intensity levels and safe positions. The disadvantages of structured routines are that they require a great deal of preparation by the instructor and take more class time to teach. Both methods, freestyle and structured, are appropriate for a dance-exercise class. Instructors usually select the method that best reflects their personal philosophies and their dance-exercise strengths. Creative instructors seeking greater program variety may choose to incorporate both methods in their dance-exercise classes.

Instructors using the structured or choreographed method should observe the following guidelines:

1. Select energetic music that is fun, and that has the appropriate number of beats per minute (this guideline also applies to the freestyle method).

2. Listen to the selected piece of music and try to visualize the style of movement as well as specific steps that might be used.

3. Count the number of beats within the phrases or verses, the chorus, and any special segments such as an instrumental section within a song.

4. Select movement patterns that fit each segment of the music.

5. Repeat steps in a regular series of counts, usually 4 or 8.

When presenting new choreographed routines or step patterns, instructors should demonstrate the entire dance or movement pattern to the class before teaching the activity. A demonstration by a good performer has a tremendous impact on observers. It motivates participants, it is an efficient time saver (a good demonstration "is worth a thousand words"), and it points to a successful level of accomplishment (Mosston 1981).

To keep track of choreographed routines or step patterns, instructors should maintain a card file or notebook that records the music, step patterns, and verbal cues. To use class time more efficiently, instructors may want to print the steps of a routine on a large poster board and display it prominently in the exercise room.

Before teaching a new routine to a class, instructors should practice the steps (preferably in front of a mirror) until the routine is completely memorized. Verbal and nonverbal cues should also be rehearsed. Practicing routines or movement patterns allows instructors to determine whether the sequence of steps flows smoothly.

TEACHING CLASS ACTIVITIES

To teach dance exercise successfully, an instructor must select an appropriate teaching style and use effective techniques for teaching movement patterns, including proper cueing. These areas are addressed in this section.

Teaching Styles

The teaching style chosen is an important factor in determining the instructor's success in effectively presenting class activities. Instructors should be familiar with a variety of styles. Mosston (1981) has identified eight specific teaching styles. Each accomplishes a different set of objectives, and it is both possible and desirable to use several styles in a dance-exercise class. The five styles directly applicable to a dance-exercise program include command, practice, reciprocal, self-check, and inclusion. Each style is described and discussed in terms of its practical application to dance exercise.

An instructor using the **command style** of teaching makes all decisions about posture, rhythm, and duration, while participants follow his or her directions and movements. This style is most appropriate when instructors want to achieve the following objectives:

- immediate participant response
- participant emulation of instructor as role model
- participant control
- safety
- avoidance of alternatives and choices
- efficient use of time
- perpetuation of aesthetic standards

The command style has been perhaps the most commonly used style in dance-exercise classes. While this style may be particularly suited to warming up, cooling down, and learning new routines and exercises, it leaves no room for individualization. The participant has little say in decisions about personal physical development and few opportunities exist for social interaction. To achieve these objectives, an instructor must rely on other teaching styles.

The **practice style** of teaching provides opportunities for individualization and includes practice time and private instructor feedback for each participant. While all dance-exercisers are working on the same task, individual participants can choose their own pace and rhythm. The practice style is particularly suited for floor exercises in classes where the fitness level of participants varies greatly. Using this style, instructors can encourage students to perform the maximum number of repetitions suitable to their skill level. The real key is that once instructors have determined the task, such as curl-ups or leg lifts, they are free to move around and give individual feedback where necessary. A disadvantage is that not all participants are sufficiently motivated to achieve their maximum potential.

The **reciprocal style** of teaching involves the use of an observer or a partner to provide feedback to each participant. This style enables everyone to receive individual feedback, an often impossible task for the instructor. The reciprocal style can best be used for screening or testing and retesting in certain areas. For example, tests evaluating posture, girth measurements, and flexibility can be quickly administered by partners. Using a criteria card that shows the nature of the test, the criteria for passing, and the performance level achieved will provide instructors with a record of participant performance and will allow students to monitor their own progress. A sample criteria card is presented in Figure 10−2. Aside from providing the participant with important feedback, the reciprocal style encourages social interaction, which is one reason people choose to participate in organized exercise

CRITERIA CARD

Name

TEST	PASSING CRITERIA	PERFORMANCE LEVEL		
		1	2	3
		Date:		

Flexibility

Hamstrings*   Leg raised to vertical

Quads*   Heel touching buttocks

Strength

Sit-ups
(1 min.)

Males		
age < 35	36-45	> 46
33+	27+	21+

Females		
age < 35	36-45	> 46
25+	18+	14+

Cardiovascular

3 min. step test

Males	Females
< 122	< 120

Body Composition

Skinfolds

Males	Females
< 16%	< 23%

*Draw the leg position of the exerciser being tested.

FIGURE 10-2 Sample criteria card

programs (Nieman 1986, Franklin 1986). One major disadvantage is that the observer or partner may not provide appropriate feedback.

The **self-check style** of teaching relies on individual participants to provide their own feedback. Participants perform a given task and then record the results, comparing their performance against given criteria or past performances. This style lends itself nicely to the recording of target heart rate, recovery heart rate, and number of floor-exercise repetitions. Instructors will need to provide a record card for each individual participant. A sample record card is presented in Figure 10-3. Because a key component of motivation and exercise compliance is self-monitoring of progress (Nieman 1986, Franklin 1986), it is desirable to incorporate the self-check style into every exercise program.

The **inclusion style** enables multiple levels of performance to be taught within the same activity. Perhaps one of the most significant problems facing the dance-exercise industry is teaching multiple skill

RECORD CARD

Name_____   Resting Heart Rate_____

                                          Target Heart Rate Zone_____ to _____

	DATE 11/23/87
ACTIVITY	
Aerobic dance-exercise HR	158
Aerobic dance recovery HR	118
Curl-ups (body weight)	20-20-20 (3 sets of 20 reps)
Leg lifts (5 lbs)	12-12-10
Shins (rubber band)	12-10-10

FIGURE 10-3 Sample record card

and fitness levels within one class. Skill and fitness level can vary in each segment of the exercise class, including stretching, strengthening, and aerobic work. Because most people tend to overestimate their ability, instructors should first administer tests to determine the skill and fitness levels of individual participants. Then the class should be designed to incorporate all levels so that each person can achieve maximum success. During the stretching and strengthening segments of the program, the instructor can offer alternate positions for the different levels. For example, during the abdominal work the participant with weak stomach muscles can choose to do pelvic tilts, while the person with stronger abdominals can perform curl-ups. The instructor can also offer different levels of difficulty during the aerobics segment. For example, beginners can perform low-impact routines using walks instead of runs, keeping the feet close to the ground and the arms below shoulder level, while advanced students can perform a more vigorous routine by using arm movements above the shoulders and taking larger steps. Instructors need periodically to demonstrate each level of aerobic dance, spending more time on the routines for beginners. Ideally the instructor would demonstrate the movements for beginners, while a teacher assistant or an experienced dance exerciser demonstrates the more advanced movements.

Teaching Movement Patterns

New movements should always be taught in their simplest form. Instructors should begin by teaching the basic footwork in place without arm movements and at a moderate tempo. As participants become more proficient, the tempo can be increased, arm movements can be added, and the step pattern can be moved in a variety of directions—namely forward, backward, sideways, diagonally, or in circles. For example, the following progression might be used for a movement pattern consisting of step touches, ponies, and jogs:

Progression

Foot pattern in place Step touch 4 times—pony 4 times—jog 4 times.

Foot pattern with arms
Step touch: Clap on each touch or swing arms across the body in the direction of movement.
Pony: One arm over head, the other arm down in front of the body moving in opposition to the feet.
Jog: Flex the elbows in opposition to the feet (bicep curl).

Foot pattern with directional movement Step touch 4 times—sideways, pony 4 times—forward, jog 4 times—backward.

Directional foot pattern with arm movements Combine above foot patterns with arm movements.

For variety, instructors can take a simple foot pattern of knee lifts and ponies and vary the sequence in the following way:

First pattern Knee lift—R, L, R, L, pony—R, L, R, L

Second pattern Double knee lifts—R, L, R, L, pony—R, L, R, L

Instructors can combine the first and second patterns and, for variety, reverse the order of each pattern.

Movements must be selected so that most participants are successful. Some participants will learn new steps more quickly than others. Instructors should be patient and supportive of the slower learners, reminding them that they will improve with practice. Instructors should always try to be available before and after class for individual help.

Instructors must select movement patterns carefully. Complex routines can slow the class down and confuse participants, particularly in a beginning or multilevel class. To avoid interfering with continuous aerobic movement in intermediate and advanced dance-exercise classes, instructors may want to teach new movement patterns or routines during the warm-up or cool-down segments when the steps can be learned at a slower pace.

A slow progression is important to learn a skill effectively and to avoid musculoskeletal injuries. Instructors must encourage beginners to start slowly and progress gradually. It is the responsibility of both the instructor and the participant to monitor exercise intensity. Beginners should take their heart rates frequently and instructors should be aware of the progress participants are making. One approach is to ask for a show of hands for those above, below, and within the target heart-rate range. Instructors should ask those participants who are above their target zone to keep their feet closer to the ground and reduce the size of their arm movements. Those students exercising below their target zone should be encouraged to take larger steps and increase the size of their arm movements *if* they are ready to do so. Instructors should make sure that exercise heart rates can be reported in a nonthreatening and noncompetitive environment to ensure honesty. Accurate reporting is particularly important for participants who are taking medications that alter heart-rate response to exercise.

It is extremely important that participants adjust the intensity of their movements to their cardiorespiratory fitness level. One way to ensure that each person is working at the appropriate fitness level is to give exercisers color-coded ribbons, wristbands, or headbands that identify their workout levels. For example, green might be beginning students, blue intermediate, and red advanced. By periodically scanning the class, instructors can readily observe whether individual participants are working at the appropriate exercise intensity.

Within a multilevel class, beginners should be encouraged to progress slowly in both the intensity and duration of exercise. After beginners have reached their aerobic goal for the day, instructors can suggest that they walk around the room while more experienced participants continue to exercise. Instructors must be very careful not to give conflicting messages to participants. If everyone is expected to work at their own level, instructors must avoid phrases such as "Get your feet up higher," "Push through it," or "Just do one more routine." Participants will feel compelled to work at higher intensities whether or not they are ready to do so.

Cueing

Cueing is a very important part of teaching dance exercise. Instructors should face the class as often as possible, using mirroring techniques such as moving to their left when directing participants to the right. Instructors can only monitor class safety by watching participants at all times. Each cue should be brief and should be called on the preceding measure to provide the participant with enough time to move smoothly from one step to the next. When beginning a routine, instructors should use rhythmic starting signals such as "Ready and," "Ready go," or "Now begin."

There are five types of cueing: footwork, directional, rhythmic, numerical, and step (Griffith 1982). **Footwork cueing** indicates which foot to move, the left or the right. **Directional cueing** tells participants which direction to move, such as forward or backward. **Rhythmic cueing** indicates the correct rhythm of the routine, such as slow (2 counts) or quick (1 count). **Numerical cueing** refers to counting the rhythm such as 1 and 2, 3, 4. Finally, **step cueing** refers to the name of the step, such as pony. When leading dance exercises, it is best to combine types of cueing. For example, the instructor might cue a sequence consisting of two schottisches and four sideways ponies as follows:

First Schottische
Step cueing: "Step, step, step, hop."

Second Schottische
Rhythmic cueing: "Quick, quick, quick, quick."

First Pony
Numerical cueing: "1 and 2."

Second Pony
Directional cueing: "Side together, side."

Third Pony
Footwork cueing: "Right, left, right."

Fourth Pony
Step cueing: "Step, ball, change."

As students become proficient at executing step patterns, they will need fewer verbal cues from exercise instructors. Instructors can then rely more on nonverbal cues, such as using the hands or head to indicate direction. Clapping the hands and snapping the fingers can help keep time with the music.

MOTIVATING PARTICIPANTS

Motivation is a key component of effective learning and thus in the continued performance of an activity. In fact a common characteristic associated with dropping out of an exercise program is lack of self-motivation (Nieman 1986). According to Magill (1980), motivation "involves the initiation, maintenance and intensity of behavior." Since motivation comes from within, it is the instructor's responsibility to create a climate that enhances participant self-motivation. The extent to which people are self-motivated depends on the degree to which they perceive they control their own behavior. The instructor therefore should involve participants in the development of personal exercise goals.

Most people are motivated by challenge, growth, achievement, and recognition (Nieman 1986). Dance-exercise instructors can enhance motivation by offering variety within their classes, by individualizing exercise programs, by giving more responsibility to participants, and by developing a warm personal relationship with each student. Instructor characteristics that encourage good relationships with participants include empathy, respect, warmth, and genuineness (Nieman 1986). Dance-exercise instructors serve as role models for their students. By being knowledgeable, cheerful, encouraging, and genuinely enthusiastic about exercise and its merits, instructors create a positive environment.

Supervised exercise programs such as dance exercise have not been successful in attracting the large percentage of people who do not exercise. Only 20% of the American population exercise regularly enough to gain or maintain cardiovascular benefits; 40% are active but less frequently and intensely, while the remaining 40% are completely sedentary (Nieman 1986). Of those who join formal exercise programs, 40%–50% drop out within 6 months to a year (Dishman 1986). Not all exercise noncompliance is medically related or behavioral; lack of support from a spouse or inaccessible program location can be unavoidable reasons for noncompliance.

Researchers have found that the people least likely to exercise in a formal program and most likely to drop out of an exercise program are blue-collar workers, smokers, and obese persons. The most common reasons given for noncompliance are inconvenient or inaccessible program location, lack of time or work conflict, and poor spouse support (Nieman 1986, Dishman 1986). There is some concern, however, that self-reports of noncompliance to exercise are not altogether accurate. People who do not exercise may be rationalizing why they are inactive. In fact, one study showed that dropouts who perceived distance from classes as a major reason for not exercising actually lived closer to exercise facilities than regular exercisers. In addition, inactive people have just as much leisure time per week (15–18 hours) as active people (Dishman 1986). In other words, removing stated barriers such as facility inconvenience may not necessarily increase exercise compliance if the stated reasons are not accurate.

While health benefits are important to people who exercise, feeling good or better as a result of participation in exercise is more important. On the basis of current research information, the following motivational strategies have been suggested to improve exercise compliance within a formal exercise program (Nieman 1986, Franklin 1986):

1. Provide good exercise leadership.
2. Conduct assessment of clients (health assessment, fitness testing).
3. Conduct periodic evaluations.
4. Provide opportunities for self-monitoring and for keeping records of progress.
5. Ensure a slow rate of exercise progression to minimize musculoskeletal injuries.
6. Provide opportunities for making social contacts.
7. Vary the exercise program.
8. Recognize individual accomplishments with extrinsic rewards such as certificates of accomplishment.
9. Provide opportunities for having fun.

Having fun is an important motivator for people to continue exercising. Dance-exercise programs provide perfect opportunities for having fun. Using a variety of music, dance styles, exercises, and props such as towels, balls, jump ropes, weights, and rubber bands, and providing opportunities for social interaction contribute to a fun exercise environment.

EVALUATING PERFORMANCE

The effective exercise leader monitors participants' progress toward personal goals through periodic testing. Each dance exerciser should be evaluated initially to establish a baseline by which to measure progress. Physiological measures such as cardiorespiratory fitness level, body composition, strength, and flexibility are described in Chapter 6.

Instructors should attempt to use valid tests that can be easily administered either by partners or by the participants themselves. Providing criteria cards that indicate the nature of the test, the criteria for passing, and the performance level achieved by the exerciser saves valuable class time and can serve as a motivation tool for participants (see Fig. 10–2). Instructors can provide perhaps 5–10 minutes of "personal time" during class for participants to work on any deficiencies discovered during testing. (See Chapter 6 for a discussion of fitness tests appropriate for a dance-exercise setting.)

In addition to periodic testing, instructors should encourage participants to monitor their daily accomplishments. A record card can be used to keep track of daily progress (see Fig. 10–3). Items such as heart rate (resting, exercise, and recovery) and the number of floor-exercise repetitions can be regularly monitored and recorded by the participants themselves. Criteria and record cards should be stored in an alphabetized file that is available to dance exercisers at each class meeting. Instructors can remind participants to pick up their cards, record the appropriate information, and refile them before leaving class.

It is important that instructors be aware of their students' progress toward their goals. They can do so by periodically examining participants' record cards and through one-on-one interaction with participants either before, during, or after class. If a participant is not showing progress, it is the instructor's responsibility to help determine the problem. It may be that unrealistic goals have been set or there has been an attendance problem. Showing genuine concern for participants encourages long-term participation in a formal exercise program.

SUMMARY

Effectively teaching an exercise class is a challenge to every dance-exercise instructor. Competent teachers carefully design their programs and employ sound teaching principles; they evaluate participant progress through initial testing and periodic retesting; and they develop sound strategies to motivate their participants to continue exercising. The extra work that is required to become an effective teacher will be repaid many times over as instructors earn their students' respect by providing safe, fun, and well-structured dance-exercise classes. Demonstrating expertise in the fitness industry will provide instructors with many professional opportunities and with the personal satisfaction of contributing to the well-being of so many dance exercisers.

REFERENCES

Dishman, R. K. "Exercise Compliance: A New View for Public Health." *The Physician and Sportsmedicine* 14, (1986): 127–43.

Fallon, D. J., and S. A. Kuchenmeister. *The Art of Ballroom Dance.* Minneapolis, Minn.: Burgess Publishing Company, 1977.

Fitts, P. M., and M. I. Posner. *Human Performance.* Belmont, Calif.: Brooks/Cole, 1967.

Franklin, B. A. "Clinical Components of a Successful Adult Fitness Program." *American Journal of Health Promotion* 1, (1986): 6–13.

Griffith, B. R. *Dance for Fitness.* Minneapolis, Minn.: Burgess Publishing Company, 1982.

Harris, J. A., A. M. Pittman, and M. S. Waller. *Dance A While.* Minneapolis, Minn.: Burgess Publishing Company, 1978.

Magill, R. A. *Motor Learning.* Dubuque, Iowa: Wm. C. Brown Company, 1980.

Mosston, M. *Teaching Physical Education.* Columbus, Ohio: Charles E. Merrill Publishing Company, 1981.

Nieman, D. C. *The Sports Medicine Fitness Course.* Palo Alto, Calif.: Bull Publishing Company, 1986.

Siedentop, D. *Developing Teaching Skills in Physical Education.* Palo Alto, Calif.: Mayfield Publishing Company, 1983.

INJURY PREVENTION
AND EMERGENCY PROCEDURES

PART III

Injuries will occur in even the best-designed classes. Although the emphasis should be on prevention—which means a safe exercise environment, proper footwear, proper exercise techniques, and good instructor supervision—an instructor must be prepared to respond to minor injuries as well as major emergencies. This section familiarizes instructors with common dance-exercise injuries and medical emergencies, provides basic procedures for proper injury management, and presents a low-impact workout that may reduce injuries related to impact stress. Because voice injury is an occupational hazard for instructors, one chapters focuses exclusively on preventing, recognizing and treating symptoms of vocal abuse. The safety of exercise classes for both instructors and participants is essential to the future of dance-exercise, and, therefore, a primary responsibility of all professionals in the field. It is hoped that dance-exercise instructors will seek additional training in injury prevention and emergency procedures.

Musculoskeletal Injuries

Marjorie J. Albohm

Marjorie J. Albohm, M.S., A.T., C., is associate director of the International Institute of Sports Science and Medicine, and she teaches at the Indiana University School of Medicine. The sixth woman in the nation certified by the National Athletic Trainers Association, she has served on the medical staff for the 1980 Winter Olympic Games and the 1987 Pan American Games.

11

IN THIS CHAPTER:

- Factors associated with injury: Floor surface, shoes, frequency and length of participation, exercise technique, quality of instruction.

- General injury guidelines: Acute and chronic injuries, warning signs, when to stop exercising and see a physician.

- Common dance-exercise injuries of the musculoskeletal system: Description, prevention, treatment.

The injuries and conditions commonly associated with aerobic dance-exercise can be extremely disabling. If not prevented or treated properly, they can stop a person from participating altogether. To prevent aerobic dance-exercise injuries, the various causes of injuries and their proper management must be thoroughly understood.

The primary cause of aerobic dance-exercise injuries is overuse—placing too much stress on one area of the body over an extended time. When stress is applied the body can either adapt by becoming stronger, or it can fail and break down (Fig. 11–1). Excessive, repeated stress causes failure, which usually results in **chronic injury.** Chronic problems have a gradual onset, without history of a specific incident of injury. They last for several weeks, often getting neither better nor worse. There may be symptoms of discomfort, swelling, or limited motion.

If a chronic injury continues to be stressed, it may become an **acute injury,** which occurs when an area already stressed and weakened is pushed beyond its limits and further injured. Acute injury has a more sudden onset, usually characterized by a specific incident. The symptoms are specific pain, specific swelling, limited motion, and inability to use the injured area normally. Shin splints, for example, are considered a chronic overuse problem. However, if they are ignored and activity levels are not reduced, the continual stress to the shin area

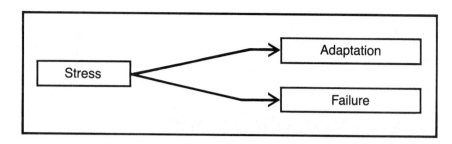

FIGURE 11–1 Overuse syndrome

can cause a stress fracture, which may become an acute problem. Acute injuries may also occur without being related to chronic injuries, as in an ankle sprain. A specific incident of injury occurs that immediately disables the person.

It is important to recognize the various causes of stress placed on the body during dance exercise so that activities can be modified to avoid stressing a particular area to failure. The locations that receive the most stress in aerobic dance-exercise are the feet, the ankles, the lower legs, and the knees.

FACTORS ASSOCIATED WITH INJURY

There are many factors associated with injury in a dance-exercise class. A class with a low rate of injury will have a safe workout environment, proper footwear, proper exercise technique, and good instructional supervision. These factors are discussed below. Other factors, such as a good warm-up and proper exercise progression, are discussed in Chapter 5.

Floor Surface

Exercising on nonresilient surfaces is a common cause of injury. Some surfaces absorb 2.5 times a person's body weight during dance exercise (Mosher 1984). An unyielding surface, such as concrete, will not absorb shock effectively, and so the feet, shins, and knees will receive more stress. The ideal floor surface provides both cushion and stability (Richie, Kelso, and Bellucci 1985). Injuries are highest on a concrete floor covered with carpet. Wood floors over airspace, which are slightly springy, are the best surfaces. Heavily padded concrete floors covered with carpet also seem to reduce injuries.

If classes must be held on inadequate floor surfaces, instructors should tailor routines accordingly. For example, on a surface such as a thick carpet that may improve shock absorption but sacrifices stability, the routine should reduce or eliminate the twisting or sliding movements that may cause participants to catch their feet in the carpet and fall or twist an ankle. On a nonresilient surface, such as linoleum over concrete in a church basement or recreation center, the instructor should use low-impact routines during the aerobics segment. (See Chapter 13 for a discussion of low-impact aerobics.) If the program budget permits, foam mats can be provided to participants for running and jumping activities. Only high-quality mats should be used, however. A slick surface, seams, or low spots resulting from point-pressure breakdown can cause participants to trip.

Shoes

Shoes are as important as floor surfaces for shock absorption and injury prevention. While running shoes and court shoes are usually better than none at all, a shoe designed specifically for aerobic dance-exercise is far preferable. A good aerobics shoe will have the following features:

1. *Shock absorption.* For aerobic dance-exercise, the most important feature of a shoe is its ability to absorb shock, especially in the forefoot where much of the impact occurs. Because shock-absorbing qualities are built into the shoe, this feature is sometimes difficult to assess in a store. The best test is to try on the shoes and jump up and down, both on the toes and flat-footed. The sensation of impact with the floor should be firm but not jarring. Ask the salesman about special shock-absorbing materials, which should extend to the toes.

Because the arch absorbs shock, shoes should also provide support to the inside long arch (inner longitudinal arch) and to the ball of the foot (metatarsal arch). (See Fig. 11–2.) Most major brands of aerobics shoes have adequate arch support, so that the choice is largely a matter of comfort and gentle support. Too high an arch will be uncomfortable, and too little will not cushion the arch against impact shock.

Participants with certain foot types or activity patterns may need additional shock-absorbing material or arch support. Inserts are available at local athletic footwear stores. It is advisable, however, to consult a podiatrist specializing in sports medicine before adding inserts to aerobics shoes. Unnecessary support or cushioning can create foot instability and cause injuries rather than prevent them.

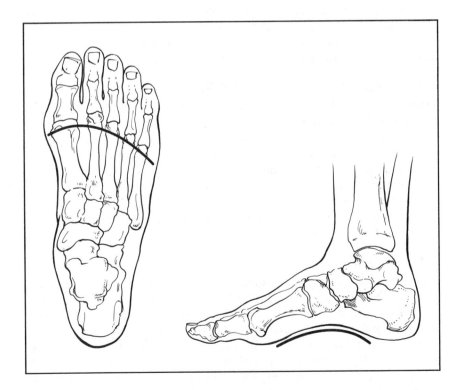

FIGURE 11–2 Arch support for aerobics shoes

AEROBIC DANCE-EXERCISE INSTRUCTOR MANUAL

2. *Lateral support and stability.* Many features of a shoe contribute to its stability. The shoe must have an outsole wide enough to provide a solid platform for the foot. A rigid heel counter is necessary to hold the foot in place and provide stability to the ankle. The upper material of the shoe should be supportive and should be reinforced at the forefoot to keep the foot from slipping sideways. The shoe should feel generally stable during all phases of dance exercise, including jumping on the toes, jumping from side to side, and twisting with the foot flat on the floor.

3. *Flexibility at the ball of the foot.* The ball of the foot is the only area in which an aerobics shoe should be flexible. General flexibility or flexibility in the rearfoot is *not* desirable. Some manufacturers add rubber toe guards to keep the toe area stable. It is important to check that these guards do not inhibit the flexibility of the shoe. An aerobics shoe should bend in the same place a foot bends—in the ball of the foot, about one-third of the way down from the toes.

4. *Fit and comfort.* Overall fit and comfort are extremely important, but they are also extremely subjective. The shoe should be long enough that the toes do not touch the end, even when the foot spreads or swells slightly during prolonged exercise. The shoe should be wide enough to accommodate the foot comfortably in both the forefoot and heel, and it should be free of irritations or pressure points.

Although high-top aerobics shoes may provide a feeling of additional support to the ankle, it is unlikely that they will significantly prevent ankle sprains. A high-top shoe may not be strong enough to keep the ankle from withstanding force and turning inward or outward.

What may be the right aerobics shoe for one person may be wrong for another. The best approach is for both instructors and participants to try on several shoes from reputable manufacturers and to buy shoes suitable for their own activity patterns, floor surfaces, and foot types.

Frequency and Length of Participation

High-intensity activity, done frequently over a long time, will have a cumulative stressful effect on the body. Injury rates increase when people dance more frequently (Richie, Kelso, and Bellucci 1985). Also, the longer someone participates in aerobic dance-exercise, the greater the chance of injury. Instructors are more affected than students because they usually teach more days, more classes per day, over a longer period. To prevent injury, it is advisable to participate in classes no longer than 1 hour and no more than 3–4 days per week. Beyond that level the risk of injury increases.

Exercise Technique

Improper dance-exercise technique may also contribute to overuse stresses. Unilateral high jumping or kicking, in excessive repetitions, may create greater stress than the lower extremities can accommodate. Instead, the instructor should emphasize lower jumps, hops, or jogging. Alternate left and right sides after each repetition during weight-bearing activities, and limit repetitions to no more than four on each side at one time. High-impact activities *do not* significantly increase aerobic output, but they do increase injury risk. Weight-bearing activities may have to be modified if injury symptoms develop.

MODIFICATIONS. It is often simple to modify dance-exercise movements to prevent injury. Any exercise that consistently causes discomfort or pain should be eliminated or modified. Assess the mechanics and technique of new exercises before they are introduced to a class. Listen to participants' comments about exercises and watch their techniques at all times. Discuss common injury problems with participants *before* they occur to emphasize prevention.

Some individual modification of movements may be necessary if a participant has a particular condition or injury. Again, movements that cause pain or discomfort to the injured area should be eliminated and alternative exercises should be provided. For example, if weight-bearing activity is painful, suggest low-impact or no-impact dance-exercise activities, as well as swimming and biking. (See Chapter 13 on low-impact aerobics.)

HIGH-RISK EXERCISES. Several high-risk exercises and techniques should never be performed in a dance-exercise class. These exercises are frequently linked with the injuries described later in this chapter:

WARNING: Figures 11–3 through 11–10 are contraindicated exercises. They may result in injury.

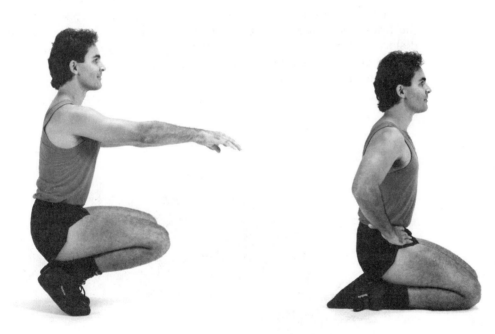

Full squats (Fig. 11–3) adversely affect the knee joint by stretching it to a fully opened position that supports the entire body. This position puts extreme stress on the supporting ligaments of the joint, weakening it over time and possibly causing chronic degenerative problems in the knee. Quarter or half squats (keeping the knees at a 90° angle or the hamstrings parallel to the floor) are much safer and are a good way to condition the thigh muscles. *Never* have less than a 90° angle at the knees when performing squats.

Knee sitting (Fig. 11–4) produces effects similar to that of full squats. The knee joint is stretched open under the stress of body weight. This position stretches the ligaments and can produce joint instability. A participant with any history of knee problems should never perform this exercise.

FIGURE 11–3 *(left)* Full squat

FIGURE 11–4 *(right)* Knee sitting

WARNING: Figures 11–3 through 11–10 are contraindicated exercises. They may result in injury.

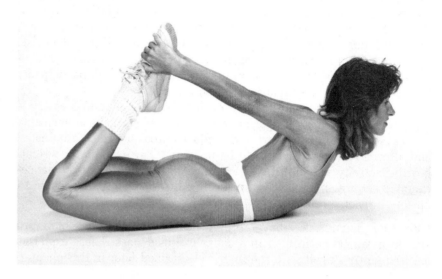

FIGURE 11–5 Back hyperextension

Back hyperextension exercises (Fig. 11–5) put abnormal stress on the low back (lumbar spine), causing possible vertebral fractures or dislocations over time. Avoid arching the back to any degree more than that produced by raising the chest while keeping the abdomen in contact with the floor.

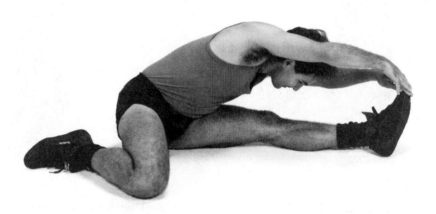

FIGURE 11–6 Hurdler's stretch

Hurdler's stretch, commonly performed in many classes (Fig. 11–6), places a great deal of stress on the medial ligament in the knee of the back leg. When the medial ligament is overstretched, pain and joint instability may occur. A modified, safer exercise can accomplish the same stretching effect: Sit with one leg in front and the opposite knee bent toward the body; lean the upper body forward until the point of tightness, and hold.

Full neck circles may cause excessive movement of the cervical vertebrae and may contribute to degenerative changes in them. This exercise may also cause dizziness in some participants. Specific flexion and side-to-side lateral movements of the low neck accomplish the same purpose as full neck circles, without the risk.

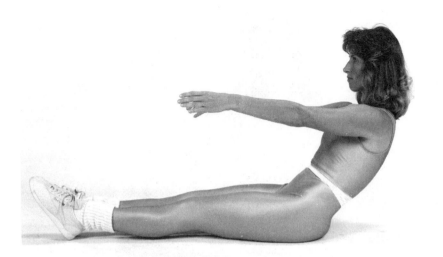

FIGURE 11–7 Straight-leg sit-ups

Straight-leg sit-ups (Fig. 11–7) should not be performed in a dance-exercise class. Sit-ups in this position place great stress on the iliopsoas muscles. Strong to begin with, their overdevelopment may cause low-back pain and the development of an abnormal lumbar curve. To strengthen the abdominals, do curl-ups with the knees bent.

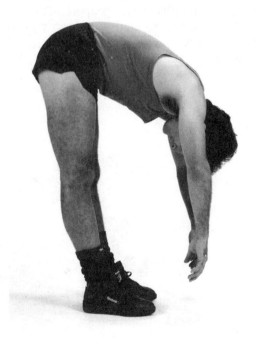

FIGURE 11–8 Forward flexion with hyperextended knees

Forward trunk flexion with hyperextended knees places the body in a potential injury-producing situation (Fig. 11–8). The hamstrings are in an extreme stretch and are pulling the knees into a hyperextended position that places them under extreme stress. The position also compresses the intervertebral discs of the spine. Low-back pain may result as well as posterior knee pain. Rotating the trunk in this position, as in windmill exercises, can be even more dangerous because it creates increased pressure on the discs. The modified hurdler's stretch or the supine hamstring stretch is safer.

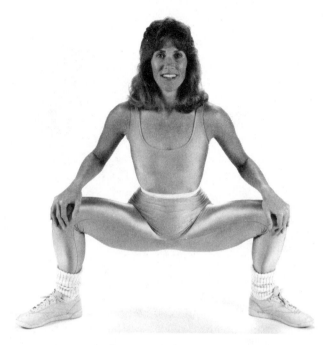

FIGURE 11–9 Grand plié

A *grand plié* may cause excessive stress on the knees and the surrounding musculature if not done correctly (Fig. 11–9). This stress may be felt on the medial side or on the anterior aspect of the knee if weight is not distributed properly. The ligaments may stretch and, over time, gradual degenerative changes may affect the bony surfaces. This exercise may be appropriate for a ballet class, but it should be avoided in a dance-exercise class.

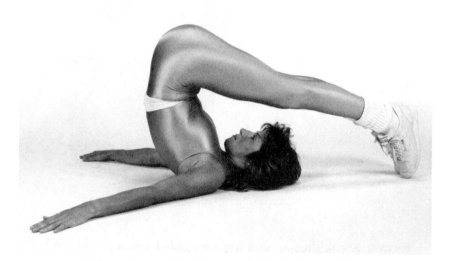

FIGURE 11–10 Plough

The *plough* puts great stress on the cervical and thoracic vertebrae (Fig. 11–10), compressing some of the vertebrae and causing the supporting ligaments of others to stretch. Extending the legs overhead adds the load of the body's weight to these stressed areas. Although some participants may choose to do this yoga exercise on their own, it is not appropriate for a large dance-exercise class.

Quality of Instruction

A good instructor is as important as all the other injury-prevention factors. Proper dance-exercise instruction and proper direct supervision of participants is of primary importance in reducing injury risk. Good instructors must be trained in exercise physiology, anatomy, kinesiology, basic first aid, and injury management. They must have a thorough understanding of all aspects of dance exercise. They determine technique, intensity, and effective injury prevention. Mirrors surrounding the dance floor are an excellent device to help participants and instructors monitor exercise technique and form. (See teaching techniques in Chapter 10.)

To ensure safety, a thorough medical history should be obtained from each participant. It should document previous significant injuries or illnesses, current medical restrictions, and problems encountered with previous exercise. At risk participants should obtain a medical release from their physician before they enter the class. (See Chapter 4.)

Each dance-exercise class should begin with a slow warm-up period emphasizing stretching and muscle flexibility. The aerobics phase should begin gradually, slowly raising the heart rate, and usually continuing for 20 to 30 minutes. For most participants, aerobic benefits are minimal after 30 minutes, and injury risk is greatly increased. Heart rate should be frequently monitored throughout the aerobic activity, and participants should often be reminded to breathe properly. Strength exercises should include biceps, triceps, abdominals, quadriceps, hamstrings, abductors, adductors, and gluteals.

A cool-down is necessary to lower the heart rate and help prevent muscle injury and soreness. A gradual decrease in intensity and a gradual change of body position are necessary during this phase to prevent lightheadedness or faintness. If the class has been exercising on the floor, they should stand up slowly. The instructor should emphasize relaxed, deep, even breathing to return heart rates to normal. (See Chapter 5 for a discussion of warm-up and cool-down.)

GENERAL INJURY GUIDELINES

Even with good aerobics shoes, a resilient floor surface, and proper exercise technique, injuries will happen occasionally in a dance-exercise class. Remember that only a physician can diagnose an injury and prescribe specific treatment. There are, however, general guidelines for managing injuries among participants.

RICE. Swelling, caused by bleeding or inflammation in and around the injured area, is the body's response to injury. If swelling is controlled and minimized, the injured area is less painful and normal movement can be resumed sooner.

Swelling is best controlled by the treatment of rest, ice, compression, and elevation (RICE). Resting may be accomplished by modifying an activity (for example, switch from weight-bearing to non-weight-bearing activities after an injury to feet or legs) until symptoms subside. Ice, compression, and elevation (ICE) should be applied for 20–30 minutes at a time, as often as possible during the first 48–72 hours after injury. If the injury is chronic, ICE should be applied after every activity session or whenever swelling occurs.

ACUTE INJURIES. When a participant has an acute (new) injury such as an ankle sprain, the instructor can recommend RICE and advise the person to see a physician immediately. Before returning to class, the participant should provide a written physician's clearance for resuming exercise activity.

CHRONIC INJURIES. A participant who has a chronic problem, with a gradual onset of symptoms, should be advised to use the RICE treatment and avoid any activity that causes pain in the affected area. If specific symptoms persist for 3–5 days or suddenly get worse, the participant should see a physician immediately. If a participant asks for the name of a physician specializing in sports injuries, the instructor should always provide two or three names, not just one. Participants should make their own choices.

WARNING SIGNS. If any of the following signs and symptoms persists for more than 3–5 days, the participant should not be allowed to continue full participation in the class without seeing a physician and obtaining a medical clearance.

1. *Specific point-tender pain on or around a bony area.* If an area of pain one or two fingers wide is located directly on or close to a bone, suspect a fracture. This principle applies to all areas of the body. The participant should have the area X-rayed as soon as possible.

2. *Radiating pain.* Any time pain moves (travels or radiates) up or down a body part, a nerve or nerves are probably involved. The pain may feel like tingling or like pins and needles. This sensation may occur any time the affected body part is used, or just during physical activity. The pain usually does not remain constant but comes and goes.

3. *Neurological signs.* Muscle weakness in a specific muscle or muscle group may indicate neurological impairment. The person will feel that one area is considerably weaker than the corresponding part. Also, any sign of disorientation, dizziness, fainting, blurred vision, or nausea may indicate a neurological problem.

4. *Swelling.* Swelling in any area, in any amount, indicates that a particular body location is being overstressed. Swelling may occur after an acute (new, fresh) injury or with a chronic injury. The amount of swelling may vary among people with the same problem. The fact that swelling is present, not the amount, is most important.

5. *Discoloration.* Common "black-and-blue" areas may be simply the result of incidental impact. If, however, there is an extremely noticeable area of discoloration associated with an acute or chronic injury, a physician should be consulted. This condition means that a considerable amount of bleeding into surrounding tissues has occurred.

6. *Movement impairment.* Any time normal movement is impaired, limiting the range of motion, the affected body part should be rested. Pain or discomfort that causes limitation of movement indicates that some problem is present. Never let anyone participate whose movement is impaired in any way, such as by limping.

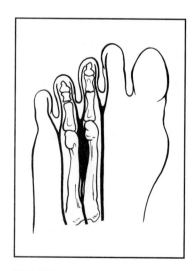

FIGURE 11–11 Neuroma

Remember, if any of these symptoms persists for more than 3–5 days, or suddenly gets worse, the participant should see a physician as soon as possible.

COMMON DANCE-EXERCISE INJURIES

Most injuries in a dance-exercise class occur to the foot, ankle, shin, low back, and knee. The following is a description of the problems an instructor will be most likely to see in class, followed by general guidelines for prevention and treatment.

Neuroma (Interdigital, Morton's)

Interdigital nerves travel between the metatarsal bones in the foot and enable the toes to function normally. A **neuroma** is an entrapment of part of an interdigital nerve that usually occurs between the third and fourth toes (Fig. 11–11), where the branches of the nerve cross in an "X" pattern. The entrapped nerve causes swelling that results in sharp, radiating pain traveling to the ends of the involved toes. The area directly over the affected nerve will be sore during weight-bearing, running, and jumping activities, and when activity is performed on the ball of the foot.

PREVENTION.   To prevent a neuroma, shoes for daily wear and exercise must be the proper width to prevent compression of the metatarsal arch and interdigital nerves. Wearing narrow dress shoes over time may cause a neuroma. Shoes worn during exercise must be well padded in the metatarsal area. Exercises should not be performed on the ball of the foot or on unyielding surfaces.

TREATMENT.   ICE should be applied for 20–30 minutes after any weight-bearing activity. It might be helpful to place a pad on the bottom of the foot, slightly behind the area of tenderness. Even with proper rest, modification of activity, and treatment, this problem often does not improve. In some cases, a podiatrist or orthopedic surgeon may recommend surgery.

Metatarsalgia

Metatarsalgia is a general term describing pain in the ball of the foot. Pain is usually felt under the second and third metatarsal heads (Fig. 11–12), caused by bruising the joints in these areas. Metatarsalgia differs from a neuroma in that the pain is more general in the area of the metatarsal heads and usually no sharp pain radiates to the end of the toes. Metatarsalgia occurs gradually and is aggravated by extreme repeated force or impact on the ball of the foot, such as in running or jumping. At first, specific pain may be felt only during activity. As this problem progresses, pain may be felt during normal weight-bearing and even non-weight-bearing activities.

PREVENTION.   Wear shoes that are well padded in the metatarsal area. Exercise on resilient surfaces and avoid repetitive impact activities, especially on the ball of the foot.

TREATMENT.   A pad placed directly behind the affected metatarsal heads may relieve some pressure to the area. ICE should be applied to the metatarsal area for 20–30 minutes after exercise. If pain continues even when not exercising, stop all running and jumping activities.

Plantar Fasciitis

The plantar fascia is a broad band of connective tissue found on the bottom of the foot, running the length of the sole of the foot (Fig. 11–13). **Plantar fasciitis** is an inflammation of this band of tissue caused by stretching or tearing, usually near the attachment at the heel.

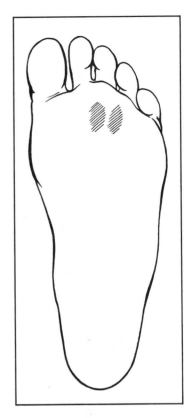

FIGURE 11–12 Metatarsalgia

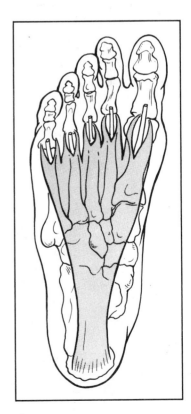

FIGURE 11–13 Plantar fascia

The plantar fascia is put under a great deal of stress during weight bearing. When weight is shifted to the ball of the foot and a push-off motion is performed, as in running or jumping, that stress greatly increases. Pain is felt in a specific area on the bottom of the foot, back toward the heel. This pain may radiate toward the ball of the foot. There is less pain during non-weight-bearing activity. Typically, the foot feels very tender the first thing in the morning and becomes gradually less painful with movement.

Repeated irritation of the plantar fascia is likely to cause the formation of a sharp, bony growth (bone spur). People with a mild high arch are more likely to experience this problem.

PREVENTION.   Shoes must have adequate arch supports to prevent this problem. The shoe and arch support should be flexible to avoid additional stress to this area. High-intensity running or jumping on unyielding surfaces should be limited. Stretching the calf and Achilles tendon daily will also help to prevent this problem.

TREATMENT.   When symptoms begin to occur, add an arch support to both activity shoes and dress shoes. Apply ICE in the arch area for 20–30 minutes after activity and whenever pain is present. Any shoe that causes pain in the arch should be avoided.

If symptoms do not improve or become worse, rest the arch until there is no pain during normal activities. Limit weight-bearing activities and substitute non-weight-bearing activities such as swimming or cycling. Persistent pain should be examined by a physician or sports podiatrist.

Stress Fractures

Stress fractures occur in major weight-bearing locations of the body, especially the foot (metatarsal bones) and lower leg (tibia). A **stress fracture** is an impending fracture due to excessive stress (overuse) of a bone. This repeated stress causes the bone to begin to break down.

Stress fractures occur gradually. There is usually a specific area of pain directly over the affected bone. Sometimes the pain will be sharp and radiating. The affected area is always tender to the touch. The pain is progressive and will gradually become more intense as weight-bearing activities continue. Pain will be most severe during running and jumping activities. Pain may also remain after exercise, during standing or walking.

Stress fractures are often difficult to diagnose accurately because they initially do not appear on X-ray. It may be necessary to obtain a bone scan to identify a stress fracture. Pain may persist in varying degrees for 4–12 weeks. If this problem is ignored, complete fractures may occur.

PREVENTION.   Avoid repetitive activities on unyielding surfaces, wear proper shoes, and increase exercise intensity gradually. If a previous injury has required rest, return to normal activity slowly and gradually.

TREATMENT.   If a stress fracture is suspected, repetitive jumping and excessive running should be avoided because they will cause increased pain. Shock-absorbing arch supports may be added to relieve stress. A doughnut-type pad placed on the area may prevent direct pressure on the point of extreme tenderness. ICE should be applied for 20–30 minutes after activity or any time pain is present. Non-weight-bearing activities may be substituted if weight-bearing activities are too painful. This type of fracture will heal gradually, and when all symptoms have disappeared, full weight-bearing activities can gradually be resumed.

Achilles Tendinitis

The Achilles tendon is a narrow tendinous extension of the calf musculature that attaches to the heel (calcaneus) (Fig. 11–14). Repeated, forceful stretching will create small tears in the fibers of the tendon, causing it to become inflamed and resulting in **Achilles tendinitis.** This chronic overuse problem has a gradual onset and is often caused by jumping and running without proper warm-up stretches. The tendon will be sore to the touch directly over the affected area and there will be pain and stiffness when the foot is dorsiflexed (toes moved toward the shin), which moves the tendon. Symptoms will get progressively worse if the problem is ignored.

PREVENTION. Changing from regular dress shoes, especially high heels, to flat aerobics shoes places a great deal of stress on the tendon. Therefore, *thorough, daily stretching* of the calf muscles (gastrocnemius/ soleus) and Achilles tendon is necessary and will help prevent this problem. Mild stretching after exercise may also help prevent muscle and tendon soreness.

TREATMENT. As soon as any symptoms are experienced, begin applying ICE to the affected area for 20–30 minutes after activity. Also, increase the amount of mild stretching to the calf area. If symptoms progress, limit activity. Do not perform any exercises that cause pain in the tendon area. Rest usually will greatly improve this condition.

Shin Splints

Shin splints is a general term applied to any pain or discomfort that occurs on the front or side of the lower leg, in the region of the shin bone (tibia) (Fig. 11–15). Shin splints may have various causes, including faulty posture, poor shoes, fallen arches, insufficient warm-up, muscle fatigue, poor running mechanics such as extensive pronation, training too fast or too soon, and exercising on unyielding surfaces. Many people consider shin splints one of the most common and disabling conditions in dance exercise.

Shin splints are characterized by pain in the shin on one or both legs. There may be a specific area of tenderness or swelling directly over the affected bone. This symptom is also common with a stress fracture. Pain and aching will be felt in the front of the leg after activity and sometimes during activity, as the condition gets worse. If shin splints are ignored and the participant attempts to "run through" them, a stress fracture will almost always occur that will present additional pain and disability and limit activity for several months.

PREVENTION. To prevent shin splints, increase activity gradually, wear shoes with good shock-absorbing features and avoid repetitive weight-bearing activities on unyielding surfaces. When running or jumping, land flat-footed or toe-heel, respectively, to minimize impact. Stretch

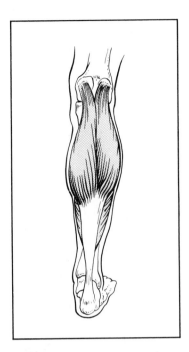

FIGURE 11–14 Achilles tendon

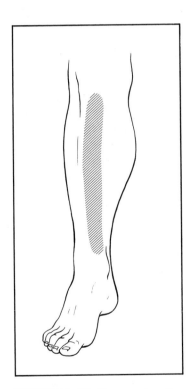

FIGURE 11–15 Common location of shin splints

the calf muscles and strengthen the anterior tibial (front shin) muscles daily and before each class.

TREATMENT. Apply ICE to the shin area for 20–30 minutes after activity. If pain persists, activity should be limited. Any time bruising, swelling, or specific point tenderness occurs in the affected area, all activity should be stopped. Any non-weight-bearing activities that do not cause pain to the shin area can be continued. Shin splints usually respond well to rest. When symptoms have subsided, activity may be resumed gradually.

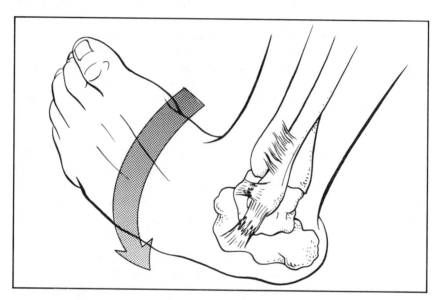

FIGURE 11–16 .Inversion ankle sprain

Ankle Sprains

A **sprain** is an injury to a ligament, which is a band of fibers connecting one bone to another bone. In the ankle, sprains usually occur on the outside of the joint, most often involving the lateral ligaments. These injuries are caused by an extreme inward (inversion) movement of the ankle, forcing it beyond its normal range of motion (Fig. 11–16). Sprains are acute injuries classified by degree of severity. A mild sprain (first degree) involves minimal stretching of ligament fibers. A moderate sprain (second degree) involves tearing of some ligament fibers, with the ligament still intact. In severe sprain (third degree), the ligament is torn completely in two or more pieces. Most ankle sprains in aerobic dance-exercise are mild or moderate.

When a sprain occurs, pain will be felt directly over the injured ligament. Swelling will occur around the injured ligament and spread throughout the joint. There may be some discoloration in the ankle and foot. Normal motion will be limited by swelling in the joint.

PREVENTION. Avoid slick dance surfaces or heavily padded surfaces where the foot sinks into the padding, causing the participant to trip. Match the shoe to the floor surface: Use a shoe with good outsole traction for smooth surfaces, and one with less traction for carpeted surfaces. If mats are used for the aerobics segment, make sure they are large enough that participants won't fall off the edge.

TREATMENT. Use RICE immediately and continue for 48–72 hours after the injury. ICE should be applied for 20–30 minutes, 3 to 4 times each day. Weight bearing should be limited. The injured person should see an orthopedic surgeon for X-rays to rule out a fracture and to receive an accurate diagnosis.

Meniscus (Cartilage) Tears

A meniscus is a gristly substance that lines the top surface of the tibia. It cushions the area where the upper leg bone (femur) rests on the tibia. There are two menisci in each knee: medial and lateral (Fig. 11–17). Tears can occur in either, although the medial meniscus seems to be injured more frequently.

Meniscus tears are commonly caused by sharp, twisting movements of the knee, forceful flexion (bending) and extension (straightening) of the knee (as in a forced squat), or a sharp hyperextension of the knee. Unstable foot plant or improper exercise technique may cause this injury.

When a meniscus is torn there is a specific incident of injury. Pain may be felt "inside" the knee. It is difficult to flex and extend the knee, which may lock or catch. It may feel as though it will give way. Movement requiring quick change of direction and squatting (deep knee-bend position) will be difficult if a meniscus is torn. There may be swelling around and behind the knee. Because the menisci have a very poor blood supply, they usually do not heal.

PREVENTION.   To prevent meniscus tears, emphasize proper body control in exercises that require balance. All change-of-direction movements must be performed in a controlled manner. Avoid squats, hurdler stretches, and other movements that bend and twist the knees. Make certain the muscles of the thigh (quadriceps and hamstrings) are well conditioned. These muscles help support the knee during various dance-exercise activities.

TREATMENT.   If a meniscus tear is suspected, limit any painful, weight-bearing exercises. Apply ICE for 20–30 minutes after activity and whenever the knee hurts. See an orthopedic surgeon to obtain a specific diagnosis and the proper treatment prescription. In some cases activity may be resumed after injury, and in others surgery may be necessary.

Chondromalacia

Chondromalacia is a gradual degenerative process in which the articular cartilage that lines the back surface of the patella, or kneecap, (Fig. 11–18) becomes softer and rougher. Although the exact cause of this problem is unknown, it may result from poor running or jumping mechanics, an abnormal position of the patella, foot pronation, excessive flexing and extending of the knee with heavy resistance (weight training), or excessive running and jumping on unyielding surfaces.

Chondromalacia may occur more frequently in girls and women because of the wider female pelvis that creates a wider angle as the femur meets the tibia at the knee. This increased angle may place the kneecap in a more outward or lateral position and cause excessive rubbing of the undersurface of the patella.

Chondromalacia produces general pain around the patella. A grating, grinding sound or sensation may be heard and felt as the affected knee is flexed and extended. Walking up and down stairs will hurt.

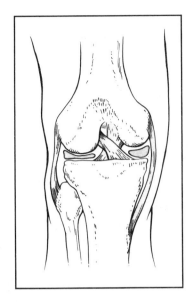

FIGURE 11–17 Medial and lateral menisci

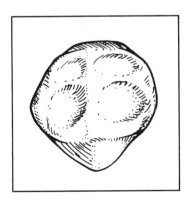

FIGURE 11–18 Undersurface of patella

Swelling may or may not be present. This condition begins gradually and progressively worsens when stressful activities are continued.

PREVENTION. To prevent chondromalacia, avoid high-resistance, lower-extremity weight training and excessive repetitive weight bearing on unyielding surfaces. Become conditioned gradually and wear shoes with good shock absorption and arch support during all weight-bearing activities.

TREATMENT. As symptoms of chondromalacia begin to appear, apply ICE for 20–30 minutes after any activity. Limit weight-bearing activities and extreme flexion and extension movements of the knee. Single straight-leg raises are recommended to maintain strength in the quadriceps (anterior thigh) without further irritating knees. Chondromalacia responds very well to rest, so decrease activity. When symptoms have subsided, resume weight-bearing exercise gradually.

Bursitis

Bursa are padlike, fluid-filled sacs located throughout the body where friction might occur, as where muscle tendons cross over bones. Bursa reduce that friction. Overuse of muscles and tendons at these friction sites, or constant pressure directly on the bursa, can irritate a bursa sac, causing **bursitis**. Bursitis can occur anywhere in the body, but it most often occurs where overuse or pressure is greatest. In aerobic dance-exercise the knees, hip, shoulder, and elbow are the most commonly affected areas. Pain and stiffness begin gradually in the area of the affected bursa. There is usually no visible swelling at first, but swelling occurs as the condition worsens.

PREVENTION. To prevent bursitis, *gradually* add any external resistance (such as hand or arm weights) when performing upper-body movements, and use proper technique with all exercise movements.

TREATMENT. Apply ICE after any activity. Try to determine what has caused the additional stress on the particular body part, and remove or reduce that stress. When normal movement is reduced and visible swelling is present, activity involving the affected area should be stopped. Bursitis responds very well to rest. Once symptoms have subsided, activity may be resumed gradually.

Low-Back Pain

The low back is composed of five lumbar vertebrae and their attaching ligaments, which provide the major support to this part of the spinal column. Extensive musculature surrounds this area to provide additional support. The low back is a site of frequent problems caused by congenital abnormalities, poor posture, postural deviations, and poor body mechanics (incorrect lifting and sitting postures). Lack of trunk flexibility and weak abdominal muscles also contribute to low-back pain.

Congenital low-back abnormalities may become apparent when abnormal stresses, such as sudden twisting, are applied to the back.

The abnormalities produce mechanical weaknesses that may make the low back vulnerable to injury during physical activity.

Faulty posture or faulty body mechanics put a tremendous strain on the muscles and ligaments of the low back. Lifting heavy objects incorrectly—using the back instead of the legs—is an example of the poor body mechanics that must be corrected to maintain a healthy back.

A sprain or strain to the low back is an acute problem with a specific incident of injury. Sudden violent twisting, extension, or hyperextension movements may injure the ligaments and muscles of the back.

Someone who once experiences an injury to the low back will usually have chronic low-back pain. The vertebrae may be misaligned or they may move in abnormal directions, putting pressure on the nerves and creating muscular weaknesses and radiating pain. These problems occur more often and become more severe with age. The numerous small injuries and postural mechanical deviations create a progressive degeneration over time and extreme low-back pain may occur, aggravated by any sudden movement. Jumping and running jar and compress the vertebrae of the back, and low-back pain may be experienced after these physical activities.

Regardless of the cause or exact structure involved, low-back pain is extremely disabling. The muscles surrounding the affected area go into spasm to protect the back, and the person experiences severe stiffness and immobility. If pain and discomfort persist, it is important to have the back thoroughly evaluated by a physician. Fractures, dislocations, or degenerative disease may be present in the vertebrae requiring that physical activity be restricted or modified.

PREVENTION. To prevent back problems, keep all of the muscles of the trunk strong. Primary movements of the back are flexion and extension, as well as lateral side-to-side movement and rotation. The musculature surrounding the back supports and protects it. The abdominal muscles and the psoas muscles flex the lumbar spine. Abdominal strength aids in maintaining proper vertebral alignment and proper postural alignment and in supporting the low back. The psoas muscles are already extremely strong, and overdevelopment could produce an abnormal lumbar curve. Instead, these muscles should be stretched to increase their flexibility. Hamstring flexibility is also extremely important to prevent postural deviations and abnormal stresses on the low back. Trunk flexibility should be emphasized to produce maximum range of motion in the back.

TREATMENT. If low-back pain is extremely severe and disabling, stretching exercises can help relieve muscle spasm. Lying down produces the least strain on the back. To relieve spasm, lie on the back, and slowly and alternately bring the knees to the chest. The pelvic tilt (Fig. 11–19) can also be helpful. Lie on the back with knees bent. Press low back to floor. Raise the hips straight up and hold for 3–5 seconds.

When acute symptoms have subsided, flexibility and strengthening exercises may be added. These may include the following:

AEROBIC DANCE-EXERCISE INSTRUCTOR MANUAL

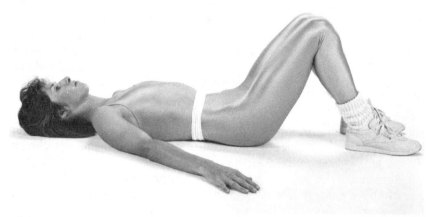

FIGURE 11–19 Pelvic tilt

a. Lie on back with knees bent.

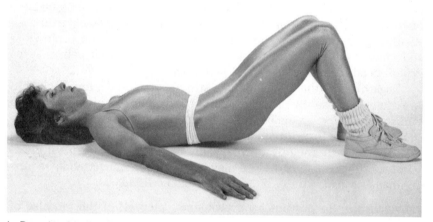

b. Press low back to floor and raise
hips straight up.

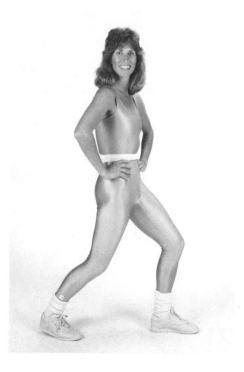

FIGURE 11–20 Hip flexor stretch

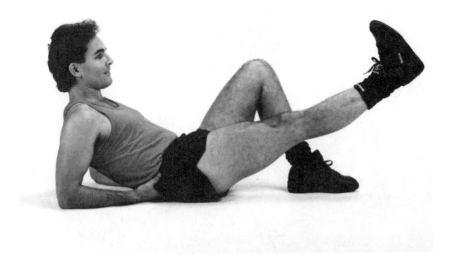

FIGURE 11–21 Single leg raise

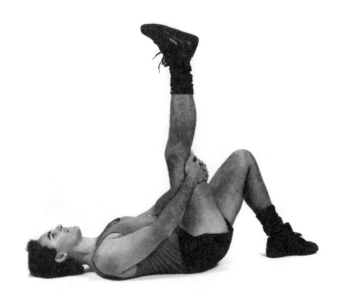

FIGURE 11–22 Hamstring stretch

1. *Hip flexor stretch (Fig. 11–20)*. Stand with one leg extended, knee bent, the other leg behind. Shift body weight downward toward extended leg.

2. *Single leg raise (Fig. 11–21)*. To strengthen the hip flexors and quadriceps, lie on the back, one knee straight and one knee bent toward the chest. Raise the straight leg as far as possible. Return slowly. Change legs after 10 repetitions. This exercise can be performed with or without weights.

Never do double leg raises lying on the back. This position puts the psoas muscles in extreme tension and causes abnormal pressure on the lumbar spine area. It may even create an abnormal lumbar curve. The low back must always be kept flat during all exercises performed while lying on the back.

3. *Hamstring stretch (Fig. 11–22)*. On the back, grasp one thigh and pull it gently toward the chest (the opposite leg is bent). Alternate legs.

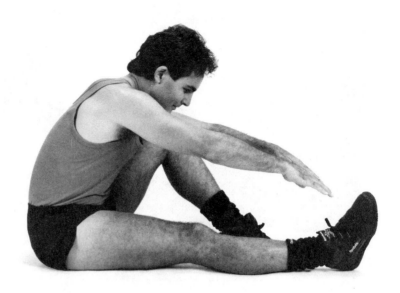

FIGURE 11–23 Alternate hamstring stretch

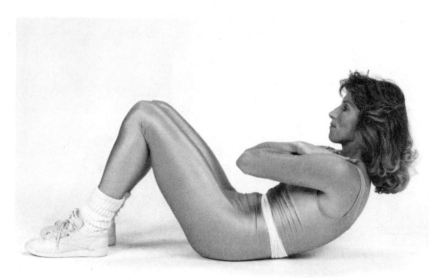

FIGURE 11–24 Abdominal curl

4. *Alternate hamstring stretch (Fig. 11–23).* Sit on the floor with one leg bent, knee toward the chest, the other leg straight. Lean forward, trying to touch your legs. All stretching must be *gradual (static), not bouncy (ballistic).* The stretch should always be felt in the belly of the muscle and not in the muscle-tendon unit. Make certain that the stretch is felt in the hamstring muscle(s) and not in the lower back.

5. *Abdominal curls (modified sit-ups) (Fig. 11–24).* On the back with knees bent, feet flat on floor, hands across chest, and elbows out straight, raise the shoulders off the floor toward your knees. Repeat. It is not necessary to raise the chest and upper trunk completely to a sitting position during an abdominal curl. These final degrees of movement are wasted effort because they do not cause further contraction of the abdominal muscles. When the hands are placed behind the head during an abdominal curl, be careful not to pull the neck and create stress on the cervical vertebrae.

Never perform an exercise that creates any pain in the low-back area. Be especially cautious during leg lifts and abdominal curls. Avoid fast, extreme twisting movements that strain the back. Practice good posture, good exercise technique, and proper body mechanics.

SUMMARY

Preventing injury and providing a safe exercise environment are the keys to the future of dance exercise.

Most aerobic-dance injuries are caused by overuse, too much stress placed on one part of the body over an extended time. The areas most frequently injured are the foot, ankle, lower leg, knee, and low back.

A chronic injury, such as shin splints, occurs gradually with no specific incident of injury. If not treated properly, a chronic injury may become acute. For example, if repeatedly stressed, a shin splint may become a stress fracture. An acute injury, such as a sprained ankle, has a more sudden onset and usually is characterized by a specific injury incident.

The best way to prevent injury is to dance on a floor surface that is both stable and resilient, wear good aerobics shoes, follow proper exercise technique (including a warm-up and cool-down), and avoid exercises with a high rate of injury.

When injuries do occur among participants, the instructor must know how to manage them properly. It is not the instructor's role to diagnose or treat injuries. Instead, the instructor should always refer the participant to a physician. The instructor may suggest that rest, ice, compression, and elevation (RICE) are helpful for many common injuries and explain how to apply the procedures. If certain warning signs (including pain, swelling, weakness in a specific muscle or muscle group, extreme discoloration, or impaired movement) persist for more than 3–5 days, the instructor should require the participant to obtain medical clearance before returning to class.

REFERENCES

Mosher, C. "Rhythm and Moves." *Women's Sports and Fitness* (December 1984): 24–27.

Richie, D. H., S. F. Kelso, and P. A. Bellucci. "Aerobic Dance Injuries: A Retrospective Study of Instructors and Participants." *The Physician and Sportsmedicine* (February 1985): 134–35.

SUGGESTED READING

Albohm, M. J. *Health Care and the Female Athlete.* North Palm Beach, Fla.: Athletic Institute, 1981.

Arnheim, D. *Modern Principles of Athletic Training.* 6th ed. St. Louis, Mo.: Times Mirror/Mosby, 1985.

Ritter, M. A., and M. J. Albohm. *Your Injury: A Common Sense Guide to the Management of Sports Injury.* Indianapolis, Ind.: Benchmark Press, 1987.

Voice Injury

Mary Anne MacLellan, Denise Grapes, and Debora Elster

12

Licensed speech pathologists Mary Anne MacLellan, M.A., C.C.C., Denise Grapes, M.A., C.C.C., and Debora Elster, M.S., C.C.C., are the founders of Voices in Motion, a program designed to train dance-exercise instructors in the proper use of the voice and in the prevention of voice injuries. Ms. MacLellan and Ms. Elster have practices in San Diego; Ms. Grapes practices in Los Angeles.

IN THIS CHAPTER:

- Symptoms of voice injury.
- Causes of voice injury.

- Techniques for preventing voice injury.

Proper care of the vocal mechanism is a crucial area of injury prevention for dance-exercise instructors because the voice is the primary tool of instruction and a key element in teaching effectiveness. Yet clinical experience and research show that as a group, instructors, although representing a high-risk population for vocal injury, are not fully aware of the problem.

Several studies document the low incidence of voice problems in the general population. Laguaite (1972) found that only 7% of 428 adults undergoing a voice screening had sufficient deviant voice quality to warrant a laryngeal examination. In speech samples taken from 112 adults at random, Brindle and Morris (1979) found only 2% had clearly abnormal voice quality.

Clinical observation has identified certain populations as high risk for abnormal voice quality and vocal cord pathology. These high-risk groups include rock singers, clergy, teachers, high school cleerleaders, and politicians. For example, Gillespie and Cooper (1973) found that the incidence of vocal cord pathology was less than half of one percent among high school girls who use their voices for normal purposes. Yet, several studies of high school cheerleaders have found chronic deviations in voice quality ranging from 37%–44%—a significantly higher percentage—of those tested.

Growing evidence indicates that the problem is even greater among dance-exercise instructors. MacLellan, Grapes, and Elster are conducting a study of 1,000 aerobics instructors to determine the inci-

291

dence of symptoms of voice injury. Preliminary findings show that 88% of the instructors interviewed report they have experienced some symptom indicative of voice injury; however, only 51% identified these symptoms as voice related. Obviously a discrepancy exists between the symptoms that the instructors are experiencing and their awareness of the symptoms of voice injury. Ignoring early warning symptoms of voice injury may lead to the development of injuries requiring long periods of rest and therapy or surgery.

SYMPTOMS OF VOICE INJURY

Vocal injuries are less readily identified than obvious physical injuries such as torn ligaments. Too often, symptoms and changes in the voice are so gradual that the dance-exercise instructor is not even aware that damage has occurred. Early symptoms can include a dry mouth and throat, frequent need to clear the throat, hoarseness, vocal fatigue, neck pain, pitch breaks, habital use of a lower pitch, and possibly a temporary voice loss. Due to the demands of different exercise programs, different work environments, and individual vocal habits, the causes of these symptoms vary from person to person.

DRY THROAT AND MOUTH.   Frequently a dry throat is caused by mouth breathing, a technique used by instructors to increase lung capacity. While nasal breathing helps to warm, filter, and moisten inhaled air, mouth breathing tends to dry out the entire vocal mechanism, especially the vocal cords. Cool, dry air from air-conditioning systems in most gyms and health clubs compounds the drying effects. This dryness causes an abrasive contact when the vocal cords close and impairs their ability to function effectively.

FREQUENT NEED TO CLEAR THE THROAT.   Needing to clear the throat more than 2–3 times per hour is excessive and abusive. This condition is caused by an irritation on the vocal cords such as increased mucus or a growth. When an upper respiratory infection or sinus drainage results in increased mucus, the phlegm can be removed by clearing the throat. However, when irritation results from swollen cords or a growth on the cords, increased mucus is produced as a protective measure to soothe and cushion the vocal cords. Persistent throat clearing cannot eliminate this irritation and actually causes further irritation, which stimulates more mucus production and further increases the need to clear the throat. The cycle perpetuates itself until only a cough is successful in eliminating the sensation that something is on the vocal cords. Clearing the throat and coughing involve a sudden, explosive closing of the cords, which is abusive to the entire vocal mechanism.

CRACKING VOICE.   Insufficient control of the vocal cords, causing them to open suddenly, results in a cracking or momentary loss of voice. Insufficient control is evident when an instructor abruptly tries to reach a pitch beyond his or her upper range. Using forced, irregular puffs to increase loudness instead of a smooth flow of air also results in unexpected loss of control with cracking and voice breaks.

VOCAL FATIGUE.   Also known as a "tired" voice, vocal fatigue is caused by unnecessary or excessive effort directed toward the production of speech. Vocal fatigue can also become a self-perpetuating cycle. Excessive effort strains the vocal muscles, which changes voice quality. To compensate for this change, the instructor exerts more effort. By the end of the week, his or her voice sounds hoarse, weak, and strained. After a weekend of rest, the voice may sound louder and clearer; the instructor is tempted to use it in the same manner, and the cycle repeats. Neck pain, often developing with vocal fatigue, is the most obvious symptom of hyperfunctional voice use. This pain is the body's way of drawing attention to the incorrect use of these muscles.

LOWERED PITCH.   Swelling or growths on the vocal cords increase their mass and weight. Consequently, the cords vibrate at a slower rate, which lowers the pitch. Most instructors may not be aware of the lowered pitch of their voice, until someone comments on the sexiness of their voice or asks if they have a cold.

A common myth in dance-exercise is that using a lower pitch projects the voice and makes it sound louder. Actually, lowering the pitch of the voice and maintaining it during class keeps the muscles in the larynx in a constant state of contraction that will lead to vocal fatigue.

HOARSENESS.   A hoarse voice is low pitched, with a breathy, gravellike quality that interferes with production of a continuous tone. Swelling or growths on the vocal cords prevent them from closing completely, thus allowing air to escape. Hoarseness limits natural projection and interferes with the overall intelligibility of speech.

Hoarseness is often confused with laryngitis, but the two are not necessarily the same. **Laryngitis** is usually a medical condition characterized by swelling of the vocal cords as a result of a cold, respiratory infection, or sinusitis. Hoarseness is a symptom of laryngitis, and voice quality returns to normal when the infection is resolved, usually in less than 2 weeks. Hoarseness that occurs without an infection is caused by continual vocal abuse or hyperfunction, resulting in swelling of the cords and the possible development of other pathologies.

The body sends out these early warning symptoms because something is wrong. If the symptoms are ignored and the muscles of the vocal mechanism continue to be used improperly, an instructor may develop vocal nodules, contact ulcers, polyps, or permanent irreparable damage to the vocal cords.

CAUSES OF VOICE INJURY

To understand the causes of voice injury, a basic knowledge of the anatomy of the vocal mechanism is necessary. Every breath we take passes through the larynx, a tube-shaped structure situated vertically in the neck between the back of the tongue and the trachea, or windpipe (Fig. 12–1). The larynx, which is made of cartilage, muscle, and connective tissues, houses the vocal cords and, thus, is sometimes called the voice box.

The **vocal cords** resemble a set of rubber sliding doors that lie horizontally across the top of the trachea at the level of the Adam's apple (Fig. 12–2). The vocal cords are a set of paired muscles about the size of a quarter, bordered by ligaments and covered with mucous membrane. They produce sound when set into vibration by the force of air exhaled from the lungs; the cords open and close hundreds of times per second.

Most voice injuries stem from a combination of factors, including the improper use of the voice, interference of muscular tension with vocalization, attempts at projection over loud music, and a poor work environment.

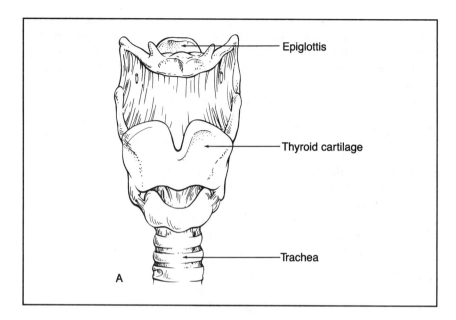

FIGURE 12–1 The larynx

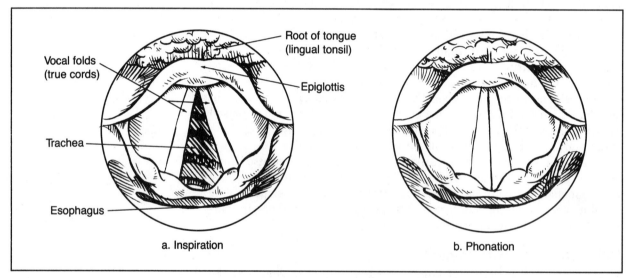

FIGURE 12–2 Normal vocal cords

The causes of injury can be divided into two categories: vocal abuse and hyperfunction. **Vocal abuse** is mistreatment of the vocal mechanism. For the dance-exercise instructor, abuses include talking continuously during a routine, scheduling 2–3 classes in a row, unnecessary vocalizing (i.e., singing with the music or making comments about the lyrics), excessive throat clearing, changing pitch (highness or lowness) and loudness abruptly, and shouting to be heard because the music is too loud or because the room has poor acoustics.

Hyperfunction is the use of excessive muscular contraction and force of movement when breathing, phonating (using the voice), or resonating (producing a sound that carries). Simply stated, it is the overuse of a particular body part, in this case, the vocal mechanism.

Many instructors demonstrate hyperfunctional breathing during the aerobics portion of a class: Because they do not have enough air to talk and exercise simultaneously, they try to speak with inadequate inhalation and exhalation. During vigorous exercise, instructors also

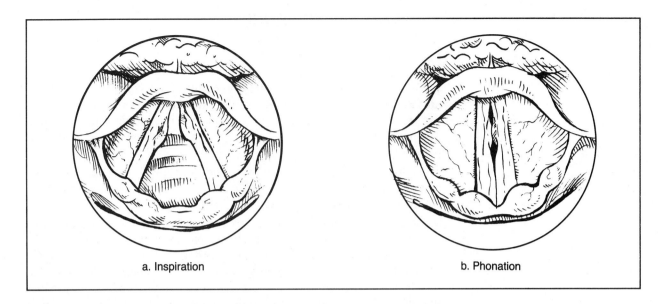

a. Inspiration   b. Phonation

tend to hold the abdominal muscles tight, which promotes clavicular or high chest breathing. Chest breathing prevents the vocal cords from functioning normally because tension is placed in the neck and in the muscles around the larynx. Chest breathing also restricts the intake of breath needed for producing the voice and makes controlling exhalation difficult.

Hyperfunctional phonation is the result of muscular tension combined with voicing. The contraction of one muscle group affects muscles throughout the body. For example, when the abdominal muscles are contracted for curl-ups or crunches, they have a tensing effect on the laryngeal muscles as well. Tension restricts the sound of the voice and the free flow of the exhaled breath stream, squeezing the sound out rather than letting it flow out effortlessly. Breath is the power source for the voice, and it cannot be used for voice production or control when it is restricted by abdominal muscle contraction during an exercise.

Other exercise positions make phonation difficult and at times dangerous to the vocal cords. During push-ups and exercises that produce upper body tension, the vocal cords close to add strength and leverage. Voicing at the same time causes the vocal cords to blow apart and slam back together. Voice quality sounds strained and the instructor tends to bark like a drill sergeant. This abrupt and forceful initiation of voice can be extremely damaging to the vocal cords.

Hyperfunctional resonance can also present problems for the dance-exercise instructor. Although looking happy while teaching is important, maintaining a permanent "Pepsodent smile" restricts jaw movement and forces the sound of the voice back down the throat. A voice that carries well requires relaxed facial muscles and a jaw that is free to move so the voice can get out.

Over time, persistent vocal abuse and hyperfunction will lead to voice injury. The most prevalent injury in the dance-exercise industry is **vocal nodules** (Fig. 12–3), benign growths that begin as tiny hemorrhages on the edges of the vocal cords. As abuse continues, fibrous tissue replaces the hemorrhage and the lesions turn white and calloused. The size of a nodule can vary from a pinhead (minimal change in voice quality) to a split pea (severe, chronic hoarseness).

FIGURE 12–3 Vocal nodules

PREVENTING VOICE INJURY

An instructor can use many techniques to prevent vocal abuse and hyperfunction.

1. *Good vocal hygiene begins with vocal warm-ups.* Just like any other muscle, the vocal mechanism can be strained or stretched beyond its limits. Warm-up exercises prepare the voice musculature for vigorous use. These exercises are best learned under the supervision of a speech pathologist.

2. *Keep cues short and meaningful and eliminate unnecessary vocalization.* Try incorporating gestures and hand signals as a substitute for counting and directional cues.

3. *Select music that does not compete with exercise cues.* Music without lyrics reduces an instructor's need to compete with the vocalist. Female instructors may find less competition with songs featuring male vocalists, and vice versa. Turning down the treble control knob on the stereo will also help deemphasize the voice on most recordings. Most important, instructors should keep the music at a decibel level that does not require them to shout to be heard.

4. *Keep the vocal mechanism lubricated.* Take small sips of water between sets of exercises. Using steam before and after class can also be helpful. A steam room or facial steamer is the best method, but the same results can be achieved by running hot water in a bathroom sink, placing a towel over the head, and inhaling the steam.

5. *Time vocalizations properly during exercise.* The best positions for voicing are standing and sitting erect or lying down on the back or side; keep the spine straight and the upper body free of neck flexion or tension. In positions that inhibit abdominal breathing (curl-ups) or constrict the vocal tract (push-ups), give cues before or immediately after the exertion of the exercise. Or, give instructions beforehand and demonstrate the exercise without verbal cues.

6. *Learn a technique called "easy onset of voice" to compensate for the tension created by certain exercises.* Mentally place an /h/ sound in front of words that begin with a vowel (up, over, extend, again). This technique softens the initiation of voice. Because the technique requires practice to be completely effective, write down the most frequent cues in a routine and add the /h/ sound lightly until it feels natural.

7. *Select a sound system carefully.* The system should have separate adjustments for the music volume and the microphone. Otherwise, each time the volume on the microphone is turned up, the volume of the music will increase as well. Monitors also can help instructors monitor their own loudness. If monitors are not available, instructors should position the sound system's speakers to help them hear their own voices.

8. *When using a microphone, remember to speak in a normal voice.* Some instructors yell into the microphone, instead of relying on it to supply the volume.

SUMMARY

With proper education, awareness of symptoms, and a willingness to modify vocal habits, instructors can maintain healthy, functional voices that will be an asset to their profession. If one or more of the early warning symptoms persist, an instructor should seek professional attention. Medical examination by an **otolaryngologist** (a physician specializing in the ears, nose, and throat), followed by voice therapy with a **speech pathologist** is the preferred course of treatment. Voice therapy helps to identify vocal abuse and hyperfunction and to replace these habits with correct vocal technique. Surgery should be considered only if therapy fails to correct the problem.

REFERENCES

Brindle, B. R., and H. L. Morris. "Prevalence of Voice Quality Deviations in the Normal Adult Population." *Journal of Communication Disorders* 12 (1979): 439–45.

Gillespie, S., and B. Cooper. "Prevalence of Speech Problems in Junior and Senior High School." *Journal of Speech and Hearing Research* 16 (1973): 739–43.

Laguaite, J. K. "Adult Voice Screenings." *Journal of Speech and Hearing Disorders* 37 (1972): 147–51.

Low-Impact Aerobics

Sylvania Reyna

Sylvania Reyna is the fitness director at Fitness Advantage in Spring Valley, California. She is also the director of operations, as well as an instructor and lecturer, for FITCAMP, an instructor-training program. Ms. Reyna lectures and consults on program design and management in dance exercise.

13

IN THIS CHAPTER:

- Safety and effectiveness of low-impact aerobics.
- Designing a low-impact routine.

- Sample routine.

Many dance-exercise instructors and participants suffer from overuse injuries caused by repeated stress to the legs, feet, hips, and lower back during high-impact aerobics routines. Low-impact aerobics provides an alternative for exercisers who want to reduce impact stress on injury-prone areas of the body, while maintaining or improving their cardiovascular conditioning.

In a low-impact routine, at least one foot is touching the floor at all times. This characteristic distinguishes **low-impact aerobics** (also known as soft, light impact, and nonpercussive aerobics) from traditional aerobics, where the routines usually include moves such as jogging or jumping jacks that bring both feet off the ground and therefore increase the stress on impact. Low impact does not mean low intensity. Although the approach is different, the goal of low-impact and traditional aerobics is the same: to improve aerobic conditioning by elevating the heart rate to a minimum of 60% of the maximal heart rate reserve for a sustained period.

A low-impact class must also be distinguished from a **nonimpact class,** in which neither foot ever leaves the floor. Although nonimpact classes may provide valuable preaerobic conditioning for unfit or special populations, the movements are probably not strenuous enough to achieve an aerobic training effect. On the other hand, low-impact classes offer an exercise alternative for a variety of participants at all levels of fitness.

Low-impact aerobics are a suitable exercise activity for the following participants:

1. Instructors and fit participants who wish to reduce stress and the likelihood of injury by alternating high-impact and low-impact classes.

2. Beginning exercisers who need to strengthen their muscles and connective tissue before moving on to traditional classes.

3. Older exercisers, who may not have the strength necessary for high-impact routines.

4. Overweight and pregnant participants who may feel more comfortable and more in control of their body's momentum with a low-impact routine.

5. People with a history of injuries, biomechanical problems, or foot deformities.

SAFETY AND EFFECTIVENESS

Because the activity is relatively new, few studies have been conducted on the safety and effectiveness of low-impact aerobics. Most instructors and participants find it to be an enjoyable and nonstressful activity and feel that they are getting a good workout. However, a preliminary study conducted in 1986 by Peter and Lorna Francis with a group of 65 participants at the IDEA International Convention in Anaheim, California, and another group of 65 at the IDEA Regional Conference in Chicago, Illinois, suggests that instructors designing low-impact classes must be particularly attuned to maintaining the intensity necessary to achieve a cardiovascular benefit.

In evaluating the responses of the two groups to low-impact activity sessions, the Francises found that 71% of the first group and 84% of the second group were working below the 65% maximal heart-rate level (equivalent to 60% maximal heart rate reserve) recommended by the American College of Sports Medicine (ACSM). They concluded that fit persons who wish to achieve cardiovascular benefits will have to increase the intensity of their low-impact routines. Another study, which evaluated energy expenditure during high-impact and low-impact aerobics (Otto et al. 1986), concluded that although high-impact aerobics offers a more intense workout, low-impact routines meet the ACSM's minimum criteria for quality and quantity of exercise.

Although generally considered to be safer, low-impact routines do have a potential for causing injury. To raise the heart rate sufficiently, some participants may indiscriminately flail their arms, causing hyperextension injuries of the shoulder. In addition, existing conditions may be aggravated by the exaggerated movements of low-impact routines. According to sports podiatrist Douglas Richie, Jr., participants with lower back and neck problems probably will not do well with low-impact aerobics (Koszuta 1986). Other researchers warn that increased knee flexion may present problems for exercisers with chondromalacia.

The challenge for aerobics instructors, therefore, is to design low-impact routines that are both safe and vigorous enough to enable participants to achieve at least a minimal training heart rate. These goals can be achieved by screening participants, designing routines carefully, observing participants to make sure they maintain proper alignment while exercising, and offering modifications as necessary.

DESIGNING A LOW-IMPACT ROUTINE

To design a safe and effective routine, keep the following guidelines in mind:

1. *Remind participants to keep one foot on the floor at all times.*

2. *Emphasize proper body alignment.* Arm movements should be controlled to avoid hyperextension. During knee bends, the knees should remain over the toes. Too much knee flexion is not desirable.

3. *Regulate the desired workout intensity by adjusting the tempo of the music,* using traveling or stationary steps, increasing arm movements, and, for the more fit participant, adding hand weights. The faster the music and the movements and the higher the arm motions, the more rapid the heart rate. However, the music should never be so fast that participants lose control of their movements and become sloppy.

Choreography also regulates intensity. As the steps move or travel, the heart rate will tend to accelerate. For example, a step-ball-change will have greater intensity if the participant is moving forward instead of staying in place. Arm movements performed at a level above the heart will also greatly increase exercise intensity. As shown in Figure 13–1, the instructor can use three different types of arm movements, depending on the needs of individual participants: (a) arms on the waist or by the side (beginners), (b) arms out to the side at shoulder level (intermediate), and (c) arms above the head (advanced).

Handheld or wrist weights (between ½ and 2 pounds) are recommended only for participants who are fit enough to maintain controlled movements and to avoid hyperextension of the joints. Never use ankle weights in a low-impact class. Even with low-impact steps, the extra weight can increase the tendency to pronate as well as cause stress fractures or Achilles tendinitis.

4. *Replace the jumping of high-impact aerobics with stepping, a slight bounce, or a knee bend.* Figures 13–2 through 13–6 illustrate ways of modifying common high-impact steps—such as jogging, jump kicks, and lunges—for a low-impact routine. Jogging is replaced by a march or stride; the jump kick becomes a step kick; and the lunge twist is performed by replacing the jumps with exaggerated steps to the sides.

5. *Monitor heart rates and encourage participants to regulate the intensity of their workouts.* More fit participants can exaggerate their movements by taking bigger steps, traveling more, and making greater use of their exercise space. Remind less fit participants to work at their own pace, if necessary by just doing the footwork and leaving their arms by their sides or at their waists.

FIGURE 13–1 Increasing heart rate with arm movements

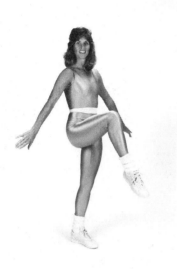 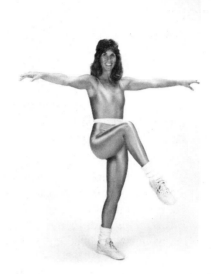 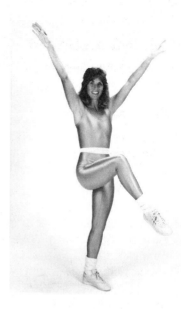

FIGURE 13–2 Jogging can be replaced by ball presses, marches, and strides.

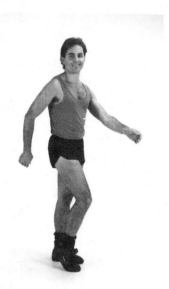 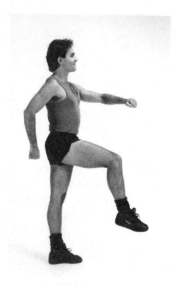 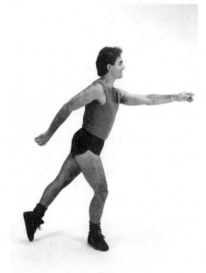

a. Ball presses: Lift the right heel. Lower it to the ground while lifting the left heel. Perform in a continuous rhythmic motion.

b. Marches: Lift one knee at a time in a military fashion.

c. Strides: Take large steps forward in a rhythmic, controlled fashion, swinging the arms at the sides.

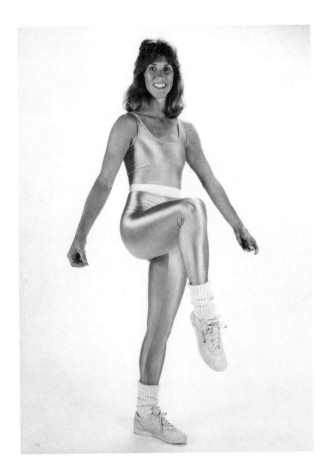

FIGURE 13–3 For knee lifts, use steps instead of hops.

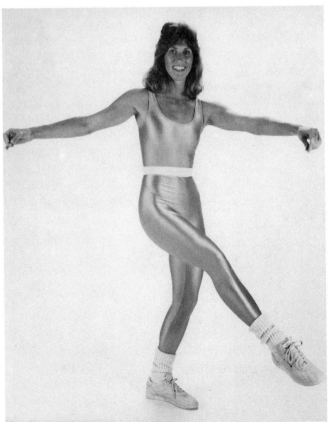

FIGURE 13–4 Use a step kick instead of a jump kick.

FIGURE 13–5 For the hopscotch, use a step instead of a straddle jump.

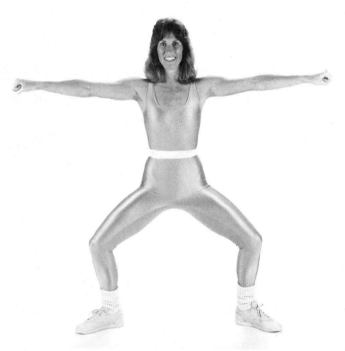

a. Bend knees. Hold arms out to the sides.

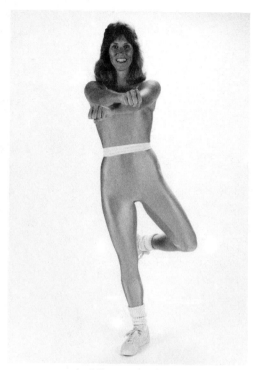

b. Lift left leg behind. Cross arms in front of body.

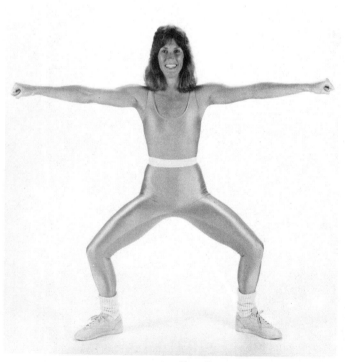

c. Bend knees. Hold arms out to the sides.

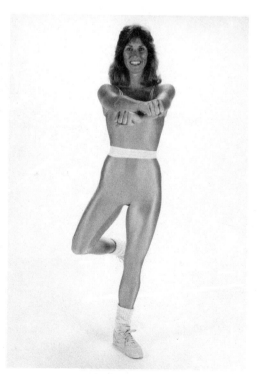

d. Lift right leg behind. Cross arms in front of body.

8

FIGURE 13–6 For the lunge twist, use exaggerated steps to the side instead of jump lunges.

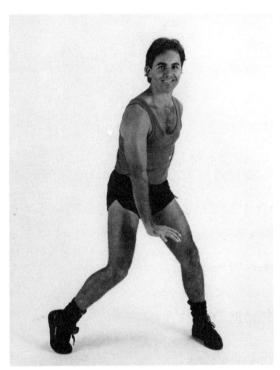

a. Lift right foot and place it to the side, turning body to left.

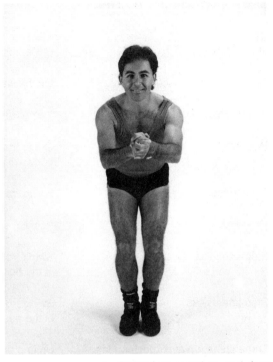

b. Bring feet together and face forward.

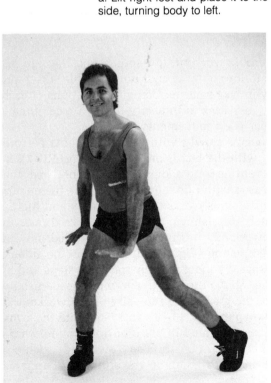

c. Lift left foot and place it to the side, turning body to right.

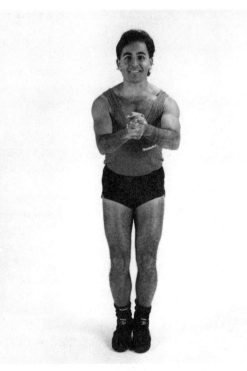

d. Bring feet together and face forward.

AEROBIC DANCE-EXERCISE INSTRUCTOR MANUAL

Table 13-1

SAMPLE LOW-IMPACT ROUTINE

STEPS (4 Repetitions)	ARM MOVEMENTS (4 Repetitions)
Step-touches in place	On the waist
Plié touches	Swing from side to side
Hopscotch	Out to the side, cross in front of body when leg bends back
Plié touches	Swing from side to side
Grapevine	Pushing up from the shoulders
Step-knee-lifts	Swing front and back by the sides of the body
Step-knee-kicks	Swing front and back by the sides of the body
Three steps forward, touch on the count of 4, reverse to back	Up and down by the sides of the body

SAMPLE ROUTINE

Like any other aerobic workout, low-impact routines are preceded by a warm-up and followed by a cool-down. Table 13-1 provides an example of a low-impact routine. Using 4 repetitions of each step, the routine gradually increases in intensity through a combination of foot patterns and upper body movements.

The routine begins slowly, with the participants performing step-touches in place, with the hands on the hips (Fig. 13-7). It is always best to begin the routine with a simple movement. Next, the intensity is gradually increased with plié touches that work the quadriceps (Fig. 13-8). Swinging the arms works the upper body and increases intensity. The hopscotch step (shown in Fig. 13-5) continues to combine the upper and lower body in rhythmical, controlled movements.

Adding the grapevine (Fig. 13-9) increases the intensity of the workout in two ways: by incorporating traveling steps and by working the arms at a level above the heart. The more space used when performing this step, the greater the intensity of the workout. Step-knee-lifts and kicks (shown in Figs. 13-3 and 13-4) with the arms swinging at the sides may be performed in place or traveling forward and backward to maintain aerobic intensity. The 3-step-and-touch combination (Fig. 13-10) continues to combine traveling with upper and lower body movements.

Participants should monitor heart rates throughout the routine and increase or decrease intensity as necessary. As with any aerobics routine, the instructor should lead the class in an aerobic cool-down before moving on to the calisthenics or stretching segments.

FIGURE 13-7 Step-touches

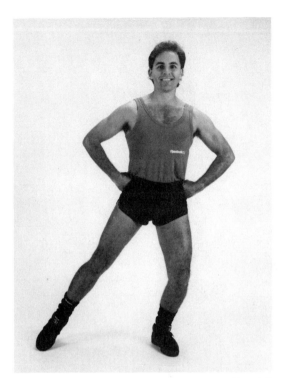

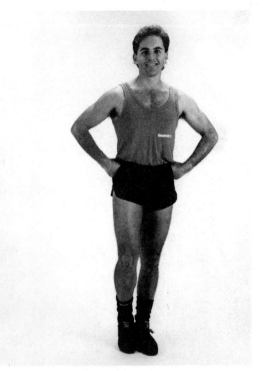

a. Step left.

b. Touch right foot by left and reverse.

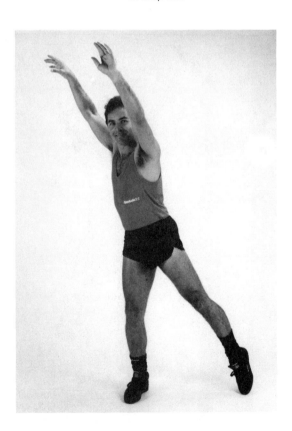

FIGURE 13-8 Plié touches. Reach arms up to right side, touching left foot out to side. Bend both knees, swing arms in front of body and reach arms up to left side, touching right foot out to side.

AEROBIC DANCE-EXERCISE INSTRUCTOR MANUAL

FIGURE 13–9 Grapevine

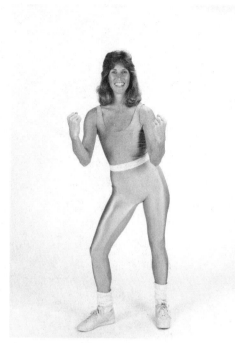

a. Step to right on right leg, arms in at the shoulders.

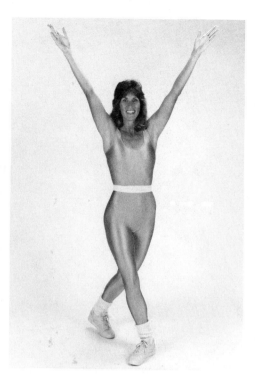

b. Step behind with the left leg, pushing arms above the head.

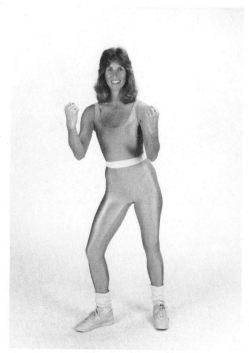

c. Step to the right on the right leg, arms in at the shoulders.

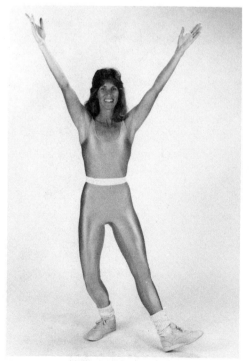

d. Touch to the left side with the left heel, pushing arms above the head. Reverse steps to other side.

FIGURE 13–10 Three-step-and-touch combination

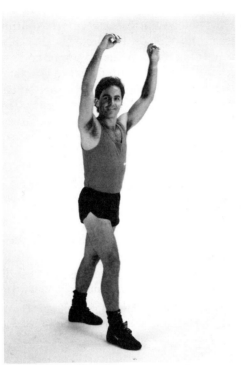

a. Step forward on the right leg, lifting arms from the sides to above the head.

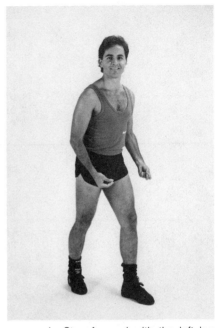

b. Step forward with the left leg, bringing arms back to the sides.

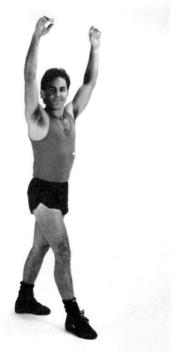

c. Step forward with the right leg, raising arms again.

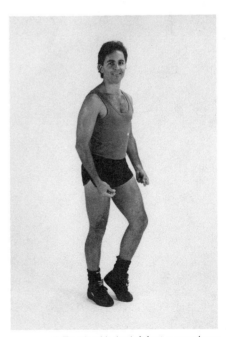

d. Touch with the left foot, arms down by the sides. Repeat, starting with left foot and moving backward.

SUMMARY

Low-impact aerobics is a good alternative for dance exercisers who want to reduce the impact stress of traditional classes and, therefore, prevent or reduce injuries. Low-impact routines reduce stress by keeping at least one foot on the floor at all times, and achieve a cardiovascular training effect by using upper body movements, adding wrist weights, and using traveling instead of stationary steps to raise the heart rate. To prevent injuries that may be caused by the upper body work, instructors should emphasize controlled movements and proper body alignment. As with all aerobics classes, participants in a low-impact class should monitor their heart rates and adjust the intensity of their workouts as necessary.

REFERENCES

Francis, P., and L. Francis. "Low-Impact Aerobics: Part 2." *Dance Exercise Today* (September 1986): 31–33.

Koszuta, L. E. "Low-Impact Aerobics: Better Than Traditional Aerobic Dance?" *The Physician and Sportsmedicine* (July 1986): 156–61.

Otto, R. M., C. A. Parker, T. K. Smith, et al. "The Energy Cost of Low Impact and High Impact Aerobic Dance Exercise." Abstract. *Medicine and Science in Sport and Exercise* 18 (1986): S23.

Emergency Procedures

Larry P. Brown and Sandra L. Niehues

Larry P. Brown, M.A., P.T., A.T.C. is director of the Sports Medicine Center at Scripps Clinic and Research Foundation. He is both a physical therapist and a certified athletic trainer and has served as assistant trainer with San Diego State University and the San Diego Chargers.

Sandra L. Niehues, M.A., A.T.C., P.T.A. is senior athletic trainer for the Sports Medicine Center at Scripps Clinic and Research Foundation. She is a lecturer for FITCAMP (Fitness Instructor Training Camps), and was a finalist in the 1984 Crystal Light National Aerobic Championships.

14

IN THIS CHAPTER:

- Emergency procedures: Equipment, assessment of an unconscious victim, assessment of a conscious victim.

- Care of sudden illness: Myocardial infarction, angina pectoris, cerebrovascular accident (stroke), seizures, diabetes mellitus, hyperventilation, shock.

- Care of wounds and bleeding: Open wounds, first aid, controlling severe bleeding, closed wounds, blisters.

- Injuries to the musculoskeletal system: Fractures, soft-tissue injuries (strains and sprains), tendinitis, bursitis, contusions.

- Physiological response to heat: Heat cramps, heat exhaustion, heat stroke.

The possibility that someone near us may become the victim of a medical emergency is a danger at all times. This potential is always present in dance exercise. By carefully screening all participants (see Chapter 4), instructors can be reasonably certain that the participants in their classes are free of medical conditions that make vigorous activity unsafe. However, some participants may have underlying disease that has not yet been identified and that appears for the first time in an exercise setting. There are also factors related to personality and motivation that can lead to sudden illness or injury. For example, unfit, sedentary participants commonly try to do too much, too soon, too fast. Even experienced exercisers may try to compete with others in the class and push themselves beyond reasonable and safe limits.

Emergencies may also result from physical hazards. A participant can be hurt while using exercise equipment or while slipping on a floor wet with sweat. Problems can occur if a class is overcrowded or if the environment is too hot or humid. A wise instructor is aware of the possible hazards and is prepared to act purposefully and appropriately when an emergency occurs.

This chapter is intended to familiarize instructors with potential medical emergencies and to provide basic guidelines for dealing with them. It is not intended as a complete resource, nor as a substitute for cardiopulmonary resuscitation (CPR) training, which is a requirement for certification through the IDEA Foundation. When faced with a medical emergency, instructors should never exceed their training and capabilities nor allow anyone in the class to do so. It is not the instructor's role to diagnose an injury or offer medical advice. If there is any doubt about the seriousness of a participant's illness or injury, it is always wise to err on the side of caution and call for help.

The authors hope that the information provided here will encourage instructors to seek basic first-aid training through the American Red Cross. Instructors who want to develop their skills even further are advised to enroll in an emergency medical technician course offered by community colleges throughout the country.

EMERGENCY PROCEDURES

Every business, no matter how large or small, should have an emergency plan for all employees. Each should receive a copy of this plan in writing, read the plan, and initial it to signify a complete understanding of the contents. The plan should include contingencies for evacuation in the event of fire or natural disaster, as well as procedures for any life-threatening situations. Telephone numbers for police, fire, emergency medical system, and poison control should be included in the written plan as well as posted in plain view near each telephone.

Equipment

There are three items every facility should have in case of an emergency. The first is a fire extinguisher that is easily accessible and in proper working order. It is important to have the extinguisher serviced at appropriate intervals and equally important for all employees to be familiar with its operation. The second item is a telephone with direct dialing capabilities. If the facility only has a pay telephone, the instructor should carry proper change in case an emergency call needs to be made. In areas where 911 emergency service is available, most pay telephones can be accessed without paying first; however, do not assume that all pay telephones can be accessed in this manner. The last item is a well-stocked and maintained first-aid kit. Each employee should be familiar with its contents and understand the use of each item. A first-aid kit should contain the following:

1. Assorted bandage materials
2. Sterile gauze pads
3. 4-inch and 6-inch elastic wraps
4. Liquid soap
5. Topical antibiotic cream
6. Tongue blades
7. Triangular bandage

8. Splinting material

9. Ammonia inhalants

10. Sphygmomanometer (blood pressure cuff)

11. Stethoscope

12. Penlight

13. Scissors

14. Paper bag

15. Chemical coldpack

Chemical coldpacks can be used immediately after an injury occurs; however, these packs do not get very cold or stay cold for very long. Ice from a nearby restaurant or market is better. Making arrangements in advance will help save time when an emergency occurs.

If an item in the first-aid kit has been used, it should be replaced as soon as possible so that it is available the next time it is needed.

Assessment of an Unconscious Victim

A rescuer who comes upon an unconscious victim must immediately be able to institute life-saving treatment. Appropriate action can only result when proper assessment is performed. The following sections will describe the primary and secondary survey of an unconscious victim.

PRIMARY SURVEY. The primary survey is designed to discover and correct any immediate life-threatening problems. A survey begins as soon as the instructor reaches the victim. During the primary survey, the instructor needs only to talk, feel, and observe.

The first 10 seconds of the primary survey should be spent assessing the scene and determining what took place and what the victim was doing before the collapse. Was the victim exercising or just finished? Try to be aware of the possible mechanism of injury. Look for medication bottles lying near the victim.

The next 50 seconds should be spent determining the status of the victim. Begin by assessing responsiveness. If the victim doesn't respond to talking or shouting, send someone to call for help right away.

The next step in the primary survey is to establish an airway. This can be accomplished by using the head-tilt method or modified jaw-thrust technique (see Appendix A on **cardiopulmonary resuscitation** [CPR]), if head or spinal injury is suspected. Next, look for signs of respiration. See whether the chest is rising and falling. Listen for sounds of breathing and feel with your cheek for respiration. Take a full 3–5 seconds to check for respiration, because well-conditioned people may breathe only 6–8 times per minute. If there are no signs of breathing, give 2 full slow ventilations.

Next, take 5–10 seconds to check the carotid artery for evidence of circulation. If there is a pulse and no breathing, begin rescue breathing. If there is no pulse, begin CPR. If the victim is bleeding severely, begin treatment immediately.

ACCESSING THE EMERGENCY MEDICAL SYSTEM. The **emergency medical system** may be activated in many areas by dialing 911. In communities without a centralized dispatch number, calling police, fire, or ambulance emergency numbers will activate the system. On the telephone, be prepared to give your name, the sex and approximate age of the victim, the nature of the condition (i.e., consciousness, unconsciousness, bleeding, convulsions, abdominal pain), as well as the location and telephone numbers of the facility. Be sure to allow the emergency dispatcher to hang up first.

SECONDARY SURVEY. Once the victim is out of immediate danger (the person is breathing and has adequate circulation; bleeding is controlled), it is time to conduct a more complete evaluation. The purpose of the secondary survey is to find additional unseen injuries that could be aggravated if mishandled. This survey begins with the head.

Check the scalp and the skull first for cuts, bruises, or depressed areas. The entire head should be gently palpated. Then check the ears and nose to make sure no fluid is draining. Palpate the neck carefully to determine whether there are any obvious fractures. Be careful not to move the victim's head. If any painful areas are found, it is wise to prevent the victim from moving until help arrives.

Next, observe the chest to determine normal rise and fall with breathing. Both sides should be symmetrical and should rise and fall simultaneously. Then gently palpate all areas of the abdomen for tenderness and spasm. Apply gentle pressure with a flat, open hand. Never poke the victim with the ends of the fingers.

Assess the pelvis for fractures by applying pressure in an inward direction against both hip bones. Once the assessment of the trunk is complete, check the lower and upper extremities for fractures and deformities by applying gentle pressure at the joints and by running the hands around the extremity, beginning at the top and moving downward. To find out whether any paralysis is present, simply ask the victim to wiggle his or her toes and grip your hand.

If the victim is lying on his or her back, injury to the buttocks and spine can only be observed by turning the victim over—a practice not recommended unless you are experienced in the assessment of spinal injuries and have adequate assistance. If a problem is suspected, palpate the areas by gently sliding your hands underneath the victim, being careful not to disturb the spine. Wait until emergency rescue teams arrive if you are afraid you might aggravate the problem. Show any medical identification tags found on the victim to the rescue team when they arrive.

DIAGNOSTIC SIGNS. Diagnostic vital signs give important clues to a victim's problem. Monitoring these signs at various intervals will give valuable information about the victim's condition and whether it is worsening or improving. Vital signs may be taken during or after the secondary survey. The specific situation will determine the appropriate time to assess diagnostic vital signs. The following is a brief description of each diagnostic sign.

The *pulse* is the wave of pressure that occurs each time the heart beats. In the adult, the average pulse is 60–80 beats per minute. In children, the rate is higher, around 80–100 beats per minute. Extremely fit persons may have resting heart rates as low as 40 beats per minute, and someone who has been exercising before collapsing may have a pulse rate as high as 200 beats per minute. Take the pulse at the carotid artery and count the number of beats in a 60-second period. If the carotid artery is not accessible, use the radial artery at the thumb side of the wrist.

Not only does the rate of the pulse need to be determined, but the quality assessed as well. Quality refers to the sensation of the pulse to the palpating fingers. In a normal person, the pulse should feel full and strong. With certain illnesses, it will feel weak. In others, it may feel bounding, similar to the sensation during exercise. Knowing whether the pulse is rapid or weak, full and bounding, absent or irregular is very important; however, knowing whether any *change* in the pulse has occurred is even more important. Therefore, the rate and quality of the pulse should be assessed and recorded initially and again at regular intervals.

The *respiratory rate* of a normal adult is usually 12–20 breaths per minute. Extremely fit persons, however, may only breathe 6–8 times per minute. Those engaged in strenuous exercise will have a much higher respiratory rate than normal. As with pulse, the number of respirations per minute is important, but knowing the quality of the respirations is equally important in establishing a diagnosis. Respirations may be shallow, deep, gasping, or labored. They may even be accompanied by coughing or frothy sputum. All these signs should be noted and recorded.

Blood pressure is the pressure against the walls of the arteries that is exerted by the circulating volume of blood. The average systolic pressure (amount present when the heart contracts) is 120 mm Hg (millimeters mercury). The average diastolic pressure (amount present when the heart relaxes) is 80 mm Hg. These figures vary with each individual. Age, sex, and disease will all affect blood pressure. Blood pressure is measured with a sphygmomanometer (blood pressure cuff) and stethoscope. With some practice, it is an easy skill to master. Instructors who do not know how to take blood pressure can ask a doctor, nurse, or someone skilled in the technique to teach them. The purpose in taking blood pressure is to aid in establishing a diagnosis. This information should be recorded initially and at regular intervals thereafter.

Skin color and temperature will be affected by various emergency conditions. A victim's skin may be a variety of shades, ranging from pale, white, grayish, and ashen to normal, blue, yellow, or bright red. To the touch, the skin may feel hot and dry, normal, or cold and clammy. Whatever condition is found should be observed and recorded.

The *pupils* of a normal person should be equal in size and react equally when exposed to light. Assess the pupils by observing their size and then observing the reaction when a light is passed across each eye. Look for constriction of the pupils when the light is present and dilation when the light is removed. If a penlight is not available, pupillary reaction can be assessed by covering the eyes one at a time and seeing whether the pupils constrict equally once they are again exposed to light.

The *level of consciousness* of a victim can range from being alert, responsive, and oriented, to a state of deep coma. It is the best indicator of the status of the nervous system. Whether the victim lost consciousness immediately, rapidly, or gradually is information the rescue team will want. This information should be recorded along with the rest of the diagnostic vital signs.

AEROBIC DANCE-EXERCISE INSTRUCTOR MANUAL

Assessment of a Conscious Victim

PRIMARY SURVEY. If the victim is awake and talking, there is a patent airway and adequate circulation. The primary survey is complete after a quick check for severe bleeding.

SECONDARY SURVEY. Before beginning the secondary survey, it is important to ask the following questions: What is the chief complaint? Pain, numbness, dizziness? If there is pain, what is the nature of it? Is it sharp, shooting, stabbing, throbbing, aching, or burning? Where is the area of the pain? What happened? Do you have any medical problems I should know about?

Once the answers are gathered, the secondary survey can be initiated and vital signs assessed as previously described.

When caring for a conscious victim, instructors should first introduce themselves and ask the victim's name. Then communicate the following:

1. *Training appropriate to the situation:* "My name is Suzie Sweatsocks, and I am trained in advanced first aid."

2. *What's going to happen next:* "I am going to check your injury. Help has been called and is on the way."

3. *What the problem is, even if it is only superficial:* "It seems you have a cut over your eye."

4. *What the victim should do:* "It is important to lie still right now. Please do not move."

Show the victim that you are in control, but never act until you have evaluated the entire situation.

CARE OF SUDDEN ILLNESS

If participants are screened properly, and if those who are at risk received medical clearance from their physicians to exercise, serious illness such as a heart attack should be rare in a dance-exercise class. However, because of the potential life-threatening nature of some medical conditions, instructors should be familiar with the signs of illness and be prepared to act quickly.

Myocardial Infarction

Myocardial infarction occurs when a blood vessel leading to the heart becomes so narrow that the muscle fibers supplied by the vessel receive inadequate oxygen and die.

SIGNS OF MYOCARDIAL INFARCTION. The most common sign of a myocardial infarction, or heart attack, is squeezing or crushing chest pain under the sternum. The victim may also feel pain between the shoulder blades or perceive the pain as radiating to the jaw, down the left arm, or down both arms. Often, the victim may assume the cause of the problem is merely indigestion. Other signs of myocardial infarction include sudden onset of weakness, nausea, and sweating without any apparent cause. In the course of the attack, it is common for complications to arise such as abnormal heart rhythms and faintness. The victim's lungs may fill with fluid, making breathing difficult, or cardiogenic shock may set in. (Cardiogenic shock occurs when damage to the heart affects its ability to pump blood through the body and adequately oxygenate tissues.) Many times, cardiac arrest (cessation of the heart's pumping action, necessitating immediate CPR) is the first sign that a heart attack has taken place.

PHYSICAL FINDINGS.   The physical findings for a myocardial infarction vary. The pulse may be elevated as a result of the injury itself, or as a normal response to fear and anxiety. In some cases, the pulse may be abnormally slow. Cardiac rhythm is usually regular but may be irregular. Frequently the victim may be short of breath, but sometimes respiration may be normal. The skin may be either dry or moist and usually will appear pale and gray. The most consistent finding in a victim experiencing a myocardial infarction is fear accompanied by an overwhelming sense of impending doom.

TREATMENT.   Call for help immediately. Place the victim in a semi-reclined position and loosen all restrictive clothing. Take vital signs, especially pulse, blood pressure, and respirations. Record the time they were taken. This information will be invaluable to the emergency rescue team. All victims of myocardial infarction will be very frightened, and so calm reassurance may be the best treatment you can render until help arrives.

Angina Pectoris

When the heart's need for oxygen exceeds the available supply because of restriction of a blood vessel, the pain that occurs is called **angina pectoris.** Angina is usually brought on by physical exertion or periods of physical or emotional stress. Unlike the pain from a myocardial infarction, the pain from angina is relieved when the heart's need for oxygen meets the available supply. Rest from the offending activity will relieve the pain because the heart's need for oxygen then decreases. **Nitroglycerin** will also relieve the pain because it diminishes the work of the heart, again reducing the need for oxygen.

In both angina pectoris and myocardial infarction, the pattern and behavior of the pain may be identical, with the exception of two major differences. First, pain from an anginal attack lasts only from a few seconds to a few minutes, but pain from a myocardial infarction can last 30 minutes or longer. Second, an anginal attack does not lead to death because no part of the heart muscle dies. Unfortunately, death is a common occurrence with a myocardial infarction. Because the signs of angina and myocardial infarction can be similar, call for emergency help whenever a participant is experiencing prolonged chest discomfort.

TREATMENT.   If a participant in an exercise class is experiencing an anginal attack, have the person stop exercising immediately. Inquire whether there is a history of heart problems and if so, find out whether any medications have been prescribed. If the victim has nitroglycerin, make sure he or she takes it. Nitroglycerin should help ease the temporary pain. However, resumption of the activity should not be allowed. A participant who is experiencing angina and is not on medication should visit a physician. It is wise not to allow a victim who has experienced an angina attack for the first time to return to class until a doctor's note is received, giving written approval to continue.

Cerebrovascular Accident

A **cerebrovascular accident,** more commonly known as a stroke, occurs when the brain loses function because of an interruption in its normal blood supply. Blood flow to the brain can be interrupted three ways: (a) when a clot forms in an artery in the brain, blocking the normal passage of blood; (b) when a clot formed elsewhere in the body lodges in a blood vessel in the brain, again blocking the normal passage of blood; and (c) when an artery in the brain ruptures, for whatever reason, causing bleeding into the tissues. This bleeding alone can cause brain damage or may trigger spasms of the ruptured artery, further interrupting blood flow.

Strokes caused by blood clots are often the result of atherosclerotic changes and usually will occur in older persons. Strokes caused by ruptured blood vessels can affect all age groups, including children.

MANIFESTATIONS OF STROKE. A stroke caused by a blood clot in an artery of the brain is manifested by a decrease in normal body functions, usually without pain or seizures. A stroke caused by a blood clot formed elsewhere is manifested by sudden loss of consciousness with possible convulsions or paralysis. If the cause of the stroke is a ruptured artery, the manifestations include headache and rapid loss of consciousness. In all cases, the final manifestations will depend on the area of the brain damaged. They may include paralysis of one or both extremities, impaired speech or vision, dizziness, convulsions, or decreased consciousness ranging from coma to simple confusion. Occasionally the only manifestation of a stroke will be a headache.

TREATMENT. Treatment for a stroke victim should begin with a call for help. If the victim is unconscious, make sure a proper airway is maintained. Place the victim on his or her side so that secretions can drain, preferably with the paralyzed side down. Take diagnostic vital signs, especially noting blood pressure and the regularity or irregularity of the pulse and respirations, because this information may give the emergency rescue team enough clues to determine the extent of the stroke. Treat the victim gently and avoid excessive handling. Do not give anything by mouth, keeping in mind the throat may be paralyzed. It is important to remember that victims of a stroke may be able to hear and understand everything going on around them, even though they may give the appearance of being unconscious and unable to speak.

Seizure Disorders

Seizures or convulsions may occur as a result of epilepsy, high fever, head injuries, allergic reactions, meningitis, hypoglycemia, eclampsia (a condition affecting pregnant women), withdrawal from alcohol or drugs, or any condition resulting in diminished oxygen to the brain. A seizure may be mild, almost impossible to notice, or it may be violent. The latter type, known as a grand mal seizure, is a dramatic event that comes on suddenly, with an abnormal burst of brain cell activity and uncontrollable jerky contractions of the skeletal muscles.

There are three phases of a grand mal seizure. During the first, or preictal phase, the victim senses a seizure is about to begin and is usually somewhat disoriented. The ictal phase, which is the actual convulsive phase, occurs next. Along with violent contractions, the victim may lose bowel and bladder control as well. The third phase, called the postictal phase, occurs after the violent contractions cease. The victim will be somewhat disoriented, usually very depressed, and often embarrassed.

TREATMENT. Emergency care during a seizure centers around preventing the victim from becoming hurt. Do not try to restrain the victim during the seizure. Instead, protect the victim's head, arms, and legs by removing surrounding objects. If help has not arrived by the time the seizure is over, try to reorient the victim. When help arrives, the rescue team will want to know what the seizure looked like and how long it lasted. They will also want to take any prescribed medications to the hospital along with the victim.

Diabetes Mellitus

Diabetes mellitus is a disease characterized by a deficiency in the body's ability to use sugar (or glucose) as an energy source, particularly following the ingestion of food. This deficiency results in a high level of glucose in the blood, a condition known as hyperglycemia. Diabetes is caused by a lack of the hormone **insulin.** In people without diabetes, insulin is released from the pancreas when glucose levels increase. This release of insulin promotes the uptake of glucose into the body's cells. In diabetics, however, insulin availability is insufficient, and the glucose level remains elevated.

There are two major classifications of diabetes: insulin dependent and non–insulin-dependent. Insulin-dependent diabetes, also known as juvenile-onset diabetes, occurs in people under 20 years of age. Non–insulin-dependent diabetes, or adult onset diabetes, occurs in people over 40 years of age, most of whom (80%) are obese. Of the 11 million diabetics in the United States, 90% are non–insulin-dependent. Insulin-dependent diabetics need daily insulin injections to control their glucose levels, while non–insulin-dependent diabetics rely on oral medication and diet.

Fortunately, diabetes mellitus can be controlled with diet, medication, and exercise. Diabetics must balance the amount of medication they take with the amount of food they ingest because some sugar is present in all foods. Diabetics must also take into consideration the amount of insulin or other oral medications in the body and the amount of exercise to be performed. When the proper balance between the level of insulin and the level of glucose in the blood changes, one of two emergency situations may occur: insulin shock or diabetic coma.

INSULIN SHOCK. **Insulin shock,** or hypoglycemia, occurs when the diabetic has taken too much insulin or oral medication, has not eaten enough food to balance the amount of insulin in the bloodstream, or has exercised excessively. In each case there is an excessive drop in the level of glucose in the blood. An emergency situation develops when the brain receives insufficient glucose. Insulin shock can occur very suddenly and although not common, unconsciousness may occur which could result in brain damage if not corrected right away.

A person in insulin shock will exhibit the following symptoms: normal respirations; pale, moist skin; a full, rapid pulse; normal blood pressure; dizziness and/or headache; disorientation or confusion; and fainting with possible unconsciousness.

DIABETIC COMA.   Although this is an emergency situation, it is rarely encountered and usually involves the insulin-dependent diabetic. **Diabetic coma,** or hyperglycemia, occurs when there is insufficient insulin available for the cells to use glucose as their energy source. As a result, cells begin to break down fat to satisfy energy needs. The breakdown of fat markedly increases the acidity of the blood and if fluid loss is sufficient, diabetic coma results. A diabetic coma will occur in the uncontrolled diabetic and in the diabetic who has not taken sufficient insulin and who has undergone some physiological stress such as infection. Unlike insulin shock, a diabetic coma develops very slowly over a period of a few days.

The victim of a diabetic coma will exhibit various levels of unresponsiveness as well as the following signs: dry, cool skin; sunken eyes due to dehydration; rapid, deep, sighing respirations; a weak, rapid pulse; normal or slightly low blood pressure; vomiting and abdominal pain; and a sweet or fruity odor on the breath.

TREATMENT.   If a diabetic participant suddenly becomes confused or changes moods, suspect insulin shock. Although both types of diabetics encounter insulin shock, insulin-dependent diabetics are most likely to experience hypoglycemia. It is important to give a fast-acting, sweet beverage or food, such as orange juice, a cola drink, or candy, to the victim. Although unconsciousness is not common in the diabetic, remember that an unconscious victim should never be given fluids. Granulated sugar can be placed under the victim's tongue to produce the desired result.

The victim of a diabetic coma needs insulin and must be transported to an emergency facility as soon as possible.

The following points are important for instructors to remember about diabetes:

1. Know who in the class is diabetic and what type of diabetes is present.
2. Look for a Medic-Alert bracelet or necklace that identifies the diabetes.
3. Insulin shock is the most common problem encountered with diabetics.
4. Always have some form of fast-acting sugar available.
5. Make sure the diabetic exerciser is regularly testing his or her blood glucose level and taking appropriate action if it is too high or too low.

Hyperventilation

Hyperventilation (rapid breathing) occurs most frequently as a response to psychological stress. The victim experiences the sensation of not being able to get enough air, even though there is a greater than normal volume of air exchanged. The main problem with hyperventilation is that carbon dioxide is being blown off very rapidly, which increases the pH of the blood and causes the body to experience **alkalosis.**

It is common for the hyperventilation victim to feel dizzy and faint or to experience numbness and tingling in the hands and feet. Stabbing chest pain is frequently a result of increased respirations. Vital signs will show increased pulse and respiratory rates, with the blood pressure remaining normal.

TREATMENT.　During an episode of hyperventilation, most people will be terrified of dying. It is important to be calm and reassuring. A simple technique to increase carbon dioxide in the blood is to have the victim breathe into a paper bag. If a bag is not available, cupping the hands over the mouth and nose will usually allow the victim to reclaim enough carbon dioxide to return the blood to its normal pH level.

It is important to know that some serious physical problems can bring on hyperventilation, because it is one of the best ways the body can decrease the acidity of the blood. Hyperventilation can occur when acid is ingested into the system, or as a result of diabetic coma when the breakdown of fat as an energy source increases the acidity of the blood. It also can occur as a result of cardiac arrest when inadequate tissue perfusion causes the acidity of the blood to rise. Hyperventilation may occur when blood clots migrate and get lodged in the lung. If you suspect that hyperventilation is caused by any of these problems, call for help immediately.

Shock

In a normally functioning person, all parts of the body receive an adequate supply of oxygen and nutrients through the cardiovascular system. For the body to function optimally, this regular perfusion of blood to the tissues must not be interrupted. Each body system has a different level of tolerance to the lack of adequate perfusion. The heart, brain, and peripheral nervous system are the most sensitive. If deprived for more than a few minutes, they can become permanently damaged. When all parts of the body receive inadequate perfusion, **shock** develops. If adequate perfusion is not restored, death will occur. Shock develops when the cardiovascular system fails (a) when damage to the heart affects its ability to pump blood through the system, (b) when severe blood loss occurs, resulting in inadequate circulating volume, or (c) when dilation of the capillaries enlarges the capacity of the cardiovascular system, making the normal volume of circulating blood insufficient to fill the system.

TYPES OF SHOCK.　There are eight different types of shock. Septic shock, which results from a severe bacterial infection, and metabolic shock, which occurs in people who have been ill for a long time, will probably never be seen in a dance-exercise class. The other six types of shock are discussed briefly below.

1. *Hemorrhagic shock*, or hypovolemic shock, results from severe blood loss. Bleeding may be external from fractures or lacerations, or it may be internal from rupture of organs or major vessels. This type of shock often accompanies severe burns because loss of plasma can also lead to loss of blood volume. Hemorrhagic shock may be seen with crushing injuries from damage to numerous blood vessels.

2. *Respiratory shock* occurs when the supply of oxygen to the tissues becomes inadequate. A blocked airway or punctured lung can produce respiratory shock, as can any other condition that hinders breathing.

AEROBIC DANCE-EXERCISE INSTRUCTOR MANUAL

3. *Neurogenic shock* occurs when blood vessels become paralyzed and then dilate as a result of spinal cord injury or head trauma. The blood vessels fill with blood, causing insufficient circulating volume.

4. *Psychogenic shock* is normally referred to as simple fainting. Fear, anxiety, bad news, severe pain, or the sight of blood may trigger fainting. There is a momentary decrease in the blood supply to the brain when a sudden dilation of blood vessels causes the blood to pool in other parts of the body. The body goes limp and falls to the ground. Immediately after collapse, the condition automatically reverses. Blood flows back to the brain and it resumes functioning. The most important concern after fainting is whether injuries were sustained by the victim during the fall.

5. *Cardiogenic shock* occurs when the efficiency of the heart as a pump significantly diminishes; that is, the pressure of the circulating blood is insufficient for the tissues to receive adequate oxygenation.

6. *Anaphylactic shock* results from a severe allergic reaction to a toxin from medication, ingestion of a food substance, an insect sting, or inhalation of dust or pollens. Signs of anaphylactic reaction include skin changes such as flushing, itching, burning, and swelling. Respiratory changes such as coughing, wheezing, and difficulty breathing may also occur. Circulatory change such as decreased blood pressure, weakened pulse, or dizziness may be noted. Treatment for anaphylactic shock should be immediate transportation of the victim to an emergency care facility.

SIGNS AND SYMPTOMS OF SHOCK. In the early stages of shock, victims may exhibit restlessness and anxiety that should be recognized immediately as a sign that shock may be developing. The victim may complain of thirst or feel nauseated and then vomit. Upon examination, the shock victim will exhibit a weak and rapid pulse. The blood pressure will be low and steadily decrease (assume systolic pressure of 100 mm Hg to be an indication of developing shock). The skin may be cool and clammy. There may be profuse sweating. Respirations will be weak, shallow, irregular or difficult. The face may turn pale or slightly blue from inadequate oxygenation. A dull, lusterless stare can be seen in a shock victim, with the pupils often dilated. The person may be unconscious.

PREVENTION OF SHOCK. Shock cannot be properly treated in the field by laypersons. However, they can give care to prevent shock by attempting to optimize the efforts of a compromised cardiovascular system. There are four steps to remember.

1. *Establish an appropriate airway.* Allow the victim to find the position in which he or she can breathe best. This will generally be supine, but in cardiogenic shock, the victim may feel more comfortable in a semireclined position.

2. *Control the bleeding.* External bleeding can be controlled with compression as described in later sections of this chapter. Internal bleeding can be controlled by splinting fractures and by avoiding excessive or rough handling.

3. *Elevate the lower extremities 12 inches to help reduce pooling of blood and encourage venous return to the heart.* A person who feels light-headed should be allowed to sit down or lie down to avoid faint-ing. If the person has been exercising rigorously and the heart rate is very high, a gradual cool-down period should be encouraged. The instructor should stay close by the participant in case fainting occurs.

4. *Cover the victim with a blanket to help maintain body temperature.*

Diagnostic vital signs should be assessed during or after the sec-ondary survey and every 5 minutes thereafter. A record of this infor-mation should be kept for the emergency rescue team. Never give a shock victim or an unconscious victim anything to eat or drink. If inadequate perfusion continues, irreversible shock will occur and the victim will die. Recognition of the development of shock, proper care and effective treatment, and prompt transportation to an emergency care facility may save the victim's life.

CARE OF WOUNDS AND BLEEDING

Wounds are breaks in the tissues, either external or internal (open or closed). An open wound is a break in the skin or mucous membrane. A closed wound involves underlying tissues without a break in the skin or a mucous membrane.

Open Wounds

Open wounds range from wounds that bleed profusely but are rela-tively free from infection to those that bleed only mildly but have greater potential for infection. Often a victim will have more than one type of wound.

An **abrasion** is a scrape of the skin, resulting in damage. Bleeding from an abrasion is usually limited to blood oozing from ruptured small veins and capillaries. However, contamination and infection are dangers because dirt and bacteria may have been ground into the bro-ken tissues.

Incisions, or cuts in body tissues, are commonly caused by sharp objects or edges. The degree of bleeding depends on the depth and extent of the cut. Deep cuts may involve blood vessels and cause exten-sive bleeding. Cuts may also damage muscles, tendons, and nerves.

Lacerations are jagged, irregular, or blunt breaks or tears in the soft tissues. Bleeding may be rapid and extensive. The destruction of tissue is greater in lacerations than in cuts.

Punctures are produced by pointed objects such as nails, pens, or pencils. External bleeding is usually minor, but the puncture object may penetrate deep into the body, damaging organs and soft tissues and causing severe internal bleeding. Puncture wounds are more likely to become infected than other wounds because they are not usually flushed out by external blood loss. Tetanus organisms and other harm-ful bacteria, which grow rapidly in the absence of air and in the pres-ence of warmth and moisture, can be carried deep into the body tissues by penetrating objects.

Avulsions involve the forcible separation or tearing of tissue from the body. Heavy bleeding usually follows immediately. A finger, toe, or in rare cases, whole limbs, may sometimes be successfully re-attached to the body by a surgeon if the severed part is sent with the victim to the hospital.

First Aid for Open Wounds

If the wound is minor and does not bleed profusely, the instructor may need only to hold the wound edges together and bandage it. At times, however, it may be difficult for the instructor to decide whether a wound needs medical care and suturing. Below is the American Red Cross list of open-wound conditions that usually require medical treatment after emergency care has been provided:

1. Blood spurting from a wound, even if controlled initially with first aid.
2. Persistent bleeding despite all control efforts.
3. An incised wound deeper than the outer layer of skin.
4. Any lacerations, deep punctures, or avulsions.
5. Severed or crushed nerves, tendons, or muscles.
6. Lacerations of the face or other body part where scar tissue would be noticeable after healing.
7. Skin broken by a bite, human or animal.
8. Heavy contamination of a wound.
9. A foreign object embedded deep in the tissue.
10. Foreign matter in a wound, not possible to remove by washing.
11. Any other open wound where there is doubt concerning the treatment needed.

Controlling Severe Bleeding

The adult human body contains approximately 6 quarts of blood, a red, sticky fluid capable of clotting normally in 6–7 minutes. A healthy adult can lose up to 1 pint of blood without harmful effects, but the loss of more than 1 quart can be life threatening. Hemorrhage from major blood vessels in the arms, neck, and thighs may occur so rapidly and extensively that death takes only a few minutes. Hemorrhage must be controlled immediately. In most medical emergencies, only restoration of breathing takes priority over the control of bleeding.

External bleeding may occur after an external injury or an internal injury in which blood escapes into tissue spaces or body cavities. External bleeding can be divided into arterial, venous, or capillary; however, such classification is of little value because with a large wound blood may escape at the same time from all three types of vessels. In capillary bleeding, such as in an area of scraped skin, blood and serum ooze to the surface. Blood from a vein is dark red with a steady flow. Arterial blood is bright red, flows in spurts, and is not likely to clot unless it is from a very small artery or blood flow is slight. When completely severed, arteries tend to constrict and seal off. In an emergency, the important consideration is the amount of bleeding and how to control it, not the source.

Internal bleeding may result from a direct blow, fractures, strains, sprains, or diseases such as bleeding ulcers. When vessels are ruptured, blood leaks into tissue spaces and body cavities. Internal bleeding should be suspected in all cases that involve penetrating or crushing injuries of the chest and abdomen.

The signs and symptoms of excessive blood loss include weakness or actual fainting; dizziness; pale, moist, and clammy skin; nausea; thirst; fast, weak, and irregular pulse; shortness of breath; dilated pupils; ringing in the ears; restlessness; and apprehension. The victim may lose consciousness and stop breathing. The number of symptoms and their severity is generally proportional to the speed and quantity of blood loss. Once bleeding has been controlled, the victim should be placed in a reclining position, be encouraged to lie quietly, and be treated for shock. Bleeding may be controlled by direct pressure, elevation, and compression of pressure points. A tourniquet should be applied only when every other method has failed to control excessive bleeding.

DIRECT PRESSURE. The simplest and preferred method of controlling severe bleeding is to place a sterile dressing over the wound, applying pressure directly to the bleeding site with the palm of the hand. If a sterile dressing is not available in an emergency, use the cleanest cloth available. In the absence of a dressing or cloth, the bare hand may be used until a dressing is available. If the first dressing becomes blood-soaked, apply another one on top of it, using firmer hand pressure. Never remove the initial dressing. To do so would disturb the clotting process, which usually takes approximately 6 minutes.

A pressure bandage can be applied over the dressing to hold it in place while additional emergency care is given. Place the center of the bandage directly over the dressing on the wound and maintain a steady pull while wrapping the ends of the bandages around the injured area. Unlike bandages for other wounds, a bandage to control severe bleeding should be tied over the dressing to provide additional pressure to the area. Do not cut off the circulation. A pulse should be felt on the side of the injured area away from the heart. If applied properly, the bandage can remain undisturbed for at least 24 hours.

ELEVATION. If a head or extremity wound is bleeding profusely, direct pressure should be applied on a dressing over the wound, with the part elevated. The force of gravity then lowers blood pressure in the affected part and reduces blood flow. Elevation should not be used on suspected fractures that are unsplinted.

PRESSURE POINTS. When direct pressure and elevation cannot control severe bleeding, pressure should be applied to the artery that supplies the area. Because this technique reduces circulation to the injury below the pressure-point site, it should be applied only when absolutely necessary and only until severe bleeding has lessened. A pressure point is a site where a main artery lies near the skin surface and directly over a bone. Although there are several pressure-point sites, the brachial artery in the arm and the femoral artery in the groin are the most effective.

The pressure point for the brachial artery is midway between the elbow and armpit of the inner arm, between the large muscles. To apply pressure, place one hand around the victim's arm with the thumb on the outside of the arm and the fingers inside the arm. Apply pressure by moving the flattened fingers and thumb toward one another.

The pressure point for the femoral artery is on the front of the upper leg at the crease between the body and the leg. Place the victim

AEROBIC DANCE-EXERCISE INSTRUCTOR MANUAL

on his or her back and apply pressure with the heel of the hand while keeping a straightened arm.

Pressure-point control of bleeding is not as satisfactory as direct pressure because bleeding rarely comes from a single major artery. Therefore, always continue direct pressure and elevation if you use a pressure point. When the bleeding stops, continue direct pressure and elevation, but slowly release the pressure point.

TOURNIQUET.   A tourniquet should be applied to control bleeding *only* when all other methods have failed. Unlike direct hand pressure, a tourniquet shuts off all normal blood circulation beyond the application site. Damage to tissues from lack of oxygen and blood may result in limb destruction or amputation. If the tourniquet is too tight or too narrow, it will damage the muscles, nerves, and blood vessels. If the tourniquet is too loose, it will increase the blood loss. A tourniquet should be applied with the thought of sacrificing the limb to save the life. Once applied, the tourniquet should remain in place. To release it will only dislodge clots, resulting in further loss of blood and increasing the danger of shock.

Tourniquets can be improvised from wide bands of cloth, folded triangular bandages, clothing, or similar material, folded approximately 2 inches wide and long enough to encircle the limb at least twice. Apply a tourniquet as follows:

1. Place slightly above the wound, fold around the limb twice, and tie a half-knot.

2. Place a piece of wood or stick (or similar material) approximately 6 inches long over the half-knot and secure it by tying two half-knots over the turnstick.

3. Twist the piece of wood several times in order to exert just enough pressure to stop the bleeding.

4. Secure the piece of wood in place with the free end of the tourniquet if it is long enough. If not, use another bandage to hold the wood in place.

5. Attach a sheet of paper to the victim's clothing or extremity, giving the location of the tourniquet and the time it was applied. Also, mark a T on the victim's forehead with blood to alert medical personnel.

6. Never cover the tourniquet with clothing or bandages, or hide it in any way.

7. Never loosen the tourniquet unless a physician advises it.

8. If a tourniquet is used, make it tight enough to shut off arterial and venous blood flow.

Closed Wounds

Most closed wounds are caused by external forces, such as falls, contusions from blunt objects, and automobile accidents. Many closed wounds are small and damage soft tissues only. Fractures of the limbs, spine, and skull, as well as damage to vital organs in the chest or abdomen, may occur in more severe wounds.

SIGNS AND SYMPTOMS.   Pain and tenderness are the most common symptoms of a closed wound. Usual signs include swelling and discoloration of soft tissues and deformity of limbs caused by fractures or dislocations. It is wise to suspect a closed wound with internal bleeding and possible rupture of a body organ whenever a powerful force exerted on the body has produced severe shock or unconsciousness. Even if signs of external injury are obvious, internal injury should be suspected when any of the following general symptoms are present:

1. Cool, pale, clammy skin.
2. Rapid but weak pulse.
3. Rapid breathing and dizziness.
4. Pain and tenderness in a body part where injury is suspected, especially if deep pain seems out of proportion to the outward signs of injury.
5. Restlessness.
6. Excessive thirst.
7. Vomiting, coughing of blood, or passage of blood in the urine or feces.

EMERGENCY CARE. Carefully examine the victim for fractures and other injuries to the head, neck, chest, abdomen, limbs, back, and spine. If internal injury is suspected, get medical care as soon as possible. If a closed fracture is suspected, immobilize the affected area before moving the victim. Carefully transport the victim in a lying position, giving special attention to the prevention of shock. Watch the victim's breathing and take measures to prevent airway blockage or uncontrolled bleeding. Do not give fluids by mouth to anyone suspected of having internal injury, regardless of how much he or she complains of thirst.

First Aid for Blisters

Blisters are caused by friction that results in separation of skin layers and accumulation of fluid between them. Avoiding friction will prevent blisters. Shoes should fit properly and be broken in gradually. Socks should always be worn to keep the feet clean and to help reduce friction. It may also be effective to dust the feet with a magnesium-carbonate-based powder, or apply a skin lubricant such as Vaseline, or apply thin adhesive felt, such as moleskin, over possible blister sites.

Blisters always carry the possibility of severe infection from contamination. A blister that appears to be infected requires medical attention. In general, a blister should be left intact and protected from further insult by either a small doughnut pad or a covering lubricant and dressing. If a large blister is in danger of tearing, it should be punctured with a sterile needle. First scrub the skin area over and around the blister with soap and water, or some other antiseptic. Then introduce a sterilized needle under the skin approximately 1/8 inch outside the raised tissue. Next, compress the blister with sterile gauze to drain fluid. The skin provides natural protection for the sensitive underskin, so leave it on for several days. An antibiotic ointment may be applied to the area and covered with a sterile dressing. Check the blister frequently for infection.

When a blister has been torn, the following approach may be indicated.

AEROBIC DANCE-EXERCISE INSTRUCTOR MANUAL

1. Cleanse the blister and surrounding area with soap and water; then rinse with an antiseptic.

2. Using sterile scissors, cut the torn blister halfway around its perimeter.

3. Apply antiseptic or antibiotic ointment to exposed tissue.

4. Lay the flap of skin back over the treated tissue and cover with a sterile dressing.

5. Within 2–3 days, or when the underlying tissue has hardened sufficiently, remove the dead skin by trimming it as close as possible to the perimeter of the blister.

INJURIES TO THE MUSCULOSKELETAL SYSTEM

Because musculoskeletal injuries are so frequent, it is important to evaluate them properly and master the skills necessary for initial emergency care. Appropriate emergency care of fractures and dislocations not only decreases immediate pain and reduces the possibility of shock, but also improves the chances for rapid recovery and early return to normal activities.

Fractures

A **fracture** is any break in the continuity of a bone, ranging from a simple crack to severe shatter of the bone with multiple fracture fragments. In the initial evaluation of a fracture, the most important factor is the integrity of the overlying skin and soft tissues. Thus, fractures are always classified as open or closed.

In an *open* fracture, the overlying skin has been lacerated by sharp bone ends protruding through the skin, or by a direct blow breaking the skin at the time of the fracture. The bone may or may not be visible in the wound. The wound may be only a small puncture or it may be a gaping hole exposing much bone and soft tissue. In a *closed* fracture, the bone ends have not penetrated the skin, and no wound appears near the fracture.

It is extremely important to determine at once whether the fracture is open or closed. Open fractures are often more serious than closed fractures because they may be associated with greater blood loss. There is greater risk of infection because the bone has been contaminated by exposure to the outside environment. For these reasons, all fractures should be described to emergency personnel as open or closed so that proper treatment can be undertaken on arrival at the hospital.

SIGNS AND SYMPTOMS.   An injured person complaining of musculoskeletal pain must be suspected of having a fracture. While bone ends protruding through the skin or gross deformity of a limb make recognizing fractures easy, many fractures are less obvious. The instructor must know the seven signs of a fracture; the presence of any one should arouse suspicion of a fracture. These seven signs include deformity, tenderness, inability to use the extremity, swelling and ecchymosis (discoloration), exposed fragments, crepitation (grating noise), and false motion.

Only the first five signs need to be present for the diagnosis of a fracture. Crepitus and false motion are extremely painful, and the limb should not be manipulated to elicit them. Inspection of the limb with clothing removed will show deformity, swelling, discoloration, or exposed bone fragments if there is a fracture. A victim's unwillingness to use the affected limb indicates guarding and loss of function. Palpation over the injured bone elicits point tenderness. Any of these signs is sufficient to assume limb fracture and initiate emergency care.

TREATMENT.   Emergency management of fractures begins after the vital functions are assessed and stabilized. All open wounds should be completely covered by a dry sterile dressing, with local pressure applied to control bleeding. Once a sterile compression dressing is applied to an open fracture, it should be managed in the same way as a closed fracture. Emergency personnel should be notified of all open wounds, dressed or splinted.

All fractures should be splinted before the victim is moved, unless life is immediately threatened. Splinting facilitates transportation of the victim and helps prevent the following:

1. Motion of fracture fragments that produces pain.
2. Further damage of muscle, spinal cord, peripheral nerves, and blood vessels by broken bone ends.
3. Laceration of skin by broken bone ends that would convert a closed fracture into an open one.
4. Restriction of distal blood flow from pressure of the bone ends on blood vessels.
5. Excessive bleeding into the tissues at the fracture site.

A splint is simply a device to prevent an injured part from moving and can be fashioned from any material; however, it is best to have an adequate supply of standard commercial splints on hand. The general rules for splinting are:

1. Remove clothing from the area of any suspected fracture or dislocation.
2. To rule out circulatory or neurological injury, check for a pulse distal to the site of injury and for sensation to a light touch or the ability to move the fingers or toes. If there is no pulse or no sensation, act as if there were a medical emergency and inform emergency personnel when they arrive.
3. A splint should immobilize the joints above and below the fracture.
4. During splint application, move the limb as little as possible.
5. Do not straighten a severely deformed limb. Splint the limb in the position of deformity.
6. In all suspected neck and spine injuries, correct the deformity only as much as necessary to eliminate airway obstruction.
7. Cover all wounds with a dry, sterile dressing before applying the splint.
8. Pad the splints to prevent local pressure.
9. Do not move or transport victims before splinting extremity injuries.
10. When in doubt, splint.

Soft-Tissue Injuries

Injuries to participants of dance exercise and other recreational sports generally involve soft tissues. Fractures occur, but far less often than sprains, strains, and overuse syndromes. Since soft tissues do not show on the X-rays, sport and recreational injuries often present diagnostic problems. Also, if ignored, athletic injuries can become increasingly disabling. Unfortunately, a victim's response to such an injury is often denial, but attempting to continue the activity in spite of the symptoms (though only slightly disabling) can result in use of compensatory mechanisms that may alter gait or other body activities. Such changes may cause problems worse than the original injury.

STRAINS AND SPRAINS. Although the terms "strain" and "sprain" are frequently used interchangeably, they are not the same. A **strain** is an overstretching or tearing of a muscle, tendon, or the musculotendinous junction. A **sprain** is an overstretching or tearing of a ligament or joint capsule.

An injury to a musculotendinous unit is usually dynamic (not requiring an outside force), caused by the victims themselves. All musculotendinous units are susceptible to strains, but those frequently strained include hamstrings, quadriceps, calf, and shoulder girdle muscles. Strains can result from poor flexibility, improper warm-up and cool-down, or sudden, violent contractions of a muscle.

Strains are classified in order of severity. First-degree strains are mild and involve a minimum of torn fibers. Mild tenderness around the area is usually accompanied by some swelling. Second-degree strains involve moderate tearing of tissue and cause greater pain, swelling, and deformity of muscle. Third-degree strains are severe, involving complete tear of the connective tissue, and require a physician's attention.

Sprains, like strains, range from minor tears or stretching to complete disruption of the ligament or joint capsule. Because ligaments attach bone to bone, sprains result when a joint is forced to move in an abnormal direction (one for which it was not designed). On the other hand, strains, which involve a muscle or tendon, usually result from an unaccustomed amount of force. Most sprains occur to hinge joints; that is, joints designed to function in one plane. The knee and ankle are the most frequently sprained joints. Preventive measures include conditioning, stretching, and avoiding overextensive muscle use. However, the excitement of participating in an exercise class may override one's caution, and thus injury may occur.

TENDINITIS. **Tendinitis** is the most common overuse syndrome, and has been described as an inflammatory response to microscopic trauma. After repetitive activity, the tendon or its sheath eventually breaks down, producing inflammation that causes pain and tenderness. Any tendon is a potential site for this injury, but the most common areas are the ankle (Achilles tendon), in and around the knee (iliotibial band and patellar tendon), the elbow, and the lower front of the leg (shin splints). Tendinitis can often be prevented through use of proper equipment such as special footwear and by preparing the musculoskeletal system for the specific demands to be placed on it. Because overuse syndromes tend to develop when demand exceeds the strength of the musculoskeletal system, proper conditioning for strength development is of great importance.

BURSITIS.   A bursa is a saclike structure that aids motion by lubricating sites of potential friction, such as where a tendon or ligament rubs over a bony prominence or other body structure. Bursae are most commonly found in the shoulder, hip, knee, and ankle.

Bursitis (inflammation of a bursa), may be caused at first by a direct blow to, or repetitive action of this fluid-filled sac. Subsequent overuse of the joint, including some activities of daily living, can cause the bursa to remain inflamed. Although this injury is less common in athletes than sprains, strains, or tendinitis, once the bursa is aggravated, recurrent irritation is far more likely.

CONTUSIONS.   A **contusion** (bruise) is an injury that crushes soft tissue but does not break the skin or bone. The usual cause is a direct blow. The intensity of a contusion can range from superficial to deep for soft tissues, and may even include underlying bone. The extent to which a person may be hampered by a contusion depends on the location and the force of the blow.

Treatment of Common Soft-Tissue Injuries

Treatment of soft-tissue injuries can be as simple as applying a Band-Aid or as complicated as requiring several operations and months of rehabilitation. Regardless of the severity of the injury, initial management includes a few simple steps to decrease pain, swelling, and inflammation. These steps are important to keep from making the injury worse and to allow better assessment of the situation because of less pain and swelling.

Proper and immediate first aid consists of **RICE**—rest, ice, compression, and elevation. After a traumatic event to the body, the area of injury swells. Swelling is a natural reaction to protect the wounded area; however, it slows healing time and can be very painful. The RICE method lessens pain and swelling, thereby speeding the healing process.

Rest the affected area, either completely (by staying off a sprained ankle, for example) or partly (by shifting from a high-impact to a low-impact exercise activity, or by refraining from exercise), depending on the nature and severity of the injury.

Ice should be applied for 20–30 minutes every 2–3 hours, immediately after soft-tissue injuries except fractures. This prolonged icing constricts the capillaries of the lymphatic system at the injured site, slowing the release of fluid, and thereby controlling the swelling. The best procedure is to put crushed ice in a moist towel, place it on the injured area, and secure it with an elastic wrap. Plastic bags filled with ice are more convenient but cooling is less effective because they are not moist.

Compression can be used with or without ice. While icing, secure the moist coldpack firmly with an elastic wrap or bandage. Between icings, apply a dry elastic wrap over a foam compression or by itself. The compression further constricts the release of excessive fluids by the body and provides the injured area with some support. It is important to wrap not only the involved area but also the area above and below it, leaving no skin exposed. Wrapping the entire area will provide even compression and greater protection to the injury. Periodically, the wrap should be released. Avoid sleeping with the wrap in place unless instructed to do so by a physician.

Elevation means getting the injured area higher than the heart, a position that allows gravity to drain fluid and prevent excess accumulation. For example, with a sprained ankle, it is far more beneficial to lie on the back with the entire leg raised and supported, than it is to sit in a chair and rest the foot on a stool. Elevation should be continued while sleeping and for as long as the swelling persists.

With acute injuries, never apply heat or wrap the area tightly enough to cause skin discoloration, numbness, or tingling. Do not attempt to walk or run off an injury. After 36–48 hours and stabilization of the injury (swelling stops), treatment may vary. That some sports-medicine advisers advocate heat and others cold (after 2 days) is confusing, but this inconsistency has nothing to do with the *initial* management, which always consists of cold. If swelling has not lessened in 48 hours, seek medical advice.

ENVIRONMENTAL STRESS

The amazingly complex human body is often compared to an engine with a thermostat, a useful analogy with one crucial difference—the human thermostat cannot "turn off the heat." We produce heat in many ways—cellular metabolism, muscular activity, ingestion of food, and hormonal actions. We pick up heat from sunrays or reflections from sand and snow.

Heat injury is 100% preventible, and yet cases of heat exhaustion and death from heat stroke continue to occur. Between 1961 and 1972, at least 60 deaths from heat stroke were reported in US sporting events. Education and constant vigilance have greatly reduced this figure since then, but cases still do occur.

Physiological Response to Heat

When it is hot, an athlete's work becomes much more difficult. Almost all athletes experience some type of heat stress, either from the external environment or from internal heat generated by their own metabolism. Most heat stress is associated with summer activities; however, it is not unusual for winter-sport participants to generate enough heat to produce a heat-stress effect.

No matter what the source, the body acts to protect itself against accumulation of heat. Thermocontrol takes place naturally by eliminating heat through loss of water, primarily as perspiration. However, sometimes the body cannot withstand the strain. A victim may feel extra tired, groggy, or thirsty. If the signs are recognized, it is simple to do the "right thing." The body must have fluid replacement, slow down, or cease activity completely. Otherwise it is prone to one of the three major heat syndromes: heat cramps, heat exhaustion, and the most serious and sometimes fatal, heat stroke.

The body is not without defenses. It possesses remarkable thermoregulatory mechanisms that adjust the inner environment to meet the demands of the outer environment, to enable the athlete to perform optimally anywhere. In the case of heat stress, however, the natural defenses have been overwhelmed, and thirst, fatigue, visual disturbances, heat cramps, and exhaustion are actual physiological cries for help.

To maintain thermal equilibrium, the heat gained by the body must be offset exactly by the amount dissipated. This delicate balance is controlled by the thermoregulatory mechanism, which includes circulation, sweating, neuroimpulses, and endocrine responses. For example, when a drop in temperature occurs, "cool" signals are transmitted to the brain that cause blood vessels to constrict, thus preserving heat. Conversely, if the temperature rises, an opposite chain of reactions is set in motion, ending with sweating and a cooling effect as the sweat evaporates.

Sweating provides the body with the main line of defense against overheating. Sweating to regulate body heat is a reflex response to a thermal stimulus. Sweat comes from sweat glands in the skin that emit a hypotonic solution (lower concentration of salt than contained in blood) on the skin for the purposes of evaporation. The total quantity of sweat produced is precisely controlled by the body's thermoregulatory requirements. It is estimated that an acceptable rate of sweating is approximately ½ quart per hour, or 3% of body weight. When this level is exceeded, the body reduces the amount of sweat it produces, particularly if fluid replacement is ignored. Cessation of sweating is a serious cautionary signal that should not be ignored. Activities should be immediately stopped, the victim moved to a cool environment, and a doctor summoned.

The circulatory system provides the lines of communication for thermoregulation, handling most heat exchange, heat distribution, and transportation of tissue fluid to the sweat glands. As the environment becomes cooler, blood vessels in the skin constrict to conserve heat. Conversely, as the temperature rises, these blood vessels dilate to increase arterial blood flow that carries heat from the core or deeper tissue to the skin, where heat is lost to the environment. Heart rate increases with rise in temperature and exposure to heat to accommodate the greater circulatory demands.

The thermoregulatory mechanism is centered in the hypothalamus, a very important part of the brain. It responds reflexively from the skin as well as directly to changes in the temperature induced by circulating blood. Hypothalamus centers control water balance, sweat glands, vasomotor activity, and inhibition of shivering. Its stimulus of hormonal activity causes the kidneys to absorb more water, thereby reducing urine output. Another hormone may have an effect in preserving salt balance, important in maintaining the water-to-electrolyte balance in the cells.

Heat Stress Syndromes

Heat injury results when demands of the environment exceed the capabilities of the body's regulatory mechanisms. The temperature regulatory system controls the body's heat to balance heat production and heat loss. If, because of thermal disturbances, the thermostat deviates from a desired condition, the regulatory center directs a response to correct the deviation.

HEAT CRAMPS.   Normal muscle contractions require a strict balance of salt and water within the muscles. Excessive perspiration may cause water and salt to be lost. Some experts believe cramps are due to excessive fluid loss (dehydration), muscle fatigue, or overheating, while others believe electrolyte (salt) imbalance causes the painful muscle spasms. **Heat cramps** occur in people who sweat profusely, and like most heat disorders, they usually take place at the beginning of a warm weather season before an acclimatization period. Cramps are most often seen in the lower leg muscles, such as the calves, but may also be seen in the hamstrings, quadriceps, and abdominal muscles.

Once the cramps have developed, treatment includes rest from the activity, gentle stretching, and cold, moist ice application to the cramp. Drinking water may help reverse the cramps.

HEAT EXHAUSTION.   **Heat exhaustion** is a more severe heat syndrome caused by a decrease in blood volume and water, or by salt depletion from excessive sweating. Normally fit persons who are involved in extreme physical exertion in a hot environment can develop heat exhaustion. Under these conditions, the muscles and brain require greater blood flow, and at the same time, the skin needs increased blood flow to radiate heat from the skin in the form of sweat. When the cardio-vascular system is inadequate to meet the demands of the muscles, brain, and skin, heat exhaustion results.

Heat exhaustion has a low mortality rate. It is characterized principally by the signs of peripheral vascular collapse or shock. Weakness, faintness, dizziness, headaches, loss of appetite, nausea, pale skin, vomiting, and postural syncope (fainting) may occur. Victims are usually sweating profusely, and their body temperature is normal or mildly elevated. The pulse is usually weak and rapid.

Replenishment of fluids and electrolytes and prolonged rest in a cool, ventilated environment are the best treatment. Rest diminishes the demands of the circulatory system. Rehydration and electrolyte replacement are best achieved over several hours. Intravenous solutions may be necessary if the victim cannot tolerate oral replacement.

HEAT STROKE.   **Heat stroke** is a true medical emergency with a high mortality rate. In this syndrome, all the mechanisms for cooling have failed to the extent that severe elevation of body temperature occurs. It may occur suddenly without being preceded by other clinical syndromes, or it may progress from water-depletion heat exhaustion.

In the other heat illnesses, body heat regulation is maintained under control of the thermoregulatory mechanism. In heat stroke, the hypothalamus loses control, and body temperature rises to levels that damage cells and organs throughout the body. The central nervous system (brain and spinal cord), however, is the most sensitive to heat damage. Central nervous system dysfunction may manifest itself initially by irritability, poor judgment, bizarre behavior, confusion, psychoses, and possibly seizures and coma. The victim may also have an unsteady gait and a glassy stare. The skin will be hot and dry as sweating ceases to avoid further dehydration, and the pulse will be rapid and strong.

Treatment of heat stroke must begin as soon as the disorder is recognized because the victim's prognosis is directly related to how quickly the body's temperature is returned to near normal. Call for help immediately. Remove the victim's clothing to allow skin exposure to air, and cool the body by using ice on the skin surface, immersing in a cool bath, or applying cool, damp towels or sheets. A fan may also be used to encourage good air circulation. Once the victim is in the hospital emergency room, physicians will provide more definitive treatment to deal with the generalized deterioration and failure that heat stroke creates.

Prevention of Heat Stress Syndromes

Heat stress syndromes are obviously related to climate, determined by temperature and humidity. Since the environment cannot be controlled, other factors must be, especially physical conditioning and acclimatization.

ACCLIMATIZATION. **Acclimatization** is the body's adaptation to heat stress and increased capacity to work in high temperatures and humidity. Since the body can adjust to the stress of repeated exposure to the heat, it is usually best to slowly increase the level of heat or intensity of the work done in a hot environment.

Most people will require 4–10 days of exposure to heat for acclimatization. When it is hot, one simple method of heat acclimatization is to reduce the normal workout by 50% on the first day. With each successive day, increase the amount of work done in the heat by 5%–10%. In this way, acclimatization should occur in 5–10 days with no major problems so long as there is proper intake of nutrients, electrolytes, and fluids.

FLUID REPLACEMENT. Over the last 10 years, producers of fluid-replacement drinks have made many claims based on a minimum of facts to promote their products. According to the advertising claims, each drink has some unique physiological quality that will replace body water and salts lost in sweat. This advertising has led to confusion among persons unable to distinguish between valid claims and unsupported promotional statements.

The single most important item in preventing heat injury is water. Small amounts of electrolytes may be added, but it is the consumption of adequate water that has radically reduced the incidence of heat-related injuries over the past few years. The role of fluids during exertion is crucial in maintaining the homeostasis of the body. With a decline in the body's water, neither the circulatory system nor the thermoregulatory system can meet the demands placed on them by the stress of exercise or a warm environment.

Sweat is quite dilute when compared with other body fluids. In other words, more water than electrolytes is removed from the body in the form of sweat. The remaining electrolytes become more concentrated in the cells of the body. As far as the cells are concerned, there is an excess of electrolyte concentration even though there has been a net loss of electrolytes in the body. So during prolonged, heavy sweating, the need to replace body water is greater than any immediate demand for electrolytes. No empirical or scientific evidence has demonstrated that electrolyte intake during exercise will enhance performance or eliminate occasional muscle cramps. Even after heavy sweating, the need to replace electrolytes is generally satisfied by a balanced diet.

Exercisers and athletes should be encouraged to take in as much fluid as desired during workouts or races, but to avoid large amounts at any one time. The drinks should be hypotonic (dilute) or just cold plain water, with little or no sugar. Fluids should be consumed in volumes of 3–10 ounces every 10–20 minutes. Prehydration of 10–20 ounces approximately 30–60 minutes before a workout is extremely beneficial. After activity, modest salting of food and ingestion of drinks with essential minerals can adequately replace the electrolytes lost in sweat.

SUMMARY

A wise instructor will be prepared to respond appropriately to emergency situations. All instructors should have training in cardiopulmonary resuscitation (CPR), and many will want additional training in first aid through the American Red Cross.

Every fitness business should have the following: (a) a written emergency plan that is read and initialed by all employees, (b) a fire extinguisher, (c) a telephone with clearly posted emergency numbers, and (d) a well-stocked first-aid kit. In a medical emergency, the instructor's first task is to discover and correct any immediate life-threatening problems and to send someone to call for help. If a victim's breathing is obstructed, first establish an airway. If there is a pulse and no breathing, begin rescue breathing. If there is no pulse, begin CPR. Next, control any severe bleeding by elevating the wound and applying direct pressure with a sterile dressing.

The most common injuries in a dance-exercise class involve the musculoskeletal system: strains and sprains, tendinitis, bursitis, contusions, and fractures. Immediate treatment for most injuries is rest, ice, compression, and elevation (RICE). The primary treatment for fractures includes splinting the injured part to prevent it from moving and then treating any open wounds for contamination. Following these steps before seeing a physician may help reduce pain and swelling and shorten the recovery time.

Although sudden, serious illness is not common in dance-exercise classes where participants have been properly screened, the potential always exists. An instructor familiar with the signs of such emergencies as a heart attack, stroke, seizure, diabetic coma, and insulin shock will be able to act quickly and effectively and perhaps save a life.

Exercising in a hot, humid environment can place great stress on the body's thermoregulatory system. All heat stress is 100% preventible through adequate fluid replacement, acclimatization, and avoiding exercise if heat and humidity exceed recommended levels. However, if body water lost through sweat is not adequately replaced, the participant may develop heat cramps, heat exhaustion, or heat stroke. Heat stroke is a medical emergency and treatment must begin immediately.

Dance-exercise instructors are not medical experts, and they should never exceed their training and capabilities. It is not the instructor's role to diagnose an injury or to offer medical advice. Instead, the instructor should be prepared to provide immediate emergency aid, call for help when necessary, and refer participants with less serious problems to their physicians. If there is any doubt about the seriousness of a participant's illness or injury, it is always wise to err on the side of caution and call for help.

SUGGESTED READING

American Academy of Orthopaedic Surgeons. *Emergency Care and Transportation of the Sick and Injured.* Chicago: American Academy of Orthopaedic Surgeons, 1977.

American Red Cross. *Advanced First Aid and Emergency Care.* 2nd ed. Washington, DC: American Red Cross, 1979.

Henderson, J. *Emergency Medical Guide.* 4th ed. New York: McGraw-Hill, 1978.

Strauss, R. H., ed. *Sports Medicine and Physiology.* Philadelphia, London, Toronto: W. B. Saunders, 1979.

Thygerson, A. L. *The First Aid Book.* Englewood Cliffs, N.J.: Prentice-Hall, 1982.

LEGAL ISSUES

PART IV

The first three sections of this book have explored the science of exercise, how to conduct a dance-exercise class, and the prevention and management of exercise-related injury. This final section is devoted to the business aspects of instruction—the legal and insurance concerns every instructor must face. Because of its rapid growth and success, dance-exercise is in the legal spotlight. Instructors must not only conduct exercise programs that measure up to the highest professional standards, they must also know how to protect participants from unnecessary hazards and themselves from potential lawsuits. Ignorance of professional responsibilities and liabilities can bring a successful career to a sudden end. It is hoped that these chapters will increase instructors' awareness in the important areas of liability, copyright law, and insurance and encourage them to consult further with their attorneys and insurance agents.

Note: These chapters do not intend to, and do not constitute, legal advice. Readers who have specific questions or problems concerning liability, copyright law, or insurance should consult their own attorneys.

Professional Responsibilities and Liabilities

David K. Stotlar

David K. Stotlar, Ed.D., is associate professor and chair of Sport Management at the United States Sports Academy, where he teaches sport law, sport administration, and finance. He has also served as a consultant to school districts, sports professionals, attorneys, and international sports administrators, as well as publishing extensively on sports law.

15

IN THIS CHAPTER:

- Definitions of liability and negligence.
- Areas of professional responsibility: health screening, fitness testing and exercise programming, instruction, supervision, facilities, equipment.

- Use of waivers and informed consent forms.

Most people who teach or administer dance-exercise programs have been trained as physical educators or exercise specialists. Often their experience with law, if they have had any, has been limited to cases involving common sports injuries. However, the rapid expansion of the dance-exercise industry has created new forms of legal liability. The purpose of this chapter is to explain basic legal concepts that concern the dance-exercise professional and to show how these concepts can be applied to reduce injuries to program participants, thus reducing the likelihood that an instructor or studio owner will be involved in a lawsuit.

LIABILITY AND NEGLIGENCE

The term "liability" refers to responsibility. Legal liability concerns the responsibilities recognized by a court of law. Every instructor who stands in front of a class faces the responsibilities of providing proper instruction, supervising the class, and knowing the physical capacities and limitations of participants before they begin an exercise program. Studio owners and managers have the added responsibility of ensuring that the facilities and equipment are appropriate and safe. Dance-exercise professionals cannot avoid liability any more than they can avoid assuming the responsibilities inherent in their positions.

The responsibilities arising from the relationship between the dance-exercise professional and the participant produce a legal expectation, commonly referred to as "standard of care." **Standard of care** means that the quality of services provided in a dance-exercise setting is commensurate with current professional standards. In the case of a liability suit, the court would ask the question, "What would a reasonable, competent, and prudent dance-exercise professional do in a similar situation?" An instructor or studio owner who failed to meet that standard could be found negligent by the court.

Negligence is usually defined as "failure to act as a reasonable and prudent person would act under similar circumstances." For the dance-exercise instructor, this definition has two important components. The first deals specifically with actions: "Failure to act" refers to acts of omission as well as acts of commission. In other words, an instructor can be sued for doing something that should not have been done, as well as for not doing something that should have been done. The second part of the definition of negligence pertains to the appropriateness of the action in light of the standard of care, or a "reasonable and prudent" professional standard. If other qualified instructors would have acted similarly under the same circumstances, a court would probably not find an instructor's actions to be negligent.

To legally substantiate a charge of negligence, four elements must be shown to exist. As stated by Arnold (1983, p. 39) they are (a) that the defendant (person being sued) had a duty to protect the plaintiff (person filing the suit) from injury, (b) that the defendant failed to exercise the standard of care necessary to perform that duty, (c) that such failure was the proximate cause of the injury, and (d) that the damage or injury to the plaintiff did occur.

Consider this situation: A participant in a dance-exercise class badly sprains her ankle while following instructions for an aerobic dance routine. The movement that led to the injury consisted of prolonged and excessive hopping on one foot, something not recommended by reasonable and prudent dance-exercise instructors. If the participant sues the instructor for negligence, the following questions and answers might surface in court: Was it the instructor's duty to provide proper instruction? Yes. Was that duty satisfactorily performed? Probably not. Did actual damages occur? The plaintiff's doctor concluded that they did. Was the instructor's failure to provide safe instruction the direct cause of the injury? It probably was.

AREAS OF RESPONSIBILITY

The duties assigned to dance-exercise professionals vary from one position to another and from organization to organization. Overall, there are six major areas of responsibility: health screening, testing and programming, instruction, supervision, facilities, and equipment. Each area poses unique questions for the professional and can be important even to the beginning instructor.

Health Screening

A dance-exercise professional's responsibility begins when a new participant walks in the door. Would a reasonable and prudent professional allow a person to begin an exercise program without having some knowledge of that person's prior activity level and health status?

Most prospective participants will be generally healthy people with the goal of improving their personal health and fitness level. Others, however, may come to recover from heart attacks or other serious health conditions. Therefore, it is imperative that a medical history be compiled for each participant (see Chapter 4) to document any existing conditions that might affect performance in an exercise program.

But a dance-exercise professional's responsibility does not end with collecting information. The health history and other data must be examined closely for information that affects programming decisions. Instructors have been charged with negligence for not using available information that could have prevented an injury. Every club or studio needs to establish policies and procedures to ensure that each participant's personal history and medical information are taken into account in designing an exercise program.

Fitness Testing and Exercise Programming

Many states require "medical prescriptions" to be developed by licensed medical doctors. Once the medical prescription is developed, a physical therapist is legally allowed to administer and supervise its implementation. As a result, dance-exercise instructors are usually limited to providing exercise programs, not exercise prescriptions which may be construed as medical prescriptions. Although the difference between the terms "program" and "prescription" may seem like a technicality, it may be important in a court of law.

Fitness testing presents similar issues. The health and fitness level of the client, the purpose of the test, and the testing methods should all be calculated before test administration. The use of relatively simple tests, such as a skinfold caliper to measure body fat, would not normally pose significant legal problems. On the other hand, the use of a graded exercise test on a treadmill with a multiple-lead electrocardiogram could expose an unqualified instructor to a charge of negligence or even practicing medicine without a license. Therefore, it is important that the test(s) be recognized by a professional organization as appropriate for the intended use, be within the qualifications and training of the instructor, and that the exact protocol (testing procedures) be followed.

Instruction

To conduct a safe and effective program, dance-exercise professionals are expected to provide instruction that is both adequate and proper. Adequate instruction refers to the amount of direction given to participants before and during their exercise activity. For example, an instructor who asks a class to perform an exercise without first demonstrating how to do it properly could be found negligent if a participant performs the exercise incorrectly and is injured as a result. "Proper instruction" refers to being factually correct. In other words, an instructor may be liable for a participant's injury resulting from an exercise that was demonstrated improperly or from an unsafe exercise that should not have been included in a dance-exercise routine.

In the courtroom, the correctness of instruction is usually assessed by an expert witness who describes the proper procedures for conducting the activity in question. Therefore, the instructional techniques used by a dance-exercise instructor should be consistent with professionally recognized standards. Proper certification from a nationally recognized professional organization can enhance an instructor's competence in the eyes of a court, should he or she ever be faced with a charge of negligence.

In addition to providing adequate and proper instruction, dance-exercise professionals should also be careful not to diagnose or suggest treatment for injuries received in an exercise program. When participants ask for advice, it is best to suggest they call their doctor. Generally, only doctors and physical therapists are allowed to diagnose, prescribe treatment, and treat injuries. An instructor can provide first aid, but only if he or she is qualified to do so. Simple advice for a sprained ankle once resulted in a nasty law suit. When a participant sprained her ankle during a fitness routine, the instructor told her to go home and put some ice on the ankle to reduce the swelling. Because the ice made the injury feel much better, the participant kept her foot in ice water for 2–3 hours. As a consequence, several of her toes had to be amputated because of frostbite.

The example may be extreme, but it serves as a valuable warning. There are several ways the instructor could have avoided this tragedy. First, the instructor could have advised the participant to see a physician. While this approach protects the instructor, it would be costly if every participant who suffered a sprained ankle had to see a doctor. Second, the instructor could have provided a more precise description of the first-aid ice treatment. The third and best approach would be a combination of the first two. The instructor would provide specific instructions (both written and verbal) on the first-aid procedures recommended by the American Red Cross and suggest that if the injury did not respond well, the participant should seek the advice of a physician.

Supervision

The instructor is responsible for supervising all aspects of a class. The standards that apply to supervision are the same as those for instruction: adequate and proper. A prerequisite to determining adequate supervision is the ratio of participants to instructors and supervisors. A prudent instructor should allow a class to be only as large as can be competently monitored. The participant/instructor ratio will, of course, vary with the activity, facility, and type of participant. A dance-exercise class of 30 may be appropriate in a large gymnasium, but too many for an aqua class. Adequate and proper supervision may be different for a class of fit 20-year-olds than for a class of 55-year-old beginning exercisers.

General or nonindividualized supervision can be used when the activity can be monitored from a position in "general" proximity to the participants. For example, in an aerobic dance-exercise class a conscientious instructor can give enough attention to all participants through general but systematic observation to keep them relatively safe. On the other hand, a series of fitness tests administered to a participant before an exercise program calls for specific, or individualized, supervision. The person qualified to administer the testing must provide continuous attention in immediate proximity to the participant in order to ensure safety. Whether general or specific supervision is required should be based on one's own judgment of the nature of the activity and the participants involved, compared with what other prudent professionals would do under the same circumstances.

Supervisory duties also include enforcing conduct and safety guidelines. Clearly written safety guidelines for each type of activity should be posted in appropriate areas of the facility and rigidly enforced by the supervisors. Of particular importance are the policies and procedures for emergencies. It is not enough that the policies exist; all employees should be thoroughly familiar with them and should have actual practice in carrying out an emergency plan. For example, every club or studio should conduct a "heart attack drill," requiring all staff to carry out emergency plans and procedures such as those recommended by the American Heart Association. Records of these simulations should be maintained by the program manager.

Many exercise programs are needlessly exposed to liability because they permit indiscriminate use of the facility. Supervisory personnel should restrict the facility to people who have a legitimate entitlement. Each staff member should have a list of the people scheduled to use the equipment and facilities during specific time periods, and the supervisor should allow access only to those people. This policy should be enforced with the same vigor as the safety procedures.

Facilities

Safety is the basic question for a fitness facility. Is the environment free from unreasonable hazards? Are all areas of the facility appropriate for the specific type of activity to be conducted in that area? For example, aerobic activity requires a floor surface that will cushion the feet, knees, and legs from inordinate amounts of stress. Similarly, workout areas or stations of a circuit should have adequate free space surrounding them to ensure that observers will not be struck by a participant.

Some facilities provide locker room and shower facilities. These areas must be sanitary, the floors must be textured to reduce accidental slipping, and areas near water must be protected from electrical shock. Although instructors may not be responsible for designing and maintaining the facilities where they teach, they should still be alert to hazards in the environment. Any problems or potential hazards an instructor observes should be communicated in writing to the person responsible for the facility. The problem should be corrected as soon as possible, and until then appropriate warning signs should be clearly posted to warn participants of the conditions.

In some cases, an instructor may be assigned to teach in an area that is unsafe or inappropriate for the activity. Under these circumstances, a prudent instructor would refuse to teach and would document that decision in writing to management so that constructive action may be taken.

Equipment

For a program that uses exercise equipment, the legal concerns center primarily on selection, installation, maintenance, and repair. Equipment should meet all appropriate safety and design standards. If the equipment has been purchased from a competent manufacturer, these standards will probably be met. However, some organizations may try to save money by using homemade or inexpensive equipment. If an injury is caused by a piece of equipment that fails to perform as expected, and the injured party can show that the equipment failed to meet basic safety and design standards, the club or studio would be exposed to increased liability.

It is also important that trained technicians assemble and install all equipment. Having untrained people assemble some types of machinery may void the manufacturer's warranty and expose the program to additional risks. A schedule of regular service and repair should also be established and documented to show that the management has acted responsibly. Defective or worn parts should be replaced immediately, and equipment that is in need of repair should be removed from service.

The best practice for an instructor or supervisor responsible for a workout area where equipment is used is to instruct each participant on equipment safety. In addition, each instructor and participant should be required to examine the equipment before each use and report any problems to the person in charge.

Another equipment-related situation arises when participants ask their instructors about which shoes to wear or what exercise equipment to purchase for home use. An exercise professional should be extremely cautious when giving such recommendations. Before an instructor is qualified to give advice, he or she should have a thorough knowledge of the product lines available and the particular characteristics of each product. If this condition cannot be met, an instructor should refer the participant to a retail sporting-goods outlet. Otherwise, the instructor could be held liable for a negligent recommendation. An instructor who makes a recommendation based solely on personal experience should clearly state that it is a personal and not a professional recommendation. Instructors who are receiving money for endorsing a particular product need to be particularly careful not to portray themselves as experts giving professional advice.

WAIVERS AND INFORMED CONSENT

The staff of many programs attempt to absolve themselves of liability by having all participants sign a liability **waiver** to release the instructor and fitness center from all liability associated with the conduct of an exercise program and any injuries that may result. In some cases, these documents have been of little value because the courts have enforced the specific wording of the waiver and not its intent. In other words, if negligence were found to be the cause of injury, and negligence of the instructor or fitness center was not specifically waived, then the waiver would not be effective. Therefore, waivers must be clearly written and include statements to the effect that the participant waves all claims to damages, even those caused by the negligence of the instructor or fitness center.

Some fitness centers use an informed consent form (see Fig. 15–1). This document looks similar to the waiver, but its purpose is different. The **informed consent** form is used to make the dangers of a program or test procedures known to the participant and thereby provide an additional measure of defense against lawsuits. The legal term is **assumption of risk,** which means that participants voluntarily expose themselves to a known danger. Two important aspects of this definition are "voluntary" and "known danger." If a program or test is not voluntarily engaged in by the participants, the assumption of risk defense

General Fitness Evaluation and Program Participation

NAME_____

ADDRESS_____

PHONE_____ AGE_____ SEX_____

I have volunteered to participate in a program of progressive
physical exercise. I waive any possibility of personal damage
which may be blamed upon such a program in the future and
accept the responsibility for requesting such exercise and
assistance. The possibility of certain unusual changes during
exercise does exist. They include: abnormal blood pressure,
fainting, disorders of heart beat, and very rare instances
of heart attack. Every effort will be made to minimize them
by preliminary examination and by observations during situations which may arise. I hereby acknowledge and accept
these risks. To my knowledge, I do not have any limiting
physical condition or disability which would preclude an
exercise program.

_____   _____
    Participant's Signature   Date

A physician's examination should be obtained by all participants
prior to involvement in the exercise program. If a participant refuses to obtain a physician's permission, he/she
must sign the following statement:

I,_____, have been informed of the
need for a physician's approval for participation in a
progressive exercise-fitness program. I fully understand
the strenuous nature of the program.

I accept complete responsibility for my health and well-being
in the voluntary exercise-fitness program and related testing
and understand that no responsibility is assumed by the leaders
of the program or sponsoring agency.

_____   _____
          Signature   Date

_____ has medical approval to
participate in a fitness program which will include progressively increasing amounts of general conditioning exercises
and jogging. I certify that the person whose name appears above
is free from infectious disease, and there appears to be no
reason why an exercise program should not be undertaken.
                                 M.D._____
_____   _____
    Physician's Signature   Date
                                 Address_____
_____
    Physician's Name   _____

FIGURE 15-1 Sample informed
consent form

cannot normally be used. Also, if participants were not informed of the risks associated with the program or test, then they cannot be held to have assumed them.

Does this mean that an instructor must describe every injury that might occur? For the most part, yes. When explaining these risks to the participants, it is important also to communicate the probability that they will occur. For instance, it is possible that someone in a dance-exercise class will have a heart attack. However, the probability of that happening is less than that same person's chances of being injured driving to class.

Obtaining informed consent is very important. It should be an automatic procedure for every person who enters the program, and it should be done before every fitness test. Nygaard and Boone (1981, p. 113) suggest the following procedures:

1. Inform the participant of the exercise program or the testing procedure, with an explanation of the purpose of each. This explanation should be thorough and unbiased.

2. Inform the participant of the risks involved in the testing procedure or program, along with the possible discomforts.

3. Inform the participant of the benefits expected from the testing procedure or program.

4. Inform the participant of any alternative programs or tests that may be more advantageous to him or her.

5. Solicit questions regarding the testing procedures or exercise program, and give unbiased answers to these inquiries.

6. Inform the participant that he or she is free at any time to withdraw consent and discontinue participation.

SUMMARY

No program, regardless of how well it is run, can completely avoid all injuries. In an attempt to reduce both injuries to participants and the accompanying legal complications, a dance-exercise instructor would be wise to adhere to the following guidelines:

1. Obtain professional education, guided practical training under a qualified exercise professional, and current certification from an established professional organization.

2. Design and conduct programs that reflect current professional standards.

3. Formulate and enforce policies and guidelines for the conduct of the program in accordance with professional recommendations.

4. Establish and implement adequate and proper procedures for supervision in all phases of the program.

5. Establish and implement adequate and proper methods of instruction in all phases of the program.

6. Post safety regulations in the facility and ensure that they are rigidly enforced by supervisory personnel.

7. Keep the facility free from hazards and maintain adequate free space for each activity to be performed.

8. Establish and document inspection and repair schedules for all equipment and facilities.

9. Formulate policies and guidelines for emergency situations, rehearse the procedures, and require all instructors to have current first-aid training and CPR certification.

By applying the recommendations presented above, dance-exercise professionals can help reduce the probability of injury to participants. Should legal action result from an injury, an examination of the facts would attempt to determine whether negligence were the cause. A properly trained, competent, and certified instructor conducting a program that was in accordance with current professional standards would probably prevail.

REFERENCES

Arnold, D. E. *Legal Considerations in the Administration of Public School Physical Education and Athletic Programs.* Springfield, Ill.: Charles C. Thomas, Publishers, 1983.

Nygaard, G., and T. H. Boone. *Law for Physical Educators and Coaches.* Salt Lake City: Brighton Publishing, 1981.

SUGGESTED READING

Herbert, D. L., and W. G. Herbert. *Legal Aspects of Preventative and Rehabilitative Exercise Programs.* Canton, Ohio: Professional and Executive Reports and Publications, 1984.

Copyright

Terry D. Avchen and Jeff Matloff

16

Terry D. Avchen is a partner in the Los Angeles law firm of Wyman, Bautzer, Christensen, Kuchel & Silbert. Mr. Avchen has extensive experience with the legal issues surrounding the dance-exercise industry.

Jeff Matloff is a production attorney with Tri-Star Pictures in Los Angeles.

IN THIS CHAPTER:

- The Copyright Act of 1976.
- Obtaining performance licenses.
- Obtaining permission to duplicate a recording.
- Exceptions under the copyright law.
- Obtaining copyright protection for original material.

One major legal responsibility of a dance-exercise instructor is compliance with the copyright law. **Copyright** is a form of protection that gives the creator of an original literary, dramatic, or musical work the exclusive right to derive profit from or control who derives profit from that work. In other words, composers, choreographers, writers, and artists have the right to financial compensation for the use of their creations. Music is the category of copyright protection most pertinent to the dance-exercise instructor.

All instructors who play music in their classes, whether music from a record or from a special aerobics tape, must pay the required royalties. On the other hand, the routines and materials an instructor develops for a class may qualify for copyright protection and be the source of substantial future income. In either case, ignorance of the copyright law can cost an instructor a substantial amount of money.

COPYRIGHT ACT OF 1976

Copyrights to musical compositions are originally owned by the person who created the composition. The owner usually assigns the copyright for licensing and income collection purposes to a **publisher.** Owning the copyright to a musical work refers to the exclusive right to do, or be compensated for allowing others to do, each of the following:

1. Perform the composition in public, as by playing the song in a nightclub or on a jukebox.
2. Reproduce the song, as on a record or tape.
3. Distribute the work publicly by sale or transfer, such as selling a record or tape at a record store.

349

4. Display the composition publicly, as in making sheet-music copies of the composition.

5. Make derivative works based on the composition, such as composing other songs or a medley that uses words or lyrics of the original composition.

6. License others to do any of the foregoing.

Under the old Copyright Act of 1909, a musical composition was protected for an initial term of 28 years from its creation or publication (distribution or sale), plus a renewal term of 28 additional years. Under the presently effective Copyright Act of 1976, a musical work created after January 1, 1978, is protected by copyright for the lifetime of the author, plus 50 years. The 1976 act also extends the copyright protection afforded to musical works created before January 1, 1978, for as long as 75 years—the initial 28-year term plus a second renewal term of 47 years. Once the musical composition is no longer protected by copyright, it falls into the **public domain,** meaning that it may be used by anyone for any purpose, free of charge. Thus, any song written more than 75 years ago may be freely used by anyone without payment to the former copyright owner.

PERFORMANCE LICENSES

Whenever someone purchases a record, a certain portion of that purchase price consists of a royalty to the copyright owner of the underlying musical composition. This royalty compensates the copyright owner for the exclusive right to distribute the work publicly. As long as the recording is for personal use only, the purchaser or other user of the recording owes no other fees to the copyright owner.

However, additional fees are required when the recording is played in a dance-exercise class, thereby constituting a public performance. The **public performance** of music occurs whenever the music is played at a "place where a substantial number of persons outside of a normal circle of a family and its social acquaintances are gathered." A health club or dance-exercise studio constitutes such a place, even though the club, studio, or instructor may limit the number of persons who may join the club or studio or enroll in a class. Since the owner of the copyright has the exclusive right to perform the composition publicly, instructors will need to obtain a public performance license enabling them to play the music in class.

It would be difficult and time-consuming to obtain permission from the copyright owner of every piece of music an instructor wanted to play in class. Fortunately, there is a convenient alternative. An instructor may obtain the performance license from one of the **performing rights societies** to which copyright owners assign the nondramatic performing rights to their music. **Nondramatic performing rights** refer to the rights to play a song on its own or with other songs, but not to accompany the song with dialogue, scenery, or costumes, or to use the song to tell a story. **Dramatic performing rights,** on the other hand, refer to the rights to use a song in conjunction with dialogue, scenery, or costumes, or to use the song to tell some form of story, as in a motion picture. The dramatic performing rights are retained by the publisher.

There are two performing rights societies in the United States: the American Society of Composers, Authors and Publishers (**ASCAP**), and Broadcast Music, Inc. (**BMI**). Together they represent approximately 80,000 composers, lyricists, and publishers who own the copyrights to virtually all of the music used in aerobics classes. A third society, the Society of European Stage Authors and Composers (SESAC, Inc.), represents less than 1% of the registered artists. Licenses from ASCAP and BMI will meet the needs of most dance-exercise instructors.

A license from ASCAP or BMI is a blanket license that permits the instructor to perform nondramatically and publicly the music of numerous artists, for profit and for an unlimited number of times. A health club or studio will usually obtain a blanket license on behalf of the instructors who are employed there. Instructors who teach as independent contractors at several different locations may need to obtain their own licenses.

For studios with no equipment or spa facilities, ASCAP has developed a fee schedule based on the number of clients who attend classes each week. For a spa or gym that includes dance exercise among its programs, the license fee is based on the number of speakers used to broadcast the music. BMI bases its fees on the square footage of each room where recorded music is used.

Both ASCAP and BMI vigorously track down studios, clubs, and instructors who violate the copyright law. Dance-exercise instructors who use music without obtaining a performance license may subject themselves to a possible copyright infringement suit by ASCAP, BMI, or the publisher of the music played in class without proper authorization. A court may require an instructor to pay statutory damages, ordinarily not less than $250 or more than $10,000 for each song played without proper authorization. An instructor who plays 10 songs during a single class could face a minimum fine of $2,500 for that one instance of use.

PERMISSION TO DUPLICATE A RECORDING

Apart from the protection afforded the creator or owner of a musical composition, the Copyright Act protects the owner of the master recording, usually the record company that manufactures and distributes records. The owner of the master recording has the exclusive right to make and distribute copies of the recording commercially.

An instructor who tapes a recording is reproducing that recording, a process altogether different from playing the music in class or purchasing a recording for home use. Because the law states that the owner of the recording has the exclusive right to reproduce the recording embodying the copyrighted musical composition, the instructor is legally required to obtain permission to tape the recording from the record company. If instructors want to duplicate more than one recording on to a tape, the law requires them to obtain permission to do so from each record company.

For example, an instructor who wants to play in class the record or commercially issued tape of "Go Home" by Stevie Wonder should obtain permission from the publisher (the entity to whom the owner has assigned the copyright for licensing and income collection purposes). This task can be accomplished by contacting the publisher directly, or by obtaining a performing rights license from the performing rights society (ASCAP or BMI) representing the publisher of that song.

On the other hand, if the same instructor wants to record all or part of "Go Home" on a tape to use in class, he or she will have to obtain permission from Motown Record Corporation, in addition to obtaining the performing rights license from ASCAP or BMI. Thus, the instructor is clearly better off playing the recording in class in the form in which it was originally purchased.

The dilemma posed by this area of copyright law is that some record companies have a practice of never granting permission to duplicate their recording on to a tape, especially with respect to popular new songs. The record companies' fear is that having tapes of their recordings accessible to the public will dilute the sales of their commercially valuable recordings. When the record companies do grant such permission, they do so with a license, either free or for a small fee.

The problem becomes more difficult when an instructor wants to duplicate the recordings of more than one artist's songs on to a single tape. To make and use the tape lawfully, the instructor has to contact the publishing company for each record label used on the tape. Since many artists are reluctant to have their music mixed with that of other artists, the instructor will probably find that obtaining such approval is time-consuming and difficult.

An instructor who wants to make and sell an exercise routine on either audio or video tape that uses music owned by others must also obtain a license from the record companies with the exclusive rights to distribute the recordings. Such a license is necessary regardless of whether the instructor plays all or part of the music, or whether the music is played without interruption or interspersed with voice-over narration or directions.

Again, it may be difficult to obtain this type of license, because permitting an instructor to distribute the same music as the record company could again dilute the record company's sales of that music. The producers of celebrity workout tapes and record albums that contain music from a variety of sources have obtained the necessary permission from each record company.

One way of avoiding the need to obtain permission is to produce "sound-alike" recordings. Several of the large exercise programs use their own musicians to record versions of popular songs for use in dance-exercise classes. In this case, the programs still need a license from ASCAP and BMI to perform the music, but they do not need permission from a recording company because they are not reproducing a record or tape.

EXCEPTIONS UNDER COPYRIGHT LAW

Certain narrow exceptions under copyright law permit public performance of music without a license from the copyright owner or performing rights organization. The first exception, known as the **"fair use" doctrine,** is designed to promote the development of the arts, science, and history, and permits the use of music for purposes of criticism, comment, news reporting, teaching, scholarship, or research. In determining whether an instructor's use of the music constitutes a fair use, courts typically examine the following four questions:

Note: At present, many readers have told the IDEA that the likelihood is not great that an individual instructor who creates a tape for class use will be sued by a record company. However, as the aerobics industry continues to grow, the practice of taping records for class use may receive more attention from record companies. Instructors and studio owners should discuss all copyright issues with their own legal advisers.

1. *Is the music being used for a noncommercial, educational purpose?* The price charged for the exercise class and the degree to which the class is part of an educational institution (such as a college classroom) would be analyzed by the court. It is unlikely that playing music in a class as part of an exercise program designed to promote physical health and fitness can be construed as a noncommercial, educational purpose.

2. *Is the music being played to teach music, geography, history, or some other subject?* Or is it merely entertaining people or providing background accompaniment to another activity? In the case of a typical dance-exercise class, music is an accompaniment to the activity.

3. *Are small portions of a song, rather than the entire song, being played?* The answer to this question will vary from class to class.

4. *Will the use of the music have any effect on the potential market for or value of the copyrighted song?* In the dance-exercise context this question could cut either way. On the one hand, the students' exposure to the music in class may encourage them to purchase the music, thereby enhancing sales of the music. On the other hand, if students' increased exposure to the music in the class lessens the likelihood of their purchasing it, the marketability of the copyrighted musical work may be diminished and its owner deprived of substantial income.

A second exception exists where the music is played as part of an instructional activity in a classroom at a nonprofit educational institution. For an instructor to become eligible for this exception, the music must be performed in classrooms or similar places devoted to systematic instructional activities (such as studios and gymnasia), and the instructional activities using the music must comprise the main activities at the nonprofit educational institution.

A third exception may apply to public exhibitions by dance-exercise instructors to promote classes or exercise techniques. To qualify for this exception, the instructor, or the entity employing the instructor, must not gain any direct or indirect commercial advantage from the exhibition. In general, to avoid a commercial gain, the instructor or the employer must not pay compensation to any performers, promoters, or organizers involved with the exhibition and must not charge admission.

In general, very few dance-exercise instructors will fall under any of the above categories. However because the guidelines issued by the courts in reviewing these situations are not always specific or evenly applied, it would be prudent for instructors to check with their attorneys before deciding whether they qualify for any exceptions.

OBTAINING PROTECTION FOR ORIGINAL MATERIAL

A dance-exercise instructor may not only be using copyrighted material, he or she may be creating original copyrightable material at the same time. There are four common ways in which an instructor may be creating works eligible for copyright protection:

1. *While simple dance routines generally cannot be protected by copyright, federal copyright law does fully protect pantomimes and choreographic works.* Thus, instructors have the exclusive right to reproduce and publicly distribute, perform, and display pantomimes or choreographic works of their own creation, as well as compose other routines based on them. As a result, instructors can derive substantial income from their creations.

To secure this form of copyright protection instructors must first publicly distribute, perform, or display their pantomime or choreographic works. Then they should register the copyright to the work by completing a copyright registration application and depositing the work in the US Copyright Office. Because only the detailed expression of an idea, and not the idea itself, can be copyrighted, instructors have to put their original work in tangible form. A choreographed routine can be documented in the form of a dance notation system (such as Benesch, Sutton, or Laban), a verbal description, a pictorial or graphic diagram, or a film or videotape. All copyrighted materials should bear a copyright notice that includes the symbol © or the word Copyright, the instructor's name, and the year the work was created.

The application may be obtained by writing the Register of Copyrights, United States Copyright Office, Library of Congress, Washington, DC 20559.

2. *A book, motion picture, or videocassette may be used to disseminate the pantomime or choreographic work that is an exercise routine or technique for meditation or relaxation.* An instructor who wants to include routines in a book should search for a publisher to purchase a description of them, print a book compiling them, and distribute the book to the public. In entering into the agreement with the publisher, the instructor will assign to the publisher the exclusive right to sell or distribute written descriptions of the routines, and the book itself will be copyrighted in the name of the publisher. (The instructor should retain, however, the rights to depict the routines in motion pictures or other media.) In return, the instructor will be compensated in the form of an advance and/or royalties on sales of the book. The amount and form of the compensation are a matter of private negotiation between the author and the publisher.

If the instructor wishes to communicate an original routine through a home videocassette, the instructor will need to find persons to produce the videocassette, finance the production, and distribute the videocassette. As with a book, the instructor will be compensated in the form of a flat fee and/or a percentage on videocassette sales or rentals. Such compensation is similarly determined after negotiations between the instructor and the company distributing the videocassette.

To exploit a routine in a motion picture the instructor may want to sell the rights to the routine to a writer, who in turn will write a screenplay incorporating the work or routine and will attempt to sell the screenplay to an independent producer or motion picture studio. If the instructor wishes to describe the routine in a book or screenplay, he or she can then try to sell the book or screenplay directly to the independent producer or studio. Alternatively, the instructor may consider licensing the use of the routine in the motion picture (in much the same way music would be licensed). Again, the instructor may be compensated in a fixed amount or as a percentage of the profits derived from the distribution of the motion picture.

3. *Dance steps or exercise routines that in themselves are too simple to be copyrighted, but that together compose an original sequence or* *program, may be eligible for copyright as a* **compilation.** The compilation may be copyrighted as long as the instructor contributes something that is *recognizably his or her own,* such as a series of exercises to be performed in a particular order for building up or toning certain muscles. An instructor who copyrights the compilation may then earn income from licensing others to perform it, from having it published in a book or depicted in a videocassette or motion picture, or from licensing it for use in a motion picture.

4. *An instructor may also copyright photographs, charts, diagrams, and other graphic and sculptural works used as instructional aids or as inducements to potential students to enroll.* Again, the applications for registering the copyrights to these items may be obtained from the US Copyright Office. These items will be accepted for copyright registration as long as they were created originally, at least in part, by the instructor.

Thus, the dance-exercise instructor may be able to copyright such items as photographs showing persons before and after attending a series of classes, charts reflecting how students have lost weight or changed their dimensions as a result of the exercise program, and diagrams explaining how to do certain routines. However, instructors who use the name, photograph, or likeness of another person in their published works must obtain a written release from any ownership, misappropriation, or other compensation claim. The display, publication or distribution of these items may translate into compensation for the instructor in two ways: increased enrollment in classes, and/or direct public sales of these items.

In sum, if dance-exercise instructors are actually creating a dance routine or exercise program as part of their teaching activities, they should seek the assistance of an attorney or the Copyright Office to obtain copyright protection for the routine or program. The potential for receiving substantial income from the ownership of these copyrights should not be ignored in the expanding field of dance exercise.

SUMMARY

Music is an important component of any dance-exercise class. According to the Copyright Act of 1976, instructors who play music in class, on record or tape, must obtain a performance license giving them the right to so use the music. The easiest way to comply with the law is to obtain blanket performance licenses from ASCAP and BMI, the two performing rights societies in the United States. Although there are several exceptions to this law, none are likely to apply to a typical dance-exercise class.

Instructors should also be aware that their original creations may be copyrightable. Copyright protection extends to original choreographic works, including exercise routines, books, or videocassettes describing or demonstrating the routines, and in some cases, photographs and other graphic works used as teaching aids or as inducements for potential students to enroll in dance-exercise classes. For all questions or problems concerning copyright law, instructors should consult with their own attorneys.

Insurance Needs

Jeffrey E. Frick

17

Jeffrey E. Frick is a partner in Howell, Murria & Frick Insurance, Solana Beach, California. He is licensed in 20 states and has worked closely with the dance-exercise industry for the past 8 years.

IN THIS CHAPTER:

- Insurance needs of individual instructors.
- Insurance needs of club and studio owners.
- Insurance market conditions.

Today's society could not function without insurance. Few people can afford to rebuild a house after a fire or pay all medical costs after a serious accident. By pooling resources, insurance companies are able to protect their clients from these and other financial disasters.

All dance-exercise instructors should assess their insurance needs and then secure the necessary protection. As professionals who work with the public, instructors should have liability coverage similar to that of doctors, architects, and lawyers. Those who own their own businesses and employ others need additional types of coverage (see Table 17–1). What follows is an overview of common insurance needs among dance-exercise instructors and a discussion of the current market conditions in the insurance business. These are general guidelines only. Before purchasing any form of insurance, instructors should carefully review their individual needs with a reputable insurance agent.

NEEDS OF INDIVIDUAL INSTRUCTORS

In our litigious society, an instructor can be held liable if a participant in a class is injured for any number of reasons. The most common type of claim is a "trip and fall" claim. Someone might slip on a wet floor or trip over a loose mat and then hold the instructor responsible for not providing a safe place to work out. A student who twists an ankle might charge an instructor with negligence for failing to demonstrate an exercise properly. Someone who pushes too hard during a workout and then collapses might claim that the instructor failed to provide adequate supervision. Although participants who sustain injuries probably have medical insurance, they still can sue an instructor

Table 17–1

INSURANCE COVERAGE

TYPE OF CLAIM	COVERAGE THAT APPLIES
A mat is left near an exercise area. A participant trips, spraining her ankle.	General Liability
Water from an air conditioner leaks onto the floor. Someone entering the studio slips and falls, breaking his arm.	General Liability
A child in a studio day care area runs into a wall and is injured.	General Liability
An instructor gives a participant a home remedy for shin splints. The problem becomes worse and is diagnosed as a stress fracture. The instructor is sued for practicing medicine without a license.	Professional Liability
An instructor allows a participant to use exercise equipment without first instructing him in its safe and proper use. The participant is injured.	Professional Liability
Because of space limitations, an instructor places an extremely overweight woman in a class for advanced exercisers. The woman tries to keep up and is injured.	Professional Liability
Jane spreads rumors that Joan is an incompetent instructor who steals routines.	Personal Injury Liability
An instructor employed at ABC Studio pulls a muscle while teaching a class and faces medical costs and loss of income while she heals.	Worker's Compensation
A studio is vandalized. The mats are ripped and the sound system is stolen.	Property Insurance
There is a fire in a studio and the business must close for three months while repairs are being made. The owner faces a loss of income while the business is closed.	Business Interruption

for the medical costs plus additional pain-and-suffering damages. The potential financial loss for an instructor without liability coverage can be enormous.

General Liability

All instructors, whether they are employees or independent contractors, should be covered by a **general liability policy.** This policy covers claims for bodily injury resulting from general negligence. For example, a participant in a dance-exercise class might trip over a loose floorboard, fall, and break an arm. A general liability policy covers any claims brought against the policy holder for this accident.

Whether or not an instructor is covered by an existing policy depends on the circumstances of his or her employment, as described below.

1. *Employees.* An instructor employed by a club or studio should ask the owner or manager what type of liability insurance the business carries. At a minimum, the club should have general liability coverage for any suits that might be brought against an employee.

2. *Independent contractors.* Some clubs hire instructors as independent contractors instead of as employees. The designation of **independent contractor** means that the instructor is just providing a service for a club and is not an employee under the law. Unlike employees, independent contractors do not receive benefits and do not have state and federal taxes withheld from their paychecks.

Independent contractors are not automatically covered by a club's general liability policy. Instructors who are hired as independent contractors instead of as employees should ask the owner of the club or studio to inform the insurance company and have them added by endorsement to the business's policy. Instructors who are not added to an existing policy should purchase their own.

3. *Instructors who teach for a nonprofit organization.* YMCAs, churches, women's clubs, and recreation centers are obligated to provide a well-maintained space, but they are usually not willing to assume responsibility should a participant in a dance-exercise class conducted in their facilities be injured. Instructors who teach for such organizations should check into existing coverage and be prepared to carry their own liability policies.

4. *Instructors who rent space on an hourly basis.* Sometimes a club will rent extra space to an instructor on an hourly basis. In this situation, instructors are neither independent contractors nor employees and must purchase their own general liability policies.

Professional Liability

In addition to the general liability policy, instructors may purchase additional kinds of coverage that broaden their protection. **Professional liability insurance** insures instructors against medical claims in a negligence suit. There can be a fine line between negligence for trip-and-fall claims and professional negligence. Instructors can be sued for negligence for everything from leading an exercise beyond the ability of participants, to failing to screen a new participant, to improperly demonstrating an exercise, to inadequate supervision. As professional standards in the dance-exercise field become established, those who fail to perform to these standards may become more susceptible to this kind of lawsuit. Therefore, instructors who want complete protection will carry a separate professional liability policy in addition to a general liability policy.

All liability policies have exclusions, and instructors must make it their responsibility to be aware of them. For example, professional liability policies do not cover an instructor for claims arising from infringement of a copyright or for actions for libel, slander, invasion of privacy, or assault. Because exclusions will vary from policy to policy, it is important to discuss them with an agent before purchasing professional liability insurance.

Personal Injury

Another liability coverage offered by most insurance companies is personal injury. This coverage offers protection against suits involving defamation of character and libel. For example, if Jeff Smith spreads rumors that Georgia Brown teaches terrible classes, has stolen all her routines from other instructors, and is a drug addict, Georgia Brown can sue Jeff Smith for defamation of character. If Jeff Smith has per-

AEROBIC DANCE-EXERCISE INSTRUCTOR MANUAL

sonal injury liability coverage, the insurance company would defend him, and if he were proven negligent, pay the necessary damages.

Professional and personal injury liability coverage is offered by most insurance companies and is usually attached to the basic liability policy for an additional 15%–20% of the total premium.

In addition to liability coverage, instructors may want to consider major medical insurance to cover their own injuries, accidents and illness, as well as disability insurance to cover lost work time from an injury or accident.

CLUB AND STUDIO OWNERS

General Liability

All clubs and studios should carry a general liability policy to protect themselves and their employees from suits by third parties. The best protection is provided by a comprehensive general liability policy with the broad form endorsement and a miscellaneous professional endorsement. Most insurance companies charge by the square footage of the facility. Others base their premiums on gross receipts or on the number of instructors. If instructors are hired as independent contractors instead of as employees, the studio owner should inform the insurance company and have them added to the general liability policy by endorsement.

It is important to determine whether the equipment in a facility and the programs being offered are covered by a liability policy. Some policies do not cover such items as suntan booths and weight machines, or exercise programs such as maternal fitness or cardiac rehabilitation. A club or studio owner should find a policy that covers all programs and facilities. If that is not possible, the club owner should seriously consider deleting the uncovered programs from the club's operation.

Property Insurance

Property insurance offers protection against the loss of a building and its contents. The standard insurance form covers only losses due to fire, smoke, wind, hail, riot, and vandalism. Those who want more extensive coverage can purchase a broader policy that covers such additional perils as theft. Instructors who lease or rent a building should review the insurance requirements included in their lease or rental contract (such as fire, legal liability, or waiver of subrogation) to determine their basic needs.

If a studio is robbed or burns down in a fire, the insurance company needs to know the **replacement cost** of the items lost. Therefore, it is advisable to supply an insurance agent with a complete list of articles that should be insured. Valuable papers, accounts receivable, signs, and many other items can be covered by the property policy. Property insurance premiums can be reduced by taking large **deductibles** (the amount the insured must pay in case of a loss), from $500 to $1,000.

Workers Compensation

Workers compensation covers the actual medical cost for injuries sustained by employees while under the supervision of the employer, as well as the wages lost as a result of the injury. Most states require businesses to have this coverage, and there are fines for noncompliance. Workers compensation does not cover employees when they are involved in activities outside the business. The annual cost for these policies is based on the size of the payroll for all employees and varies from state to state.

Business Interruption Insurance

Each business has an earning potential that needs to be protected in case of a fire loss or vandalism loss. Business interruption coverages, which reimburse a studio owner for loss of earnings and extra expenses while the building is being repaired or rebuilt, can provide this protection. An insurance agent must know the income and expenses of a business to provide the proper coverage.

INSURANCE MARKET CONDITIONS

Instructors and studio owners can purchase insurance policies from local independent insurance agents, professional associations, and direct-writing insurance agents. Many insurance companies write major medical, property, and life insurance. The numbers reduce drastically when it comes to liability, workers compensation, and disability. These coverages are available, but the instructor must shop around to find the best deal. While it is preferable to find one insurance firm that can handle all insurance needs, it is often necessary to purchase one type of coverage from one source and another type of coverage from another source. The cost of insurance varies from one location to another. It is usually more expensive to buy insurance in cities such as New York and Los Angeles than in rural areas.

The current liability crisis in the insurance industry affects all dance-exercise instructors. Many studios have seen their liability insurance premiums increase by as much as 1,000 percent, and some have had their policies canceled entirely. The problem is not unique to the fitness industry. Local governments, as well as businesses and professionals throughout the nation, are facing the same escalating rates and loss of coverage.

There are three issues to consider in an attempt to understand this problem. First, it is difficult to set liability rates for different classes of businesses. How does an insurance company price the potential risk of an underground contractor, a manufactured product, or a dance-exercise studio? How can a company anticipate what the courts may award an injured party for pain and suffering or **punitive damages**? These questions have always been difficult ones for insurance companies, but with the high dollar amounts now being awarded by the courts, the problem has increased.

A second issue is the status of the insurance industry. Insurance companies can write as much insurance as they wish, as long as they keep within certain ratios. One of these ratios obligates the companies to have a surplus of funds equaling one-third of their written premiums. At present, some companies have no funds to expand, others are discontinuing operations in the United States, and many are short of the surplus necessary to handle all classes of liability insurance.

Companies also want an **underwriting** profit and, thus, are becoming more selective in the types of businesses they insure. The result is that certain classes of businesses are suddenly out in the cold, with-

AEROBIC DANCE-EXERCISE INSTRUCTOR MANUAL

out liability insurance. The accounts that are written are spread through fewer businesses, and therefore the premium costs for each business are higher.

A third issue in the liability crisis is the number of liability suits in the courts and the size of the awards. In 1985, there was a civil suit for one out of every 15 families in the country. In 1983 alone, 360 personal injury awards were settled for over $1 million, 13 times the number in 1975 (Andresky, Kuntz, and Kallan 1985). For example, an overweight man with a history of coronary disease suffered a heart attack while attempting to start a lawnmower. He sued Sears, charging that too much force was required to yank the mower's pull rope. A jury in Pennsylvania awarded him $1.2 million, plus $550,000 for delays in settling the claim.

Another widely quoted example is that of the 41-year-old body builder who entered a foot race with a refrigerator strapped to his back to demonstrate his strength. He alleged that during the race one of the straps broke, and he was badly injured. He sued everyone he could, including the manufacturer of the strap. Jury award: $1 million.

Suits like these are being defended by insurance companies when there isn't really any just cause for the suit. Since insurance companies are in business to make a profit, it is not too difficult to understand why an insurance company might be reluctant to insure a business they consider to be high risk, or if they do, to charge a high premium.

SUMMARY

Today, almost everyone is suffering from the high cost of liability insurance. What should the dance-exercise instructor do? First, instructors and studio owners should maintain the highest professional standards. Second, an instructor should shop carefully to find the broadest possible coverage at the lowest possible rates. Because there is safety in numbers, insurance purchased through a large group, such as a professional association, will probably have broad coverage at the lowest rates. Third, instructors must thoroughly review their liability and other insurance needs with the insurance agent before purchasing a policy. All policies have some exclusions, so it is up to the instructor to make sure a policy provides adequate protection for his or her own situation.

REFERENCES

Andresky, J., M. Kuntz, and B. Kallan. "A World Without Insurance." *Forbes Magazine* (July 15, 1985): 40.

Appendix A

Standards and Guidelines for Cardiopulmonary Resuscitation (CPR) and Emergency Cardiac Care (ECC)

Adult Basic Life Support

Basic life support (BLS) is that particular phase of emergency cardiac care that either (1) prevents circulatory or respiratory arrest or insufficiency through prompt recognition and intervention or (2) externally supports the circulation and ventilation of a victim of cardiac or respiratory arrest through cardiopulmonary resuscitation (CPR).[1] The major objective of performing CPR is to provide oxygen to the brain, heart, and other vital organs until appropriate, definitive medical treatment (advanced cardiac life support) can restore normal heart and ventilatory action. Speed is critical—the key to success. The highest hospital discharge rate has been achieved in those patients for whom CPR was initiated within four minutes of the time of the arrest and who, in addition, were provided with advanced cardiac life support measures within eight minutes of their arrest.[2] Early bystander CPR intervention and fast emergency medical system (EMS) response are therefore essential in improving survival rates[3-5] and good neurological recovery rates.[6-7]

INDICATIONS FOR BLS
Respiratory Arrest

When there is primary respiratory arrest, the heart can continue to pump blood for several minutes, and existing stores of oxygen in the lungs and blood will continue to circulate to the brain and other vital organs.[9] Early intervention for victims in whom respirations have stopped or the airway is obstructed can prevent cardiac arrest. Respiratory arrest can result from drowning, stroke, foreign-body airway obstruction, smoke inhalation, drug overdose, electrocution, suffocation, injuries, myocardial infarction, injury by lightning, and coma of any cause leading to airway obstruction.

Cardiac Arrest

When there is primary cardiac arrest, oxygen is not circulated, and oxygen stored in the vital organs is depleted in a few seconds. Cardiac arrest can be accompanied by the following electrical phenomena: ventricular fibrillation, ventricular tachycardia, asystole, or electromechanical dissociation.

THE SEQUENCE OF BLS: ASSESSMENT OF THE *ABCs* of CPR

The assessment phases of BLS are crucial. No victim should undergo any one of the more intrusive procedures of cardiopulmonary resuscitation (i.e., positioning, opening the airway, rescue breathing, and external chest compression) until the need for it has been established by the appropriate assessment. The importance of the assessment phases should be stressed in the teaching of CPR.

Each of the *ABCs* of CPR, *A*irway, *B*reathing, and *C*irculation, begins with an assessment phase: "determine unresponsiveness," "determine breathlessness," and "determine pulselessness," respectively. Assessment also involves a more subtle, constant process of observing and interacting with the victim.

Airway

1. Assessment: Determine Unresponsiveness. The rescuer arriving at the scene of the collapsed vic-

AEROBIC DANCE-EXERCISE INSTRUCTOR MANUAL

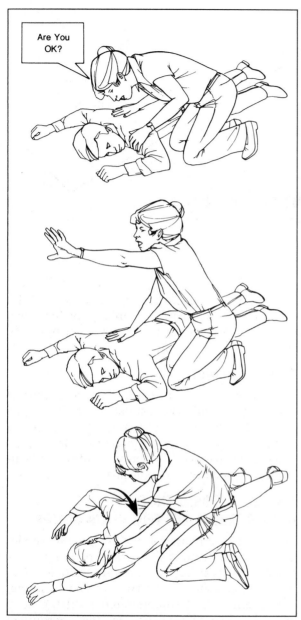

Figure 1 Initial steps of cardiopulmonary resuscitation. *Top*, Determining unresponsiveness; *center*, calling for help; *bottom*, positioning the victim.

tim must quickly assess any injury and determine whether the individual is unconscious (Fig. 1, top). If the victim has sustained trauma to the head and neck, the rescuer should move the victim only if absolutely necessary because improper movement may cause paralysis in the victim with a neck injury.

The rescuer should tap or gently shake the victim and shout, "Are you OK?" This precaution will prevent injury from attempted resuscitation of a person who is not truly unconscious.

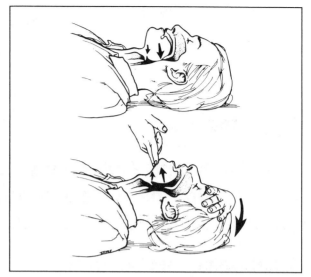

Figure 2 Opening the airway. *Top*, Airway obstruction produced by tongue and epiglottis; *bottom*, relief by head-tilt/chin-lift.

2. Call for Help. If the victim does not respond to attempts at arousal, call out for help (Fig. 1, center). When someone responds, send that person to activate the EMS system.

3. Position the Victim. For CPR to be effective, the victim must be supine and on a firm, flat surface (Fig. 1, bottom); even flawlessly performed external chest compressions will produce inadequate blood flow to the brain if the head is positioned higher than the thorax. If the victim is lying face down, the rescuer must roll the victim as a unit so that the head, shoulders, and torso move simultaneously with no twisting. The head and neck should remain in the same plane as the torso, and the body should be moved as a unit. Once the body is supine, the victim's arms should be placed alongside the body. The victim is now appropriately positioned for the next step in CPR.

4. Rescuer Position. By kneeling at the level of the victim's shoulders, the rescuer can perform, in turn, rescue breathing and chest compression without moving the knees.

5. Open Airway. The most important action for successful resuscitation is immediate opening of the airway. In the absence of sufficient muscle tone, the tongue and/or the epiglottis will obstruct the pharynx and the larynx, respectively (Fig. 2, top).[10-14] The tongue is the most common cause of airway obstruction in the unconscious victim. Since the tongue is attached to the lower jaw, moving the lower jaw forward will lift the tongue away from the back of the throat and open the airway.

Either the tongue or the epiglottis,[13] or both, may produce obstruction also when negative pressure is created in the airway by inspiratory effort, causing a valve-type mechanism to occlude the entrance to the trachea.

The rescuer should use the head-tilt/chin-lift maneuver, described below, to open the airway (Fig. 2, bottom). If foreign material or vomitus is visible in the mouth, it should be removed. Excessive time must not be taken. Liquids or semiliquids should be wiped out with the index and middle fingers covered by a piece of cloth; solid material should be extracted with a hooked index finger. The mouth can be opened by the "crossed-finger" technique.[15]

HEAD-TILT/CHIN-LIFT MANEUVER. Head-tilt/chin-lift is more effective in opening the airway than the previously recommended head-tilt/neck-lift.[16] Head-tilt is accomplished by placing one hand on the victim's forehead and applying firm, backward pressure with the palm to tilt the head back. To complete the head-tilt/chin-lift maneuver, place the fingers on the other hand under the bony part of the lower jaw near the chin and lift to bring the chin forward and the teeth almost to occlusion, thus supporting the jaw and helping to tilt the head back. The fingers must not press deeply into the soft tissue under the chin, which might obstruct the airway. The thumb should not be used for lifting the chin. The mouth should not be completely closed (unless mouth-to-nose breathing is the technique of choice for that particular victim). When mouth-to-nose ventilation is indicated, the hand that is already on the chin can close the mouth by applying increased force and in this way provide effective mouth-to-nose ventilation.[13] If the victim has loose dentures, head-tilt/chin-lift maintains their position and makes a mouth-to-mouth seal easier.[16] Dentures should be removed if they cannot be managed in place.

JAW-THRUST MANEUVER. Forward displacement of the mandible can be accomplished by grasping the angles of the victim's lower jaw and lifting with both hands, one on each side, displacing the mandible forward while tilting the head backward.[15,17] The rescuer's elbows should rest on the surface on which the victim is lying. If the lips close, the lower lip can be retracted with the thumb. If mouth-to-mouth breathing is necessary, the nostrils may be closed by placing the rescuer's cheek tightly against them.[15] This technique is every effective in opening the airway[18,19] but is very fatiguing and technically difficult.[16]

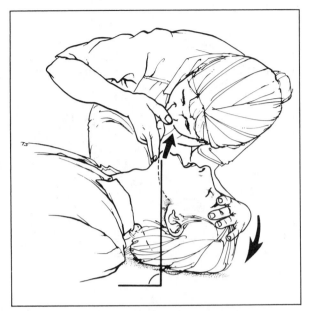

Figure 3 Determining breathlessness.

The jaw-thrust technique without head-tilt is the safest first approach to opening the airway of the victim with suspected neck injury because it usually can be accomplished without extending the neck. The head should be carefully supported without tilting it backward or turning it from side to side. If jaw-thrust alone is unsuccessful, the head should be tilted backward very slightly.

Breathing

6. Assessment: Determine Breathlessness. To assess the presence or absence of spontaneous breathing, the rescuer should place his or her ear over the victim's mouth and nose while maintaining an open airway (Fig. 3). Then, while observing the victim's chest, the rescuer should (1) *look* for the chest to rise and fall; (2) *listen* for air escaping during exhalation; (3) *feel* for the flow of air. If the chest does not rise and fall and no air is exhaled, the victim is breathless. The evaluation procedure should take only 3 to 5 seconds.

It should be stressed that, although the rescuer may notice that the victim is making respiratory efforts, the airway may still be obstructed and opening the airway may be all that is needed. If the victim resumes breathing, the rescuer should continue to help maintain an open airway.

7. Perform Rescue Breathing. (*Mouth-to-Mouth.*) Rescue breathing using the mouth-to-mouth technique is a quick and effective way of providing the necessary oxygen to the victim's lungs (Fig. 4, top).[20] The rescuer's exhaled air contains suf-

AEROBIC DANCE-EXERCISE INSTRUCTOR MANUAL

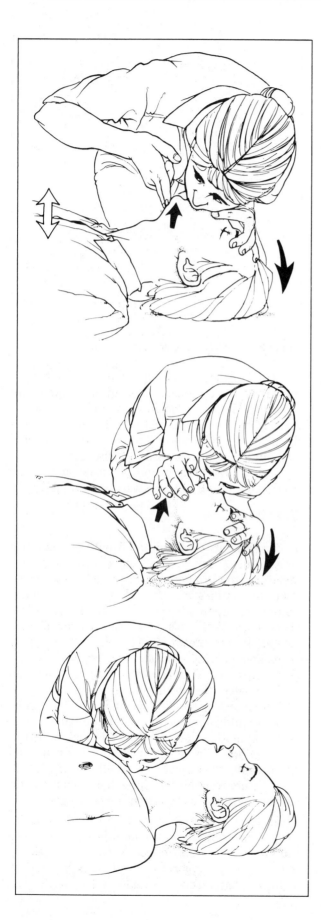

Figure 4 Rescue breathing. *Top,* Mouth-to-mouth; *center,* mouth-to-nose; *bottom,* mouth-to-stoma. (Adapted from *Cardiopulmonary Resuscitation.* Washington, DC, American National Red Cross, 1981, pp 16-17. Used by permission.)

ficient oxygen to supply the victim's needs. Rescue breathing requires that the rescuer inflate the victim's lungs adequately with each breath. Keeping the airway open by the head-tilt/chin-lift maneuver, the rescuer gently pinches the nose closed using the thumb and index finger of the hand on the forehead, thereby preventing air from escaping through the victim's nose. The rescuer takes a deep breath and seals his or her lips around the outside of the victim's mouth, creating an airtight seal; then the rescuer gives two full breaths.

Adequate time for the two breaths (1 to 1½ seconds per breath) should be allowed to provide good chest expansion and decrease the possibility of gastric distention. (Measurements of time "per breath" given herein are, more precisely, measurements of the victim's inspiratory time.) The rescuer should take a breath after each ventilation, and each individual ventilation should be of sufficient volume to make the chest rise. In most adults, this volume will be 800 mL (0.8 L). Adequate ventilation usually does not need to exceed 1,200 mL (1.2 L). An excess of air volume and fast inspiratory flow rates are likely to cause pharyngeal pressures that exceed esophageal opening pressures, allowing air to enter the stomach and, thus, resulting in gastric distention.[21–23] Indicators of adequate ventilation are (1) observing the chest rise and fall and (2) hearing and feeling the air escape during exhalation.

If the initial attempt to ventilate the victim is unsuccessful, reposition the victim's head and repeat rescue breathing. Improper chin and head positioning is the most common cause of difficulty with ventilation. If the victim cannot be ventilated after repositioning the head, proceed with foreign-body airway obstruction maneuvers (see "Foreign-Body Airway Obstruction, below).

MOUTH-TO-NOSE. This technique is more effective in some cases than mouth-to-mouth (Fig. 4, center).[24] The technique is recommended when it is impossible to ventilate through the victim's mouth, the mouth cannot be opened (trismus), the mouth is seriously injured, or a tight mouth-to-mouth seal is difficult to achieve. The rescuer keeps the victim's head tilted back with one hand on the forehead and uses the other hand to lift the victim's lower jaw (as in head-tilt/chin-lift) and close the mouth. The rescuer then takes a deep breath, seals the lips around the victim's nose, and blows into the nose. The rescuer's mouth is then removed, and the victim exhales passively. It may be necessary to open the victim's mouth intermittently or separate the lips (with the thumb) to allow air to be exhaled since nasal obstruction may be present during exhalation.[25]

MOUTH-TO-STOMA. Persons who have undergone a laryngectomy (surgical removal of the larynx) have a permanent stoma (opening) that connects the trachea directly to the skin.[26] The stoma can be recognized as an opening at the front base of the neck. When such an individual requires rescue breathing, direct mouth-to-stoma ventilation should be performed (Fig. 4, bottom). The rescuer's mouth is sealed around the stoma and air is blown into the victim's stoma until the chest rises. When the rescuer's mouth is removed from the stoma, the victim is permitted to exhale passively.

Other persons may have a temporary tracheostomy tube in the trachea. To ventiallate these persons, the victim's mouth and nose usually must be sealed by the rescuer's hand or by a tightly fitting face mask to prevent leakage of air when the rescuer blows into the tracheostomy tube. This problem is alleviated when the tracheostomy tube has a cuff that can be inflated.

Circulation

8. Assessment: Determine Pulselessness. Cardiac arrest is recognized by pulselessness in the large arteries of the unconscious victim (Fig. 3). The pulse check should take 5 to 10 seconds, and the carotid artery should be used. It lies in a groove created by the trachea and the large strap muscles of the neck. While maintaining head-tilt with one hand on the forehead, the rescuer locates the victim's larynx with two or three fingers of the other hand. The rescuer then slides these fingers into the groove between the trachea and the muscles at the side of the neck where the carotid pulse can be felt. The pulse area must be pressed gently—to avoid compressing the artery. This technique is usually more easily performed on the side nearest the rescuer. Adequate time should be allowed since the pulse may be slow, irregular, or very weak and rapid. This is the most accessible, reliable, and easily learned technique for locating the pulse in adults and children. The pulse in the carotid artery will persist when more peripheral pulses (e.g., radial) are no longer palpable. For health care professionals, or in the hospital set-

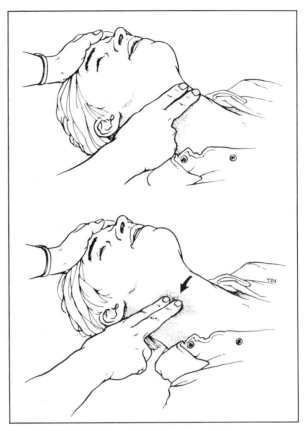

Figure 5 Determining pulselessness.

ting, determining pulselessness using the femoral pulse is also acceptable; however, this pulse is difficult to locate in a fully clothed patient.

Proper assessment of the victim's condition must be made since performing external chest compressions on a patient who has a pulse may result in serious medical complications. If a pulse is present but there is no breathing, rescue breathing should be initiated at a rate of 12 times per minute (once every 5 seconds) after initial two breaths of 1 to 1½ seconds each.

If no pulse is palpated, the diagnosis of cardiac arrest is confirmed. If not yet done, the EMS system should be activated and external chest compression begun after the initial two breaths.

9. Activate the EMS System. The EMS system is activated by calling the local emergency telephone number (911, if available). This number should be widely publicized in each community. The person who calls the EMS system should be prepared to give the following information as calmly as possible[27]; (1) where the emergency is (with names of cross streets or roads, if possible); (2) the telephone number from which the call is made; (3) what happened—heart attack, auto accident, etc; (4) how many persons need help; (5)

AEROBIC DANCE-EXERCISE INSTRUCTOR MANUAL

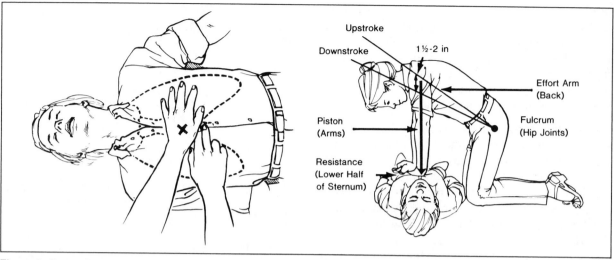

Figure 6 External chest compression. *Left,* Locating the correct hand position on the lower half of the body; *Right,* Proper position of the rescuer, with shoulders directly over the vic- tim's sternum and elbows locked (Adapted from *Cardiopulmonary Resuscitation.* Washington, DC, American National Red Cross, 1981, p 25. Used by permission.)

condition of the victim(s); (6) what aid is being given to the victim(s); (7) any other information requested. To ensure that EMS personnel have no more questions, the caller should hang up last.

If no one responds to the call for help and the rescuer is alone, CPR should be performed for about one minute and then help should be summoned. The decision when to leave the victim to telephone for help is affected by a number of variables, including the possibility of someone else arriving on the scene. If the rescuer is unable to activate the EMS system, the only option is to continue with CPR.

10. External Chest Compressions. Cardiac arrest is recognized by pulselessness in the large arteries of the unconscious, breathless victim. All the *ABCs* of CPR are required in rapid succession to optimize the chances for survival.

The external chest compression technique consists of serial, rhythmic applications of pressure over the lower half of the sternum (Fig. 5).[28] These compressions provide circulation to the heart, lungs, brain, and other organs as a result of a generalized increase in intrathoracic pressure and/or direct compression of the heart. Blood circulated to the lungs by external chest compressions will receive sufficient oxygen to maintain life when the compressions are accompanied by properly performed rescue breathing.[29]

During cardiac arrest, properly performed external chest compressions can produce systolic blood pressure peaks of more than 100 mm Hg, but the diastolic blood pressure is low, the mean blood pressure in the carotid arteries seldom exceeding 40 mm Hg. The carotid artery blood flow resulting from external chest compressions on a cardiac arrest victim usually is only one fourth to one third of normal.

The patient must be in the horizontal supine position when external chest compressions are performed. Even during properly performed external chest compressions, blood flow to the brain is reduced. With any elevation of the head above the heart, blood flow to the brain is further reduced or even eliminated. If the victim is in bed, a board, preferably the full width of the bed, should be placed under the back of the patient. Elevation of the lower extremities, while keeping the rest of the body horizontal, may promote venous return and augment artificial circulation during external chest compressions.

PROPER HAND POSITION. Proper hand placement is established by the following guidelines (Fig. 6, left):

1. With the middle and index finger of the hand nearest the victim's legs, the rescuer locates the lower margin of the victim's rib cage on the side next to the rescuer.

2. The fingers are then moved up the rib cage to the notch where the ribs meet the sternum in the center of the lower part of the chest.

3. With the middle finger on this notch, the index finger is placed next to it on the lower end of the sternum.

4. The heel of the hand nearest the patient's head (which had been used on the forehead to maintain head position) is placed on the lower half of the sternum, close to the index finger that is next to the middle finger in the notch. The long axis of the heel of the rescuer's hand should be placed on the long axis of the sternum. This will keep the main force of compression on the sternum and decrease the chance of rib fracture.

5. The first hand is then removed from the notch and placed on top of the hand on the sternum so that both hands are parallel to each other.

6. The fingers may be either extended or interlaced but must be kept off the chest.

7. Because of the varying sizes and shapes of different persons' hands, an alternate acceptable hand position is to grasp the wrist of the hand on the chest with the hand that has been locating the lower end of the sternum. This technique is helpful for rescuers with arthritic problems of the hands and wrists.

PROPER COMPRESSION TECHNIQUES. Effective compression is accomplished by attention to the following guidelines (Fig. 6, right):

1. The elbows are locked into position, the arms are straightened, and the shoulders of the rescuer are positioned directly over the hands so that the thrust for each external chest compression is straight down on the sternum. If the thrust is other than straight down, the torso has a tendency to roll, losing part of the force, and the chest compression may be less effective.

2. The sternum must be depressed 1.5 to 2 in (3.8 to 5.0 cm) for the normal-sized adult.

3. The external chest compression pressure is released to allow blood to flow into the heart. The pressure must be released completely and the chest allowed to return to its normal position after each compression. The time allowed for release should equal the time required for compression.

4. The hands should not be lifted from the chest or the position changed in any way, lest correct hand position be lost.

Rescue breathing and external chest compression must be combined for effective resuscitation of the cardiopulmonary arrest victim.

CPR PERFORMED BY ONE RESCUER AND BY TWO RESCUERS

CPR Performed by One Rescuer

A lay person should learn only one-rescuer CPR. The previously recommended two-rescuer technique is thought to cause too much confusion and to be infrequently used by laypersons in actual rescue situations. Teaching only one-rescuer CPR should result in better skill retention and possibly better performance. One-rescuer CPR is effective in maintaining adequate circulation and ventilation but is more exhausting than two-rescuer CPR. When trained professionals arrive at the scene of an emergency, they will proceed with two-rescuer CPR and advanced cardiac life support, as appropriate for the situation. The lay rescuer is relieved of responsibility at this point.

One-rescuer CPR should be performed as follows:

A. Airway. (1) Assessment: determine unresponsiveness (tap or gently shake and shout), (2) call for help, (3) position the victim, and (4) open the airway by the head-tilt/chin-lift maneuver.

B. Breathing. Assessment: determine restlessness. *If the victim is breathing,* (1) monitor breathing, (2) maintain an open airway, and (3) activate the EMS system (if not done previously). *If the victim is not breathing,* perform rescue breathing by giving two initial breaths. If unable to give two breaths, (1) reposition the head and attempt to ventilate again, and (2) if still unsuccessful, perform the foreign-body airway obstruction sequence. If successful, continue to the next step.

C. Circulation. (1) Assessment: determine pulselessness. If pulse is present, continue rescue breathing at 12 times per minute and activate the EMS system. (2) If pulse is absent, activate the EMS system (if not previously done) and continue to the next step. (3) Begin external chest compression: (a) Locate proper hand position. (b) Perform 15 external chest compressions at a rate of 80 to 100 per minute. Count "one and, two and, three and, four and, five and, six and, seven and, eight and, nine and, ten and, eleven and, twelve and, thirteen and, fourteen and, fifteen." (Any mnemonic that accomplishes the same compression rate is acceptable.) (c) Open the airway and deliver two rescue breaths. (d) Locate the proper hand position and begin 15 more compressions at a rate of 80 to 100 per minute. (e) Perform four complete cycles of 15 compressions and two ventilations.

D. Reassessment. After four cycles of compressions and ventilations (15:2 ratio), reevaluate the patient.

Check for return of the carotid pulse (5 seconds). If it is absent, resume CPR with two ventilations followed by compressions. If it is present, continue to next step.

Check breathing (3 to 5 seconds). If present, monitor breathing and pulse closely. If absent, perform rescue breathing at 12 times per minute and monitor pulse closely.

If CPR is continued, stop and check for return of pulse and spontaneous breathing every few minutes. Do not interrupt CPR for more than 7 seconds except in special circumstances.

One-Rescuer CPR With Entry of a Second Rescuer

When another rescuer is available at the scene, it is recommended that this second rescuer should activate the EMS (if not done previously) and perform one-rescuer CPR when the first rescuer, who initiated CPR, becomes fatigued.

The following steps are recommended for entry of the second rescuer. The second person should identify himself or herself as a qualified rescuer who is willing to help. If the first rescuer is fatigued and has requested help, the logical sequence is as follows: (1) The first rescuer stops CPR after two ventilations. (2) The second rescuer kneels down and checks for pulse for 5 seconds. (3) If there is no pulse, the second rescuer gives two breaths. (4) The second rescuer commences external chest compressions at the recommended rate and ratio for one-person CPR. (5) The first rescuer assesses the adequacy of the second rescuer's ventilations and compressions. This can be done by watching the chest rise during rescue breathing and by checking the pulse during the chest compressions.

"Standards and Guidelines for Cardiopulmonary Resuscitation (CPR) and Emergency Cardiac Care (ECC), Part II—Adult Basic Life Support." *Journal of the American Medical Association*, 255 (1986): 2915-21, 2931. Reproduced with permission from the American Heart Association.

REFERENCES

1. *A Manual for Instructors in Basic Life Support*. Dallas, American Heart Association, 1977.

2. Eisenberg MS, Bergner L, Hallstrom A: Cardiac resuscitation in the community. Importance of rapid provision and implications for program planning. *JAMA* 1979;241:1905-1907.

3. Cobb LA, Werner JA, Trobaugh GB: Sudden cardiac death: Parts 1 and 2. *Med Concepts Cardiovasc Dis* 1980;49: 31-36, 37-42.

4. Eisenberg MS, Copass MK, Hallstrom AP, et al: Treatment of out-of-hospital cardiac arrest with rapid defibrillation by emergency medical technicians. *N Engl J Med* 1980;302: 1379-1383.

5. Myerburg RJ, Kessler KM, Zaman L, et al: Survivors of prehospital cardiac arrest. *JAMA* 1982;247:1485-1490.

6. Abramson N, Safar P, Detre K, et al: An international collaborative clinical study mechanism for resuscitation research. *Resuscitation* 1982;10:141-147.

7. Longstreth WT, Diehr P, Inui TS: Prediction of awakening after out-of-hospital cardiac arrest. *N Engl J Med* 1983;308: 1378-1382.

8. *Risk Factors and Coronary Disease: A Statement for Physicians*. Dallas, American Heart Association, 1980.

9. Safar P: The pathology of dying and reanimation, in Schwartz G, Safar P, Stone J, et al (eds): *Principles and Practice of Emergency Medicine*, ed 2. Philadelphia, WB Saunders Co, 1985.

10. Safar P: Ventilatory efficacy of mouth-to-mouth artificial respiration. Airway obstruction during manual and mouth-to-mouth artificial respiration. *JAMA* 1958;167:335-341.

11. Safar P, Escarraga L, Change F: A study of upper airway obstruction in the unconscious patient. *J Appl Physiol* 1959;14:760-764.

12. Morikawa S, Safar P, DeCarlo J: Influence of head position upon upper airway patency. *Anesthesiology* 1961;22:265.

13. Ruben H, Elam JO, Ruben AM, et al: Investigation of upper airway problems in resuscitation. *Anesthesiology* 1961;22:271-279.

14. Boidin MP: Airway patency in the unconscious patient. *Br J Anaesth* 1985;57:306-310.

15. Safar P: *Cardiopulmonary Cerebral Resuscitation*. Philadelphia, WB Saunders Co, 1981.

16. Guildner CW: Resuscitation—opening the airway: A comparative study of techniques of opening an airway obstructed by the tongue. *JACEP* 1976;5:588-590.

17. Esmarch F: *The Surgeon's Handbook*. London, Sampson Low Marston Searle & Rivington, 1978, pp 114-118.

18. Elam JO, Greene DG, Schneider MA, et al: Head tilt method of oral resuscitation. *JAMA* 1960;172:812-815.

19. Safar P, Lind B: Triple airway maneuver, artificial ventilation and oxygen inhalation by mouth-to-mask and bag-valve-mask techniques, in *Proceedings of the 1973 National Conference on CPR*. Dallas, American Heart Association, 1975.

20. Elam JO, Greene DG: Mission accomplished. Successful mouth-to-mouth resuscitation. *Anesth Analg Curr Res* 1961; 40:440-442, 578-680, 672-676.

21. Ruben H, Knudsen EJ, Carugati G: Gastric inflation in relation to airway pressure. *Acta Anaesth Scand* 1961;5:107-114.

22. Melker R: Asynchronous and other alternative methods of ventilation during CPR. *Ann Emerg Med* 1984;13(pt 2): 758-761.

23. Melker R: Recommendations for ventilation during cardiopulmonary resuscitation. Time for change? *Crit Care Med* 1985;13:882-883.

24. Ruben H: The immediate treatment of respiratory failure. *Br J Anaesth* 1964;36:542-549.

25. Safar P, Redding J: 'Tight jaw' in resuscitation. *Anesthesiology* 1959;20:701-702.

26. *First Aid for (Neck Breathers) Laryngectomees*. New York, American Cancer Society, 1971.

27. *Instructors Manual for Basic Life Support*. Dallas, American Heart Association, 1985.

28. Kouwenhoven WB, Jude JR, Knickerbocker GG: Closed-chest cardiac massage. *JAMA* 1960;173:1064-1067.

29. Safar, P, Brown TC, Holtey WH, et.al: Ventilation and circulation with closed-chest cardiac massage in man, *JAMA* 1961; 176: 574-580.

Appendix B

Guidelines for Training of Dance-Exercise Instructors

The IDEA Foundation has prepared this position statement to offer a uniform set of standards and guidelines for training and certifying all dance-exercise instructors. These guidelines have been developed by the Committee on Standards and Certification in Dance Exercise, a group of more than 50 industry leaders actively involved with training, research, and education in fitness and health. The work of this committee represents a consensus within the dance-exercise industry on the recommended level of proficiency for an instructor leading a dance-exercise class. The implementation of the committee's guidelines will ensure quality control within the dance-exercise industry.

I. CORE KNOWLEDGE AND SKILLS FOR TEACHING DANCE-EXERCISE CLASSES

A. Exercise Physiology

The dance-exercise instructor will demonstrate an understanding of the basic principles of exercise physiology.

1. GENERAL PHYSICAL FITNESS

a. List the major components of physical fitness: muscular endurance, flexibility, muscular strength, cardiovascular endurance, and body composition.

b. Identify the musculoskeletal, cardiorespiratory and psychological benefits of participating in an aerobic dance-exercise program, such as increased efficiency of heart and lungs, increased bone density, increased stroke volume, or change in body composition.

c. Identify the benefits of regular exercise on specific disease conditions, such as adult-onset diabetes, arthritis, coronary heart disease, obesity, and asthma.

d. Define and explain the following terms: specificity, overload, adaptation, progression, frequency, intensity, and duration.

e. Identify primary and secondary risk factors for coronary heart disease and list those that may be favorably modified by regular and appropriate physical activity.

2. PHYSIOLOGY OF CARDIOVASCULAR ENDURANCE

a. Define the following terms: aerobic, anaerobic, cardiovascular endurance, oxygen consumption, heart rate, cardiac output, stroke volume, myocardial infarction, angina pectoris, ischemia, Valsalva maneuver, hyperventilation, interval training, continuous training, metabolism, hemoglobin, and recovery heart rate.

b. Describe the normal cardiorespiratory responses to aerobic exercise in terms of heart rate, blood pressure, and oxygen consumption.

c. Discuss recommendations to improve cardiovascular endurance for the general population with reference to type of activity, intensity, frequency, and duration.

d. Explain the differences between aerobic and anaerobic metabolism in terms of exercise intensity, exercise duration, oxygen availabil-

AEROBIC DANCE-EXERCISE INSTRUCTOR MANUAL

ity, fuel substrates used, and metabolic by-products produced.

  e. Discuss the importance of a proper warm-up and cool-down with respect to cardiovascular and musculoskeletal response.

3. **PHYSIOLOGY OF MUSCULAR STRENGTH AND ENDURANCE**

  a. Define the following terms: muscular strength; muscular endurance; isotonic, isometric, and isokinetic contractions; progressive resistance; concentric and eccentric contractions; and muscular atrophy and hypertrophy.

  b. Describe the common theories of acute muscle soreness and delayed onset muscle soreness (24–48 hours post-exercise).

  c. Discuss the disadvantages and/or advantages of exercising to muscular exhaustion/fatigue ("going for the burn") in a dance-exercise class.

  d. Describe the pros and cons of using hand and ankle weights to improve muscular strength, muscular endurance and cardiovascular fitness.

4. **PHYSIOLOGY OF FLEXIBILITY**

  a. Define and explain range of motion.

  b. Define and compare static and dynamic (ballistic) stretches for the purpose of improving flexibility. Discuss the risks and benefits of each method.

  c. Describe the muscle stretch reflex.

  d. List and describe the limitations to range of motion.

5. **ENVIRONMENTAL CONSIDERATIONS**

  a. Describe the physiological responses to exercising in the cold, heat, humidity, and altitude.

  b. Give precautions and guidelines for exercising in heat, humidity, and cold.

B. Basic Anatomy and Kinesiology

The dance-exercise instructor will be able to demonstrate knowledge of human anatomy and kinesiology.

1. **ANATOMY**

  a. Define the following terms with respect to anatomical position: anterior, posterior, lateral, medial, supination, pronation, supine, prone, dorsal, plantar, superior, inferior.

  b. Describe the general anatomy of the heart, cardiovascular system, and respiratory system.

  c. Explain the properties and function of bone, muscle, nerve tissue, ligaments, and tendons.

  d. Identify major muscle groups and bones.

  e. Describe and locate the following types of joints in the body: hinge, ball and socket, saddle.

2. **KINESIOLOGY**

  a. Define the following terms: flexion, extension, adduction, abduction, hyperextension, supination, pronation, inversion, eversion, balance, center of gravity, stability (in relation to base of support), equilibrium, and leverage.

  b. Identify good postural alignment for the standing position.

  c. Identify and define the abnormal curvatures of the spine: lordosis, scoliosis, and kyphosis.

  d. Describe the action of major muscle groups: trapezius, pectoralis major, latissimus dorsi, biceps, triceps, rectus abdominus, internal and external obliques, transverse abdominus, erector spinae group, gluteus maximus, quadriceps, hamstrings, gastrocnemius, tibialis anterior, tibialis posterior, hip adductors, hip abductors, deltoids, iliopsoas, soleus. Identify examples of exercises for these muscle groups.

  e. Identify major muscles involved in specific exercise movements, such as push-ups, sit-ups, jumping jacks, side-lying leg raises, and standing knee lifts.

3. **INJURY PREVENTION**

  a. Define and describe the common orthopedic problems associated with dance exercise: shin splints, stress fractures, plantar fasciitis, Morton's neuroma, metatarsalgia, achilles tendonitis, chondromalacia patella, ankle sprains, meniscus tears, bursitis, and low back pain.

  b. Identify precautions to take during the cooldown phase of a dance-exercise class to prevent fainting or lightheadedness.

  c. Discuss common causes of dance-exercise injuries.

  d. Explain the role of abdominal strength, hamstring flexibility and hip flexor length in the prevention of lower back pain. Identify common exercises advocated to prevent or treat this problem.

  e. Discuss common causes of low back pain.

f. Identify exercises contraindicated for persons with low back conditions.

g. Describe the potential risks associated with the following exercises: straight leg sit-ups, double leg raises, full squats, grand plié, full neck circles, hurdler's stretch, plough exercise, and back hyperextension.

h. Describe desirable floor surfaces for dance exercise.

i. Identify ways to modify dance-exercise movements to reduce impact stress and improve safety.

j. Identify the features of a shoe preferred for aerobic dance exercise.

k. Identify symptoms and common causes of voice injury. Be able to discuss techniques for preventing injury.

C. Exercise Programming Skills

The dance-exercise instructor will demonstrate competence in program design for group exercise programs.

1. BASIC PROGRAMMING

a. Demonstrate an understanding of the components of a typical aerobic dance-exercise class (warm-up, cool-down, aerobic phase, calisthenics) and be able to put these components in sequence to design a safe and effective program. Justify the sequence used.

b. Describe how to individualize an exercise program on the basis of information obtained through health screening, progress made in class, or fitness evaluations; for example, by raising or lowering exercise intensity, placing someone into a beginning or advanced program, or modifying specific exercises.

c. Recommend proper exercises for improving range of motion of all major joints.

d. Describe the types of exercises or activities used for developing cardiovascular endurance.

e. Describe exercises appropriate in dance-exercise classes for the improvement of muscular strength or endurance.

f. Explain modifications and restrictions in the dance-exercise class for persons suffering from the following musculoskeletal problems: arthritis, overweight, chondromalacia patella, and lower back discomfort.

g. Explain modifications that a physician might recommend for persons in dance-exercise programs who are suffering from acute illness (colds and flu), diabetes, hypertension, and cardiovascular disease.

h. Describe the signs and symptoms of over-exercising (acute responses), both during and after exercise, that would indicate the need to decrease the intensity, duration, or frequency of an excercise session.

i. Describe the signs and symptoms of over-training (chronic response) that would indicate the need to modify the intensity, duration, or frequency of an exercise session.

j. Discuss reasons for using physical fitness assessments in exercise programs.

k. Identify field testing methods you might use to measure each of the following: cardiovascular fitness, muscular strength, muscular endurance, flexibility, and body composition.

2. PROGRAMMING FOR SPECIAL POPULATIONS

a. *Older Adult*

1. Describe the natural aging changes in the sedentary adult that occur in the following: skeletal muscle, bone structure, maximal oxygen uptake, grip strength, flexibility, heart rate, body composition.

2. Identify common orthopedic problems of the older participant and explain how an exercise program could be modified to avoid aggravation of these problems.

3. Describe the physiological, psychological, and social benefits of regular exercise for the older adult.

b. *Pre/postnatal Woman*

1. Be familiar with the American College of Obstetricians and Gynecologists' guidelines for exercise during pregnancy and the postpartum period, especially with reference to: cardiovascular response (specifically blood volume and cardiac output), connective tissue changes, postural changes, hydration, temperature control, exercise guidelines and contraindications, special exercises for pregnancy and post partum, and warning signs and symptoms for exercise during pregnancy.

2. List recommendations for acceptance of previously exercising and nonexercising prenatal women into regular dance-exercise classes.

AEROBIC DANCE-EXERCISE INSTRUCTOR MANUAL

3. Identify social and emotional advantages of participation in specialized pre/post-natal classes rather than regular dance-exercise classes.

4. Describe how to adjust frequency, duration, and intensity of exercise for pregnant women who stay in regular dance-exercise classes.

5. Discuss the limitations of using heart rate as an indicator of exercise intensity during pregnancy. Describe other measures that can help gauge exercise intensity.

D. Leadership Techniques

The dance-exercise instructor will demonstrate an understanding of principles and practices of teaching and monitoring physical activity.

1. MONITORING TECHNIQUES

a. Describe how the heart rate is determined by palpitation at radial and carotid sites. Describe the precautions in the application of these techniques.

b. Demonstrate the ability to measure pulse rate accurately at rest, during exercise and immediately following.

c. Calculate a target heart rate using the Karvonen formula.

d. Give precautions and ranges of error when using an estimated target heart rate.

e. Describe methods, other than heart rate, for monitoring physical effort, such as respiration and perceived exertion.

2. TEACHING SKILLS AND PRACTICES

a. Identify inappropriate exercise responses from a participant that indicate the need to stop exercising.

b. Discuss techniques for accommodating various fitness levels within the same class.

c. Demonstrate an ability to recognize common student errors to employ instructional techniques for making individual corrections in a class structure.

d. Demonstrate an understanding of verbal and nonverbal instruction techniques: voice, movement, timing, eye contact.

e. Understand the principles of movement progression used in choreographing and teaching routines: slow to fast, simple to complex.

f. Describe appropriate exercise apparel for a variety of activities and environmental conditions.

g. Identify motivational strategies and adherence techniques to encourage regular participation in exercise.

h. List traditional dance step patterns that can be used to provide movement variety in a dance-exercise class, such as skip, polka, Charleston, and pony.

i. Define basic music terms: tempo, meter, rhythm.

II. OPERATION AND ADMINISTRATIVE SKILLS

A. Emergency Training

The dance-exercise instructor will demonstrate competence in basic life support and be able to implement first aid procedures, should the need arise, either during or after exercise. An instructor should possess a current cardiopulmonary resuscitation (CPR) card or equivalent credentials.

1. Outline emergency procedures appropriate for an exercise facility should an accident occur.

2. Describe basic first aid procedures for heat cramps, heat exhaustion, heat stroke, lacerations, abrasion, contusion, simple and compound fractures, bleeding, shock, hypoglycemia, hyperglycemia, convulsions and seizures, sprains, strains, fainting, cardiac arrest, angina, and blisters.

3. Explain the use of rest, ice, compression, elevation (RICE), and heat in treating athletic injuries.

B. Health Screening

The dance-exercise instructor will demonstrate an ability to screen participants and identify health problems and risk factors that may require consultation with health professionals prior to participation in physical activity.

1. Identify health information that should be obtained prior to admitting a participant into a class: past and present medical history (especially with regard to cardiovascular, respiratory, and musculoskeletal systems), prescribed medication, current activity patterns, family history of heart disease, and smoking history.

2. Identify health problems or risk factors that interfere with a participant's ability to exercise safely in class and that may warrant physician referral, such as recent surgery, diabetes, obesity, pregnancy, orthopedic problems (including arthritis), history of cardiovascular or respiratory disease (including hypertension and asthma), and previous difficulty with exercise (including exercise-related chest discomfort, dizzy spells, and extreme breathlessness).

3. Be familiar with the effects the following substances may have on heart rate response: beta blockers (beta-adrenergic blocking agents), diuretics, antihypertensives, antihistamines, tranquilizers, alcohol, diet pills, cold medications, caffeine, and nicotine.

C. Legal Issues

The dance-exercise instructor will understand the legal responsibilities of a professional in the field.

1. Explain the 1976 U.S. copyright act and procedures for:

    a. Recording music.

    b. Playing music in class.

    c. Selling tapes of copyrighted music with voice-overs.

2. Describe the professional responsibilities and liabilities of a dance-exercise instructor with respect to responsibility for exercise programming, fitness testing, and medical clearance.

3. Discuss common insurance needs and practices of dance-exercise instructors.

III. RELATED KNOWLEDGE

A. Nutrition

The dance-exercise instructor will demonstrate basic knowledge of good nutrition as it relates to exercise.

1. BASIC NUTRITION

a. Define the following terms: high-density lipoprotein cholesterol (HDL-C), low-density lipoprotein cholesterol (LDL-C), and total cholesterol/HDL cholesterol ratio.

b. Be familiar with the U.S. Dietary Goals.

c. Identify the four food groups and give an example of each.

d. List the six classes of essential nutrients and describe their general role.

e. Discuss the importance of an adequate iron intake for active women.

f. Explain the potential risk of toxicity with oversupplementation of vitamins.

2. NUTRITION AND EXERCISE

a. Be aware of common areas of nutrition misinformation as they relate to exercise: salt tablets, diet pills, protein powders, sugar, caffeine, and nutritional supplements.

b. Explain the relationship between a high complex carbohydrate/low fat diet and exercise performance.

c. Describe the procedures for maintaining normal hydration at times of heavy sweating; contrast plain water replacement with the use of special electrolyte drinks.

d. Describe the chronic effect of diet and aerobic exercise as they relate to changes in coronary risk factors.

e. Identify dietary and exercise measures that can be taken to reduce risk of developing osteoporosis. Given common food sources of calcium.

B. Weight Loss and Weight Control

The dance-exercise instructor will demonstrate basic knowledge of safe and effective methods for weight loss.

a. Define the following terms: obesity, overweight, underweight, percent body fat, lean body mass, bulimia, and anorexia nervosa.

b. Discuss the misconceptions of spot reduction.

c. Contrast the effectiveness of the following practices for fat weight loss and/or body composition change: diet and exercise combined, diet alone, and exercise alone.

d. Identify problems with using standard height-weight charts to determine ideal body weight.

e. Explain the concept of energy balance as it relates to weight control.

f. Explain the set point theory of weight control.

g. Describe the myths and dangers concerning the following as they pertain to body composition changes and weight loss: saunas, vibrating belts, body wraps, electric muscle stimulators, and sweat suits.

h. Discuss misconceptions surrounding the term "cellulite."

i. List the approximate number of kilocalories in 1 gram of fat, carbohydrate, protein, and alcohol.

j. Identify the generally recommended minimum number of calories for men and women for consumption in a safe, unsupervised weight loss program.

k. Identify the maximum number of pounds per week recommended for safe, unsupervised weight loss as identified by the American College of Sports Medicine.

Reprinted in part from the "Guidelines for Training of Dance-Exercise Instructors". San Diego: The IDEA Foundation, 1986.

Glossary

Abduction Movement of a body part away from the body's midline.

Abrasion Injury to the skin, usually from scraping the surface.

Acclimatization The act or process whereby the body physiologically adapts to an unfamiliar environment, such as a high altitude or a hot climate.

Achilles tendinitis A chronic overuse injury characterized by inflammation of the Achilles tendon resulting from small tears in its fibers.

Acidosis A condition characterized by an increase of blood acidity above normal.

Acute injury An injury having a sudden onset, characterized by specific pain and swelling and the inability to use the injured area normally.

Adduction Movement of a body part toward the body's midline.

Adenosine diphosphate (ADP) One of the chemical products of the breakdown of ATP during muscle contraction.

Adenosine triphosphate (ATP) The high-energy phosphate molecule required to provide energy for cellular function. One of the phosphagens.

Adipocyte A single fat cell.

Adipose tissue A conglomeration of adipocytes (fat cells) forming the major depot of body fat.

Age-predicted maximal heart rate A mathematical formula for estimating a person's maximal heart rate: 220 − age.

Aerobic With or in the presence of oxygen.

Aerobic cool-down The period at the end of the aerobics segment of a dance-exercise class in which intensity is reduced to begin lowering the heart rate.

Aerobic dance-exercise A method of exercising to music that conditions the cardiovascular system by using movements that create an increased demand for oxygen over an extended time.

Aerobic fitness Cardiovascular or cardiorespiratory endurance.

Aerobic glycolysis The metabolic pathway that, in the presence of oxygen, uses glucose (or glycogen) for energy production (ATP).

Affective domain One of the three domains of learning, which involves the learning of emotional behaviors.

Afferent neurons Receptors that transmit impulses to the spinal cord and brain.

Agonist A muscle that is directly engaged in contraction.

Alkalosis A condition characterized by a decrease in acidity or hydrogen ion concentration of the blood and extracellular fluids.

Alveoli The air sacs in the lungs, where carbon dioxide and oxygen are exchanged with the surrounding pulmonary capillaries.

Amino acids Nitrogen-containing compounds that are the building blocks of proteins.

Amphiarthrodial A type of synovial joint that has very limited mobility because both the ligaments and the capsule are taut, and the articular surfaces are tough (e.g. the sacroiliac joint).

Anaerobic Without the presence of oxygen. Not requiring oxygen.

Anaerobic glycolysis The metabolic pathway that uses glucose (or glycogen) for energy production (ATP) without requiring the presence of oxygen. This pathway produces lactic acid.

Anaerobic threshold The point during high-intensity activity when the body can no longer meet its demand for oxygen and anaerobic metabolism predominates.

Anatomical position Standing erect with the feet and palms facing forward.

Anemia See iron-deficiency anemia.

Angina pectoris Chest pain caused by inadequate blood flow, and thus oxygen supply, to the heart. Often aggravated or induced by exercise or stress.

Anorexia nervosa An eating disorder characterized by extreme weight loss, distorted body image, and an intense fear of becoming obese.

Antagonist A muscle that acts in opposition to the action produced by an agonist muscle.

Anterior The front side or to the front side of the body.

Aorta The main artery coming out of the left ventricle of the heart.

Apical pulse A pulse point located at the apex of the heart.

Appendicular skeleton The bones of the upper and lower extremities of the body.

Arrhythmia An abnormal rhythm of the heart beat.

Arteries Vessels that carry oxygenated blood to the tissues from the heart.

Arterioles Smaller divisions of arteries.

Arteriosclerosis A generic term that encompasses any arterial disease that leads to thickening and hardening of arteries.

Arthritis See Osteoarthritis and Rheumatoid arthritis.

Articulations The joints of the body where bones come together and where all movement of the skeletal system takes place.

ASCAP The American Society of Composers, Authors and Publishers. One of two performing rights societies in the United States that represents music publishers in negotiating and collecting fees for the nondramatic performance of music.

Associative stage The second stage of learning in which performers, having learned the basic fundamentals or mechanics of the skill, can now concentrate on refining their skills.

Assumption of risk A defense used to show that a person has voluntarily accepted known dangers by participating in a specific activity.

Asthma A disease of the lungs characterized by episodes of dyspnea (difficult breathing) due to constriction of bronchial smooth muscle.

Atherosclerosis A specific form of arteriosclerosis, characterized by the accumulation of fatty material on the inner walls of the arteries.

ATP See Adenosine triphosphate.

Atrium One of the two (left or right) upper chambers of the heart (atria). Also called auricle.

Atrophy A reduction in muscle size resulting from inactivity or immobilization.

Autonomous stage The third stage of learning in which the skill has become automatic or habitual to performers.

Avulsion A wound involving forcible separation or tearing of tissue from the body.

Axial skeleton The bones of the head, neck, and trunk.

Balance The state of the body when its center of gravity is above the base of support.

Ballistic stretching A technique to improve flexibility using rigid, bouncy, explosive movements.

Basal metabolic rate The minimum energy required to maintain life processes in the resting state.

Basic four food groups A framework for making dietary selections. It groups together foods with similar nutrients and recommends the number of servings that should be eaten daily from each group to achieve a balanced diet.

Basic locomotor steps Steps that use the feet as the base of support and only include walking (or stepping), running (or leaping), hopping, and jumping.

Beats Regular pulsations that have an even rhythm and occur in a continuous pattern of strong and weak pulsations.

Beta blockers (beta-adrenergic blocking agents) Medications, used for cardiovascular and other medical conditions, that "block" or limit sympathetic nervous system stimulation.

Biarticulate A muscle that crosses two articulations (joints).

Blood pressure The pressure exerted by the blood on the walls of the arteries. Measured in millimeters of mercury by the sphygmomanometer.

BMI Broadcast Music, Inc. One of two performing rights societies in the United States that represents music publishers in negotiating and collecting fees for the nondramatic performance of music.

Body composition The makeup of the body in terms of the relative percentage of lean body mass and body fat.

Bronchioles The smallest tubes that supply air to the alveoli in the lungs.

Bulimia An eating disorder characterized by episodes of binge eating, followed by self-induced vomiting, fasting, or the use of diuretics or laxatives.

Bursitis Irritation of a bursa, which is a padlike fluid-filled sac located at friction sites throughout the body. Bursitis occurs most often in the knees, hips, shoulders, and elbows.

Calcium The most abundant mineral in the body. Involved in the conduction of nerve impulses, heart function, muscle contraction, and the operation of certain enzymes. An inadequate supply of calcium contributes to osteoporosis.

Calcium-channel blockers (calcium-channel blocking agents, or antagonists) Medications, used primarily for cardiovascular disorders, that reduce movement of calcium ions across cell membranes.

Calisthenics Exercises to increase muscular strength and endurance which use the weight of the body or body parts for resistance.

Calorie The amount of heat necessary to raise the temperature of 1 gram of water 1°C. Often used incorrectly in place of kilocalorie. (1 kilocalorie = 1000 calories.)

Capillaries The smallest blood vessels that supply blood to the tissues.

Carbohydrates A primary foodstuff used for energy. Dietary sources include sugars (simple) and grains, rice, potatoes and beans (complex). Carbohydrate is stored as glycogen in the muscles and liver and is transported in the blood as glucose.

Cardiac arrest The cessation of cardiac output and effective circulation.

Cardiac output The amount of blood pumped by the heart per minute. Usually expressed in liters of blood per minute.

Cardiopulmonary resuscitation (CPR) A technique that artificially produces blood flow and air exchange in a pulseless, nonbreathing victim, by mouth-to-mouth respiration and rhythmical compression on the chest.

Cardiovascular endurance The ability to perform large muscle movement over a sustained period. The capacity of the heart-lung system to deliver oxygen for sustained energy production. Also called cardiorespiratory endurance.

Carotid pulse Pulse point located on the carotid artery in the neck about 1 inch below the jaw line, next to the esophagus.

Cartilage A smooth, semi-opaque material that provides a frictionless surface of a joint.

Cellulite A name for subcutaneous fat with a dimpled appearance, commonly found on the thighs and buttocks.

Center of gravity An imaginary point around which the masses of the body segments are balanced. It is located just below the navel in most people.

Cerebrovascular accident (CVA) A loss in function resulting from impaired blood supply to part of the brain. More commonly known as a *stroke*.

Cervical vertebrae The seven vertebral bones of the neck.

Cholesterol A fatty substance found in the blood and body tissues and in certain foods. Its accumulation in the arteries leads to narrowing of the vessels (atherosclerosis).

Chondromalacia A gradual degeneration of the articular cartilage that lines the back surface of the patella (kneecap), causing pain and sometimes swelling, or a grinding sound or sensation when the knee is flexed and extended.

Chronic injury An injury that recurs or lasts a long time, usually beginning gradually without a specific incident of injury.

Circumduction Movement of a segment in a circular pattern.

Coccyx The four small vertebral bones making up the "tailbone."

Cognitive domain One of the three domains of learning, which describes intellectual activities and involves the learning of knowledge.

Cognitive stage The first stage of learning in which performers make many gross errors and have highly variable performances.

Command style A teaching style in which the instructor makes all decisions about posture, rhythm, and duration, while participants follow the instructor's directions and movements.

Compilation An original, and hence copyrightable, sequence or program of dance steps or exercise routines that may or may not be copyrightable in themselves.

Complete protein A protein containing all nine amino acids essential to health.

Concentric contraction Contraction of a muscle in which the muscle shortens, or the proximal and distal attachments of the muscle come closer together.

Connective tissue The tissue that binds together and supports various structures of the body. Ligaments and tendons are connective tissue.

Contraindication Any condition that renders some particular movement, activity or treatment improper or undesirable.

Contusion Slight bleeding into soft tissue as a result of a blow. More commonly known as a *bruise*.

AEROBIC DANCE-EXERCISE INSTRUCTOR MANUAL

Cool-down A period following moderate to heavy exercise during which activity tapers off and the heart rate and body temperature gradually return to resting levels.

Copyright The exclusive right, for a certain number of years, to perform, make, and distribute copies and otherwise use an artistic, musical, or literary work.

Coronary heart disease (CHD) The major form of cardiovascular disease; almost always the result of atherosclerosis.

Coronary heart disease risk ratio The ratio between high-density lipoprotein (HDL) cholesterol and total cholesterol, used to predict the risk of developing heart disease. The lower the ratio, the lower the risk.

Corrective feedback statement Used when a response is incorrect, the statement identifies the error and tells the learner how to correct it.

CPR *See* cardiopulmonary resuscitation.

Creatine phosphate (CP) A high-energy phosphate molecule that is stored in cells and can be used to resynthesize ATP immediately. One of the phosphagens.

Cueing A verbal technique using only a few words, to inform exercise participants of upcoming movements.

Deductible The amount the insured must pay in the event of an insurance loss.

Dehydration The condition resulting from excessive loss of body fluids.

Diabetes mellitus A disease of carbohydrate metabolism, in which an absolute or relative deficiency of insulin results in an inability to metabolize carbohydrates normally.

Diabetic coma A state of deep unconsciousness as a result of uncontrolled diabetes.

Diarthrodial A type of articulation (joint) that is movable (as opposed to immovable or slightly movable).

Diastolic blood pressure The pressure exerted by the blood on the vessel walls when the heart is relaxed between contractions.

Directional cueing A verbal technique that tells participants in which direction to move.

Distal Farthest from the midline of the body, or from the point of attachment of a body part.

Diuretics Medications that produce an increase in urine volume and sodium (salt) excretion.

Dorsal Referring to the top or upper surface, as in the top of the foot.

Dorsiflexion Movement of the foot up toward the shin. Also called *flexion* of the foot.

Dramatic performing rights The right to use a song in conjunction with dialogue, scenery, or costumes, or to tell a story, as in a motion picture.

Dry bulb temperature The temperature of the air.

Duration The total time of each exercise session.

Dyspnea Difficult or labored breathing.

Dyspnea scale A scale used to monitor exercise intensity as determined by respiration effort.

Eccentric contraction A muscle contraction in which the muscle lengthens against a resistance.

Efferent neurons Nerves that carry impulses away from the central nervous system to the tissues.

Elasticity The property of a material to return to its original length after being stretched.

Elastic limit The place beyond which a tissue that is stretched does not return to its original shape.

Electrocardiogram (EKG or ECG) A recording of the electrical activity of the heart.

Emergency Medical System (EMS) A system found in many areas to provide fast, easy contact with police, fire, and emergency rescue teams.

Emphysema A disease of the lungs characterized by overexpansion of the lungs and dyspnea (difficulty breathing).

Endurance *See* Muscular endurance.

Endurance fitness Same as cardiovascular or cardio-respiratory endurance.

Energy balance The principle that body weight will stay the same when caloric intake equals caloric expenditure and that a positive or negative balance will cause a weight gain or weight loss.

Equilibrium The state of a system whose motion is not being changed. A balanced body is in *static* equilibrium; a body moving at a constant speed is in *dynamic* equilibrium.

Essential body fat The amount of fat thought to be necessary for the maintenance of life and reproductive function

Eversion Rotation of the foot to direct the plantar surface outward.

Exercise progression The increase in total work and/ or exercise intensity as a person becomes increasingly fit.

Exercise specificity principle A principle of training, which states that physiological adaptations are specific to the systems that are overloaded (stressed) with exercise.

Extension Movement that increases the angle at a joint, such as straightening the elbow.

Fair Use Doctrine An exception to the requirement of obtaining a license for the public performance of a copyrighted musical composition, where the musical composition is used for the purpose of criticism, comment, news reporting, teaching, scholarship, or research.

Fast twitch fiber Type of muscle fiber characterized by its fast speed of contraction and a high capacity for anaerobic glycolysis.

Fats One of the six classes of nutrients; a compound containing glycerol and fatty acids that is used as a source of energy. Stored in the body as adipose tissue.

Fatty acid The building block of the fatty compound. An important nutrient for the production of energy during low-intensity exercise.

Fatty acid oxidation The aerobic (oxygen-requiring) breakdown of fatty acid for the production of ATP.

Feedback An internal response within a learner. During information processing, it is the correctness or incorrectness of a response that is stored in memory to be used for future reference.

Femoral torsion Rotation of the femur inward relative to the tibia.

Fetus The developing and growing baby in the uterus.

Field tests Fitness tests that can be used in mass testing situations.

FITT principle Using the criteria of frequency (F), intensity (I), time (T), and type of activity (T) to individualize an exercise program.

Flexibility The range of motion possible about a joint.

Flexion The movement at an articulation that decreases the angle between two bones.

Footwork cueing A verbal technique that tells exercisers which foot to move.

Four food groups See Basic four food groups.

Freestyle method A way of designing the aerobics segment of a class that uses movements randomly chosen by the instructor.

Frequency Refers to the number of exercise sessions per week needed to reach a training effect.

Frontal plane A plane that divides the body into front and back.

General liability insurance Insurance for bodily injury or property damage resulting from general negligence, such as wet flooring, an icy walkway, or poorly maintained equipment.

Glucose A simple sugar; the form in which all carbohydrates are used as the body's principal energy source.

Glycogen The storage form of glucose found in the liver and muscles.

Glycolysis The metabolic process whereby glucose is chemically broken down to produce energy (ATP). Glycolysis occurs with or without the presence of oxygen (aerobic or anaerobic).

Golgi tendon organ A sensory organ within a tendon which, when stimulated, causes an inhibition of the entire muscle group.

Hand grip dynamometer An instrument to measure static gripping strength of the hands. The scores provide an estimate of general strength.

Heart rate The number of beats of the heart per minute.

Heart-rate reserve The result of subtracting the resting heart rate from the maximal heart rate. It represents the working heart-rate range between rest and maximal heart rate within which all activity occurs.

Heat cramp A muscle spasm induced by physical work in intense heat, or at the onset of warm weather before acclimatization takes place.

Heat exhaustion A reaction to heat marked by weakness and collapse as a result of water or salt depletion.

Heat stroke The final stage in heat exhaustion. An extremely dangerous condition, normally manifested by cessation of sweating and dangerously high body temperature.

Hemoglobin Protein molecule in red blood cells specifically adapted to carry (bond) oxygen molecules.

High-density lipoprotein cholesterol (HDL-C) A plasma complex of lipids and proteins that contains relatively more protein and less cholesterol and triglycerides. High levels of HDL-C are associated with a low risk of coronary heart disease.

Homeostasis State of dynamic equilibrium or stability of physiological function.

Hydrostatic weighing An underwater test used to measure the percentage of lean body weight and body fat, based on the principle that fat floats and muscle and bone sink.

Hyperextension Extension of an articulation beyond anatomical position.

Hyperfunction Overuse of a particular body part involving excessive muscular contraction and excessive force of movement.

Hyperhydration The state obtained by consuming several cups of water 2–3 hours before exercising in the heat, and again shortly before exercising.

Hypertension High blood pressure, or the elevation of blood pressure above the normal range.

Hypertrophy An increase in muscle size resulting from an increase in contractile proteins.

Hyperventilation A greater-than-normal rate of breathing, resulting in an abnormal loss of carbon dioxide from the blood. Dizziness may occur.

Hypoglycemia Low blood sugar (glucose), characterized by such symptoms as dizziness, confusion, headache, and anxiety.

Hypothermia A life-threatening reduction in body core temperature.

Incision A cut into body tissue caused by a sharp object or edge.

Inclusion style This teaching style enables multiple levels of performance to be taught within the same activity.

Independent contractors People who conduct business on their own on a contract basis and are not employees of an organization.

Inferior Below.

Informed consent Voluntary acknowledgement of the purpose, procedures, and specific risks of an activity in which one intends to engage.

Insulin A hormone, secreted into the bloodstream by the pancreas, that helps regulate carbohydrate metabolism.

Insulin shock The condition produced when an excessive amount of insulin is present in the bloodstream. Characterized by pale, moist skin; a full, rapid pulse; dizziness or headache; disorientation; and fainting with possible unconsciousness.

Intensity The physiological stress on the body during exercise. Indicates how hard the body should be working to achieve a training effect. Heart rate is generally a reliable way to assess exercise intensity in dance exercise.

Interval training Short, high-intensity exercise periods alternated with periods of rest. Example: 100-yard run, 1-minute rest, repeated 8 times.

Inversion Rotation of the foot to direct the plantar surface inward.

Iron A mineral crucial in the formation of hemoglobin, the oxygen-carrying pigment within red blood cells.

Iron-deficiency anemia A disorder caused by a low hemoglobin content in the blood, which reduces the amount of oxygen available to the body's tissues. Symptoms include fatigue, breathlessness after exercise, giddiness, and loss of appetite.

Isokinetic contraction A muscle contraction that occurs when resistance to movement is altered as the limb moves through the normal range of motion. The force developed by the muscle remains the same as the muscle changes in length, and the speed of contraction remains constant throughout the range of motion.

Isometric contraction A muscle contraction in which the muscle length remains static or unchanged.

Isotonic contraction A shortening or concentric muscle contraction that results in limb movement. Also referred to as a dynamic contraction.

Karvonen formula The mathematical formula that uses heart-rate reserve (maximal heart rate minus resting heart rate) to determine target heart rate.

Kegel exercises Exercises designed to gain control of and tone the pelvic floor muscles by controlled isometric contraction and relaxation of the muscles surrounding the vagina.

Kilocalorie (kcal) The amount of heat needed to increase the temperature of 1 kilogram of water 1°C. One kcal equals 1,000 calories. Kcal is the appropriate term to express energy intake and energy expenditure in nutrition and exercise.

Knowledge of results (KR) Feedback from external sources such as the instructor.

Kyphosis Exaggerated sagittal curvature of the thoracic (upper) spine.

Laceration A wound in the soft tissue that has rough edges from tearing or cutting.

Lactic acid A by-product of anaerobic glycolysis known to cause localized muscle fatigue.

Laryngitis Inflammation of the larynx.

Lateral Away from the midline of the body, or the outside.

Lateral flexion Bending of the vertebral column to the side.

Lateral rotation Rotation of a body part away from the midline of the body.

Lean body mass The metabolically active part of the body. The muscles, bones, nerves, skin, or organs of the body. That part of the body excluding fatty tissue.

Learning Internal changes in a person inferred from an external improvement in performance as a result of practice.

Liability Legal responsibility.

Ligament Strong, fibrous tissue that connects one bone to another.

Lipid Fat.

Lipoproteins A complex of lipid and protein molecules, which transports cholesterol and other lipids throughout the body. Includes high-density lipoproteins (HDLs), low-density lipoproteins (LDLs), and very low-density lipoproteins (VLDLs).

Lordosis An exaggerated forward curvature of the lumbar spine. Often referred to as *swayback*.

Low-density lipoprotein cholesterol (LDL-C) A plasma complex of lipids and proteins that contains relatively more cholesterol and triglycerides and less protein. High levels of LDL-C are associated with an increased risk of coronary heart disease.

Low-impact aerobics An aerobic workout in which at least one foot remains on the floor at all times to reduce impact and upper body movements are used to increase intensity.

Lumbar vertebrae The five vertebrae in the low back, just below the thoracic vertebrae and just above the sacrum.

Maximal exercise test A test that continues until a person has reached a maximal level ($\dot{V}O_2$ max) or voluntary exhaustion. The most accurate way to evaluate cardiovascular fitness.

Maximal heart rate (max HR) The highest heart rate a person can attain.

Maximal heart rate formula A formula for determining target heart rate based on a percentage of the maximal heart rate.

Maximal oxygen consumption ($\dot{V}O_2$ max) The highest volume of oxygen (measured in ml/kg · min^{-1}) a person can consume during heavy exercise. Also referred to as *maximal functional capacity*.

Measure One group of beats in a musical composition marked by the regular occurrence of the heavy accent.

Medial Toward the midline of the body, or the inside.

Medial rotation Rotation of a body part toward the midline.

Medical clearance Indication by a physician that a person can safely participate in a specific exercise program.

Meniscus tears An acute injury characterized by tears in either the medial or lateral meniscus, a gristly substance (cartilage) lining the top surface of the tibia (lower leg bone).

Metabolism The chemical and physical processes in the body that provide energy for the maintenance of life.

Metatarsalgia A general term describing pain in the ball of the foot, usually under the second and third metatarsal heads, caused by bruising the joints of the foot.

Meter The organization of beats into musical patterns or measures.

MET system A simplified system for classifying physical activities using metabolic equivalents, or METS. One MET is equal to the resting oxygen consumption, which is approximately 3.5 milliliters of oxygen per kilogram of body weight per minute (3.5 ml/kg · min^{-1}).

Minerals Inorganic compounds that serve a variety of important functions in the body.

Mitochondria Specialized, subcellular structures located within body cells that contain oxidative enzymes needed by the cell to metabolize foodstuffs into energy sources. Glycolysis and fatty acid oxidation occur within the mitochondria.

Mobility The degree to which an articulation is allowed to move before being restricted by surrounding tissues.

Motor domain One of the three domains of learning, which involves the learning of motor skills.

Motor end plate The synaptic connection between a motor neuron and a skeletal muscle cell.

Motor neuron A neuron that sends electrochemical impulses from the spinal cord to the muscle fibers causing muscular contraction.

Motor unit A motor neuron and all of the muscle fibers it innervates.

Movement pair A movement of a segment away from anatomical position and the opposite movement back to anatomical position.

Multiarticulate A muscle that crosses more than two articulations.

Muscle spindle The sensory organ within a muscle that is sensitive to stretch.

Muscular endurance The capacity of a muscle to exert force repeatedly, or to hold a fixed or static contraction over time.

Muscular strength The maximum force that can be exerted by a muscle or muscle group against a resistance.

Myocardial infarction Death of a portion of the heart muscle from interruption of the blood supply. Commonly called *heart attack*.

Myocardial ischemia Deficiency of blood supply to the heart muscle.

Negligence Failure of a person to perform as a reasonable and prudent professional would perform under similar circumstances.

Neuroma (Interdigital or Morton's) Entrapment of part of an interdigital nerve, usually between the third and fourth toes, causing sharp, radiating pain and swelling.

Neuron A nerve cell.

Neutral feedback statement Feedback to the student that acknowledges performance but does not judge or correct the performance.

Nitroglycerin A drug that dilates the blood vessels; used to treat angina pectoris.

AEROBIC DANCE-EXERCISE INSTRUCTOR MANUAL

Nondramatic performing rights The right to play a song on its own or with other songs, but not to accompany the song with dialogue, scenery, or costumes, and not to use the song to tell a story.

Nonimpact aerobics An exercise class in which neither foot ever leaves the floor. Usually not strenuous enough to achieve an aerobic training effect.

Numerical cueing A verbal technique used by instructors to count the rhythm of the exercise, such as "1 and 2, 3, 4."

Nutrients Components of food needed by the body. There are six classes of nutrients: water, minerals, vitamins, protein, carbohydrates, and fats.

Nutrition The study of nutrients in foods and of their digestion, absorption, metabolism, interaction, storage, and excretion.

Obesity The accumulation and storage of excess body fat. Usually defined as over 20% above ideal weight, or over 30% body fat for women and over 23% body fat for men.

Osteoarthritis A degenerative joint disease, found chiefly in older adults, caused by a degeneration of the cartilage of the joints.

Osteoporosis A disorder, primarily affecting women past menopause, in which bone mass decreases and susceptibility to fracture increases.

Otolaryngologist A physician specializing in diseases of the ear, nose, and throat.

Overload principle The principle that a physiological system or organ subjected to a greater-than-normal load (stress) will respond by increasing in strength or function.

Overuse injury An injury caused by activity that places too much stress on one area of the body over an extended period.

Overweight A weight above average for a person's height and frame size, as defined by standard scales.

Oxygen consumption The rate at which oxygen is used to produce energy for cellular work. Also called *oxygen uptake.*

Oxygen debt The temporarily elevated oxygen consumption that follows immediately after cessation of exercise.

Oxygen deficit The difference between actual oxygen consumption and the total oxygen requirement for energy production.

Palpate To examine by touch, as in determining the heart rate by feeling the pulse at the radial or carotid arteries.

Palpitations A rapid throbbing or fluttering of the heart of which the person is aware.

Part teaching approach Teaching a skill part by part instead of all at once.

Performing rights society An organization to which the copyright or publisher assigns the nondramatic performing rights in the musical composition. The two performing rights societies in the United States are ASCAP and BMI.

Perfusion Pumping of a fluid through an organ or tissue.

Phosphagens Adenosine triphosphate (ATP) and creatine phosphate (CP), two high-energy phosphate molecules that can be broken down for immediate use by the cells.

Physical fitness The physical aspects of well-being that enable a person to function at an optimal level.

Placenta The vascular organ in mammals that unites the fetus to the maternal uterus and mediates its metabolic exchanges.

Plantar The bottom, as in the bottom or sole of the foot.

Plantar fascitis Inflammation of the plantar fascia, a broad band of connective tissue running along the sole of the foot. This inflammation is caused by stretching or tearing the tissue, usually near the attachment at the heel.

Plantar flexion Movement of the foot toward the sole of the foot. Also called *extension* of the foot.

Plaque A deposit of fatty or fibrous material inside arterial walls, causing the arteries to narrow and lose their elasticity.

Plasma The liquid portion of the blood.

Posterior Toward the back or dorsal side.

Postpartum The period of time after childbirth.

Practice style A teaching style that provides opportunities for individualization and includes practice time and private instructor feedback for each participant.

Primary bronchi The two main branches of the trachea or windpipe.

Primary risk factor A characteristic or behavior that, by itself, is significantly associated with a major health problem.

Prime mover A muscle responsible for a specific movement.

Professional liability insurance Insurance to protect against professional negligence or failure of an instructor to perform as a competent and prudent professional would under similar circumstances.

Progression *See* Exercise progression.

Pronation Rotating the palm downward; a combination of ankle dorsiflexion, subtalar eversion, and foot abduction.

Prone Facing downward.

Protein A compound composed of amino acids that is the major structural component of all body tissue.

Proximal Nearest to the midline of the body or point of attachment of a body part.

Public domain A term referring to an artistic, musical, or literary work that is no longer protected by copyright and, therefore, may be used by anyone for any purpose, free of charge.

Public performance Playing a recording of a copyrighted musical composition at a place where a substantial number of persons outside of a normal circle of a family and its social acquaintances are gathered.

Publisher The entity to which the owner of a copyrighted artistic, musical, or literary work assigns such copyright for licensing and income collection purposes.

Pulmonary function The functional capacity of the lungs, including lung volume, breathing rate, and vital capacity.

Pulse The wave of pressure in the arteries that occurs each time the heart beats.

Puncture A penetrating wound caused by a pointed object.

Punitive damages Damages awarded to a plaintiff in excess of normal compensation, to punish a defendant for a gross wrong.

Quadriceps angle (Q-angle) The angle formed between the quadriceps muscle and the patellar tendon.

Quality of life Overall positive feeling and enthusiasm for life, without fatigue from routine activities.

Radial flexion Movement of the hand toward the radius or thumb side. Also called *radial deviation*.

Radial pulse A pulse point located on the thumb side of the wrist.

Range of motion (ROM) The number of degrees that an articulation will allow one of its segments to move.

Rating of perceived exertion (RPE) A scale that correlates the subjective perception of exercise effort with the actual intensity level.

Receptor Nerve tissue that is sensitive to changes in its environment.

Reciprocal style A teaching style that involves using an observer or partner to provide feedback to the performer.

Recommended Dietary Allowance (RDA) The daily amount of a nutrient recommended for practically all healthy persons to obtain optimal health.

Recovery heart rate The number of heartbeats per minute following the cessation of vigorous physical activity. As cardiorespiratory fitness improves, the heart rate returns to resting levels more quickly.

Rehearsal effect A learning principle. Rehearsing motor patterns in the warm-up enhances performance when the same patterns are used later in the class.

Relaxin A hormone of pregnancy that softens connective tissue.

Repetitions The number of successive contractions performed during each weight-training exercise.

Replacement cost An insurance term referring to the cost of replacing an item at the current cost in today's marketplace.

Respiration The exchange of oxygen and carbon dioxide between the cells and the atmosphere.

Resting heart rate The number of heartbeats per minute when the body is at complete rest; usually counted first thing in the morning before any physical activity.

Reversibility principle The principle which states that training adaptations will gradually decline if the altered system or organ is not sufficiently stressed on a regular basis.

Rheumatoid arthritis An autoimmune disease that causes inflammation in the connective tissues in the joints.

Rhythm A regular pattern of movement or sound that can be felt, seen, or heard.

Rhythmic cueing A verbal technique that indicates the correct rhythm of an exercise or step pattern, such as slow (2 counts) or quick (1 count).

RICE An immediate treatment for injury: rest, ice, compression, elevation.

Risk factor A characteristic symptom, or behavior related to the presence or development of a condition or disease.

Rotation Movement of a body part around its longitudinal axis.

Sacrum The five vertebrae that join the vertebral column to the pelvis.

Sagittal plane A plane that divides the body into right and left parts.

Saturated fats Fatty acids carrying the maximum number of hydrogen atoms. These fats are solid at room temperature and are usually of animal origin.

Scoliosis A lateral curvature of the vertebral column, usually in the thoracic area.

Secondary risk factor A characteristic symptom, behavior, or condition that, by itself, has a weak association with a disease, but increases the risk when other risk factors are present.

AEROBIC DANCE-EXERCISE INSTRUCTOR MANUAL

Seizure An attack, such as a convulsion.

Self-check style A teaching style that relies on individual performers to provide their own feedback.

Sensory neuron A neuron that sends electrochemical impulses from a sensory organ to the spinal cord. Responsible for sensation.

Set The number of repetitions performed for each weight-training exercise.

Setpoint theory A theory of weight control that explains the tendency of the body to maintain a certain level of body fat, or setpoint.

Shin splints A general term for any pain or discomfort on the front or side of the lower leg, in the region of the shin bone (tibia). A common, chronic dance-exercise injury with several causes.

Shock A circulatory disturbance produced by severe injury or illness, in which there is inadequate perfusion of blood through the body tissues.

Sit and reach test A test that uses a flexibility box to evaluate the flexibility of the low back.

Skinfold caliper An instrument used to measure the thickness of skinfolds at various sites on the body. The measurements are used to estimate the percent of body fat.

Slow twitch fiber A type of muscle fiber characterized by its slow speed of contraction and a high capacity for aerobic glycolysis.

Specificity *See* Exercise specifity principle.

Speech pathologist A specialist in diagnosis and remediation of speech, language, and voice disorders.

Spot reducing The effort to reduce fat at specific sites by exercising the muscles at those sites. A popular but false concept.

Sprain Overstretching or tearing of a ligament or joint capsule, resulting in discoloration, swelling, and pain.

Stability The ability of an articulation to maintain its integrity; the extent to which it is difficult for a body to lose its balance.

Standard of care Appropriateness of an exercise professional's actions, in light of current professional standards and based on the age, condition, and knowledge of the participant.

Static stretching A technique to increase flexibility by holding a steady position with the desired muscles at their greatest possible length.

Step cueing A verbal technique that refers to the name of the step in an aerobic dance-exercise routine, such as "step, ball, change."

Step test (submaximal) A test for cardiovascular fitness which requires the subject to step up and down from a bench at a prescribed rate for a given period. There are several different step test protocols.

Strain Overstretching or tearing of a muscle or tendon.

Strength *See* Muscular strength.

Stress fracture A fracture caused by excessive stress (overuse) to a bone. Most common in the foot (metatarsal bones) and lower leg (tibia).

Stretch reflex An involuntary muscle contraction initiated by stimulation of a muscle spindle within that muscle.

Stroke *See* Cerebrovascular accident.

Stroke volume The volume of blood pumped from the left ventricle during one heartbeat.

Structured method A way of designing the aerobics segment of a class that uses formally arranged step patterns, repeated in a predetermined order.

Subcutaneous fat Fat stored beneath the skin.

Submaximal exercise test A test to evaluate cardiorespiratory fitness, performed at less than maximal effort and terminated before exhaustion.

Substrate A fuel source for energy metabolism.

Superior Located above.

Supination A combination of ankle plantar flexion, subtalar inversion, and foot adduction.

Supine Face up.

Synarthrodial A type of articulation that is immovable.

Synergist A muscle that aids another muscle in its action.

Systolic blood pressure The pressure exerted by the blood on the vessel walls during ventricular contraction.

Talk test A method for measuring exercise intensity using observation of respiration effort and the ability to talk while exercising.

Target heart rate The number of heartbeats per minute that indicate appropriate exercise intensity levels for each person. Also called *training heart rate*.

Target heart-rate range The exercise intensity that represents the minimum and maximum intensity for safe and effective exercise. Also referred to as *training zone*.

Task complexity The number of parts or components within a task and the level of information processing required to complete the task.

Task organization The extent to which the parts of a task are interrelated. In a task that is high in organization, the parts that constitute the task are closely related to one another. In a task low in organization, the parts are independent.

Tempo The rate of speed at which a musical composition is played.

Temporal pulse Pulse point located on either temple.

Tendinitis An inflammatory response to microtrauma from overuse of a tendon.

Tendon Strong, fibrous connective tissue that attaches a muscle to a bone.

Thoracic vertebrae The twelve vertebrae to which the ribs are attached.

Tibial torsion Outward rotation of the tibia relative to the femur, causing the feet to toe out.

Tidal volume The amount of air that passes in and out of the lungs in an ordinary breath.

Total cholesterol The total of all forms of cholesterol in the body, including high-density lipoprotein cholesterol (HDL-C) and low-density lipoprotein cholesterol (LDL-C).

Training effect The physiological changes leading to increased functional capacity resulting from participation in regular and vigorous exercise.

Training zone The exercise intensity range that represents the minimum and maximum intensity for safe and effective exercise. Also called target heart-rate range.

Transverse plane A plane that divides the body into upper and lower parts.

Triglycerides The storage form of fat consisting of three free fatty acids and glycerol.

Ulnar flexion Movement of the hand toward the ulna or little finger.

Underwriting Evaluation of a risk and the potential responsibility of becoming answerable for a specific loss.

Uniarticulate A muscle that crosses one articulation.

Unsaturated fats Fatty acids that contain double bonds between carbon atoms and thus are capable of absorbing more hydrogen. These fats are liquid at room temperature and usually of vegetable origin.

US dietary goals Dietary guidelines established by the US Senate Select Committee on Human Needs to improve the eating habits of US citizens.

$\dot{V}O_2$ max *See* Maximal oxygen consumption.

Valgus Tending outward from proximal to distal.

Valsalva maneuver Increased pressure in the thoracic cavity caused by forced exhalation with the breath held.

Value feedback statement Feedback that projects a feeling about a performance, using such words as "good," "well done," or "poor job."

Varus Tending inward from proximal to distal.

Vein A blood vessel that carries blood to the heart.

Ventilation The movement of air into and out of the lungs.

Ventricle One of the two (left or right) lower chambers of the heart.

Vertebrae The bones that form the spinal column.

Vertebral disc The spongy, disc-shaped fibrous cartilage that lies between the vertebrae and acts as a shock absorber.

Vital signs Measurable bodily functions, including pulse rate, respiratory rate, blood pressure, skin color, and temperature.

Vitamins Organic compounds that function as metabolic regulators in the body. Classified as water soluble or fat soluble.

Vocal abuse Mistreatment of the vocal mechanism by talking for prolonged periods, excessive throat clearing, changing pitch abruptly, and shouting to be heard.

Vocal cords Paired set of muscles that vibrate to produce voice and serve as a valve for breathing and swallowing.

Vocal nodules Benign growths on the edge of the vocal cords that occur at the juncture of the anterior thirds.

Waiver Voluntary abandonment of a right to file suit.

Walk/run test (1.5 miles) A test for cardiovascular fitness based on the time it takes a subject to complete the 1.5-mile distance.

Warm-up The preparatory portion of a workout or exercise session designed to ready the body for vigorous motion. A warm-up period consists of stretching, walking, and general exercises designed to stimulate the muscles, heart, and lungs.

Wet bulb temperature A temperature that combines the temperature of the air and the humidity into one reading. When humidity is low, the wet bulb temperature is below air temperature. When humidity is high, the wet bulb temperature is similar to air temperature.

Whole teaching approach Teaching an entire skill all at once, instead of part by part.

INDEX